```
QR           Cytokin
188.3        autoimmun
.R65         [edited b
             Fionula M
             Brennan,
```

MEDICAL INTELLIGENCE UNIT

CYTOKINES IN AUTOIMMUNITY

Fionula M. Brennan
Marc Feldmann

Kennedy Institute of Rheumatology
Hammersmith, London

CHAPMAN & HALL
ITP An International Thomson Publishing Company

New York • Albany • Bonn • Boston • Cincinnati • Detroit • London • Madrid • Melbourne •
Mexico City • Pacific Grove • Paris • San Francisco • Singapore • Tokyo • Toronto • Washington

R.G. LANDES COMPANY
AUSTIN

MEDICAL INTELLIGENCE UNIT
CYTOKINES IN AUTOIMMUNITY

R.G. LANDES COMPANY
Austin, Texas, U.S.A.

U.S. and Canada Copyright © 1996 R.G. Landes Company and Chapman & Hall
International Copyright © 1996 Springer-Verlag, Heidelberg, Germany

All rights reserved.
No part of this book may be reproduced or transmitted in any form or by any means, electronic or mechanical, including photocopy, recording, or any information storage and retrieval system, without permission in writing from the publisher.
Printed in the U.S.A.

Please address all inquiries to the Publishers:
R.G. Landes Company, 909 Pine Street, Georgetown, Texas, U.S.A. 78626
Phone: 512/ 863 7762; FAX: 512/ 863 0081

North American distribution:
Chapman & Hall, 115 Fifth Avenue, New York, New York, U.S.A. 10003

International distribution (except North America):
Springer-Verlag GmbH & Co. KG, Tiergartenstrasse 17, D-69121 Heidelberg, Germany

U.S. and Canada ISBN: 0-412-10271-4
International ISBN: 3-540-60687-4

While the authors, editors and publisher believe that drug selection and dosage and the specifications and usage of equipment and devices, as set forth in this book, are in accord with current recommendations and practice at the time of publication, they make no warranty, expressed or implied, with respect to material described in this book. In view of the ongoing research, equipment development, changes in governmental regulations and the rapid accumulation of information relating to the biomedical sciences, the reader is urged to carefully review and evaluate the information provided herein.

Library of Congress Cataloging-in-Publication Data

Role of cytokines in autoimmunity / [edited by] Fionula M. Brennan, Marc Feldman.
      p. cm.—(Medical intelligence unit)
    Includes bibliographical references and index.
    ISBN 0-412-10271-4 (alk. paper)
      1. Autoimmunity. 2. Cytokines—Pathophysiology. 3. Autoimmune disease—Pathophysiology. I. Brennan, Fionula M., 1957-. II. Feldmann, Marc. III. Series.
    [DNLM: 1. Autoimmune Diseases—immunology. 2. Cytokines—immunology. 3. Cytokines—genetics. WD 305 R745 1996]
QR188.3.R65 1996
616.97'8—dc20
DNLM/DLC
for Library of Congress
95-49399
CIP

Publisher's Note

R.G. Landes Company publishes six book series: *Medical Intelligence Unit, Molecular Biology Intelligence Unit, Neuroscience Intelligence Unit, Tissue Engineering Intelligence Unit, Environmental Intelligence Unit* and *Biotechnology Intelligence Unit.* The authors of our books are acknowledged leaders in their fields and the topics are unique. Almost without exception, no other similar books exist on these topics.

Our goal is to publish books in important and rapidly changing areas of bioscience for sophisticated researchers and clinicians. To achieve this goal, we have accelerated our publishing program to conform to the fast pace in which information grows in bioscience. Most of our books are published within 90 to 120 days of receipt of the manuscript. We would like to thank our readers for their continuing interest and welcome any comments or suggestions they may have for future books.

Deborah Muir Molsberry
Publications Director
R.G. Landes Company

CONTENTS

1. **The Role of Cytokines in Normal and Pathological Situations 1**
   Marc Feldmann, Steve Dower and Fionula M. Brennan
   Introduction 1
   Cytokine Networks 2
   Properties of Cytokines 3
   Cytokine Receptors 6
   Soluble Cytokine Receptors 16
   Cytokine Production by Cells in Inflammation and Immunity 17
   Regulation of Cytokine Action 19
   What Happens to Cytokines in Disease Processes? 19

2. **Cytokines in Rheumatoid Arthritis 25**
   Fionula M. Brennan, Ravinder N. Maini and Marc Feldmann
   Abstract 25
   Introduction 25
   Cytokine Analysis 26
   Cytokine Expression in Rheumatoid Synovial Tissue 27
   Regulation of Cytokine Responses in Rheumatoid Arthritis 33
   Cytokine Inhibitors 34
   Immunoregulatory Cytokines 38
   Concluding Remarks 41

3. **Cytokines in Diabetes 49**
   Janette Allison, Jacques Miller and Nora Sarvetnick
   Introduction 49
   The Role of Cytokines in Autoimmune Diabetes 51
   Regulation of Autoimmunity by Cytokines 65
   Discussion 66

4. **Cytokines in Multiple Sclerosis 77**
   David Baker, Lawrence Steinman, and Koenraad Gijbels
   Disease Course of Multiple Sclerosis 77
   Analysis of Cytokines in MS 80
   Cytokines in Disease Initiation 81
   Cellular Recruitment During Neuroimmunological Disease 82
   Role of TNFα as an Important Pathogenic Mediator
     of Cellular Recruitment 83
   Cytokines in Myelin Pathology 84
   Cytokine Induced Regulation of Disease 88
   Inhibition of the Progression of Multiple Sclerosis with Interferons 89
   Conclusions 90

5. **The Role of Cytokines in Thyroid Health and Disease** 101
   Beatrix Grubeck-Loebenstein
   Introduction 101
   Production of Cytokines in the Thyroid Gland 102
   Effects of Cytokines in the Thyroid Gland 106
   Role of Cytokines in Graves' Ophthalmopathy 110
   Conclusion 111

6. **Cytokines in Sjögren's Syndrome** 121
   F. N. Skopouli and H. M. Moutsopoulos
   Introduction 121
   The Histologic Lesion 121
   B Lymphocyte Hyperactivity 122
   Etiopathogenesis 123
   Cytokine Studies 124
   Concluding Remarks 131

7. **Cytokines in Systemic Lupus Erythematosus** 137
   Josef S. Smolen, Winfried B. Graninger, Andrea Studnicka-Benke and Günter Steiner
   Lymphokines 139
   Monokines 142

8. **Scleroderma** 153
   Carol M. Black and Christopher P. Denton
   Introduction 153
   Cellular Sources for Cytokines in the Pathogenesis of SSc 155
   Cytokine Mediated Modulation of Cell-Cell Contact in SSc 156
   Direct Evidence for the Role of Cytokines in the Initiation
      or Maintenance of the SSc Fibroblast Phenotype 157
   Circulating Cytokines and Adhesion Molecules in SSc 158
   Therapeutic Implications 160
   Summary of the Evidence for a Role
      of Individual Cytokines in SSc 161

9. **Psoriasis** 175
   Stephen M. Breathnach and William G. Phillips
   Introduction 175
   The Skin Immune System 178
   The Skin Immune System and Psoriasis 182
   The Effect of Exogenous Cytokines on Psoriasis 186
   The Effects of Therapies for Psoriasis on Cytokines 186
   Conclusion 188

10. **What Can We Learn From 'Gene Knockout' Mice?** 201
    Andrew P. Cope
    Introduction 201
    Why Study Cytokine Knockout Mice? 202
    Nature's "Knockouts" 203
    "Knockout" Technology 204
    Cytokine Gene Knockouts and Autoimmunity 207
    What the Future Holds in Store 218

11. **What Can We Learn From Transgenic Mice?** 227
    George Kollias
    Introduction 227
    Cytokines and the T Cell Component in Autoimmunity 228
    Cytokines and the B Cell Component in Autoimmunity 229
    Cytokine Overexpression Can Be Causal in the Development
        of Chronic Inflammatory Disease 230
    Tumor Necrosis Factor Specifically Triggers Inflammatory
        Arthritis in Transgenic Mice 231
    Chemokine Transgenics 232
    Immunoregulatory Cytokine Transgenics 233
    Concluding Remarks 233

12. **What Are the Prospects for Therapy Based on
    Cytokines and Anticytokines in Rheumatoid Arthritis?** 239
    Michael J. Elliott and Ravinder N. Maini
    Introduction 239
    Cytokine Blockade in RA 240
    What Are the Prospects for Long-Term Cytokine Blockade? ... 247
    Cytokines as Therapy 249
    Colony Stimulating Factors in RA 249
    Erythropoietin 250
    Summary 250

Index 257

EDITORS

Fionula M. Brennan, B.Sc., Ph.D.
The Mathilda & Terence Kennedy Institute of Rheumatology
Hammersmith, United Kingdom
Chapters 1, 2

Marc Feldmann, M.B., B.S., B.Sc., Ph.D., F.R.C.Path.
The Mathilda & Terence Kennedy Institute of Rheumatology
Hammersmith, United Kingdom
Chapters 1, 2

CONTRIBUTORS

Janette Allison, B.Sc., Ph.D.
The Walter and Eliza Hall Institute
 of Medical Research
Royal Melbourne Hospital
Victoria, Australia
Chapter 3

David Baker, B.Sc., Ph.D.
Department of Clinical
 Ophthalmology
Institute of Ophthalmology
University College London
London, United Kingdom
Chapter 4

Carol M. Black, M.D., F.R.C.P.
Rheumatology Unit
Royal Free Hospital
London, United Kingdom
Chapter 8

Stephen M. Breathnach, M.A.,
 M.D., Ph.D., F.R.C.P.
St. John's Institute of Dermatology
St. Thomas's Hospital
London, United Kingdom
Chapter 9

Andrew P. Cope, M.B., B.S., B.Sc.,
 Ph.D., M.R.C.P.
Department of Microbiology
 and Immunology
Stanford University
 School of Medicine
Stanford, California, U.S.A.
Chapter 10

Christopher P. Denton, B.Sc.,
 M.R.C.P.
Rheumatology Unit
Royal Free Hospital
London, United Kingdom
Chapter 8

CONTRIBUTORS

Steve Dower, B.A., D.Phil.
Department of Medicine
  and Pharmacology
University of Sheffield
Royal Hallamshire Hospital
Sheffield, United Kingdom
Chapter 1

Michael J. Elliott, M.B., B.S.,
  Ph.D., F.R.A.C.P.
The Mathilda & Terence Kennedy
  Institute of Rheumatology
Hammersmith, London,
  United Kingdom
Chapter 12

Koenraad Gijbels, M.D., Ph.D.
Department of Neurology
  and Neurological Sciences
Stanford University Medical Center
Stanford, California, U.S.A.
Chapter 4

Winfried B. Graninger
Department of Rheumatology
University of Vienna
Vienna, Austria
Chapter 7

Beatrix Grubeck-Loebenstein, M.D.
Institute for Biomedical Aging
  Research
Austrian Academy of Sciences
Innsbruck, Austria
Chapter 5

George Kollias, Ph.D.
Department of Molecular Genetics
Hellenic Pasteur Institute
Athens, Greece
Chapter 11

Ravinder N. Maini, B.A., M.B.,
  B.Chir., F.R.C.P., F.R.C.P.(E)
The Mathilda & Terence Kennedy
  Institute of Rheumatology
Hammersmith, London,
  United Kingdom
Chapters 2, 12

Jacques Miller, M.D., Ph.D.,
  D.Sc., F.R.S.
The Walter and Eliza Hall Institute
  of Medical Research
Royal Melbourne Hospital
Victoria, Australia
Chapter 3

H. M. Moutsopoulos, M.D.,
  F.A.C.P., F.R.C.P.(Edin)
Department of Pathophysiology
University of Athens Medical School
Athens, Greece
Chapter 6

William G. Phillips, M.A., (Cantab.)
  M.R.C.P., M.R.C.G.P.,
  Dip.R.C.Path.
St. John's Institute of Dermatology
St. Thomas's Hospital
London, United Kingdom
Chapter 9

CONTRIBUTORS

Nora Sarvetnick, Ph.D.
Department of Neuropharmacology
The Scripps Research Institute
La Jolla, California, U.S.A.
Chapter 3

F. N. Skopouli, M.D.
Department of Internal Medicine
University of Ioannina
 Medical School
Athens, Greece
Chapter 6

Josef S. Smolen, M.D.
2nd Department of Medicine
 at Lainz Hospital
Ludwig Boltzmann Institute
 for Rheumatology and
Department of Rheumatology
University of Vienna
Vienna, Austria
Chapter 7

Günter Steiner, Ph.D.
Ludwig Boltzmann Institute
 for Rheumatology
University of Vienna
Vienna, Austria
Chapter 7

Lawrence Steinman, M.D.
Department of Neurology
 and Neurological Sciences
Stanford University Medical Center
Stanford, California, U.S.A.
Chapter 4

Andrea Studnicka-Benke, M.D.
2nd Department of Medicine
 at Lainz Hospital
University of Vienna
Vienna, Austria
Chapter 7

PREFACE

Cytokines are the powerful local protein mediators which are now known to be of major importance in virtually every biological process such as immunity, inflammation, cell growth, repair and fibrosis. These proteins were first identified in the late 1960s, biochemically purified in the 1970s, and finally came of age scientifically in the 1980s with the cDNA cloning and expression of abundant cytokine proteins. This led to a dramatic augmentation of the pace of progress, and permitted the evaluation of the role of cytokines in diseases, and clinical trials of cytokines. The first success of cytokines in the clinic were the hemopoietic growth factors, particularly erythropoietin and granulocyte colony stimulating factor, and then the interferons.

With these new molecular tools, it has been possible to demonstrate the involvement of numerous autoimmune diseases. The field of cytokines in autoimmunity is young, but it is rapidly growing. The importance of this field is now apparent, as our work in defining that TNFα was a major proinflammatory cytokine in rheumatoid arthritis has now led to successful clinical trials of anti-TNFα antibody in these patients. These are the first unequivocally (and reproducible) successful trials of an anticytokine therapy, and suggest that with more knowledge of the cytokine networks in a variety of diseases, more therapeutic successes may be attained. This book, by emphasizing what is known and what is yet to be learned, aims to promote the rational therapeutic application of this field.

Our work in this field has depended on the help, encouragement, friendship and support of numerous colleagues, the most important of which is Professor Ravinder Maini. We gratefully acknowledge the enormous assistance generously donated by numerous academic and industrial colleagues.

CHAPTER 1

THE ROLE OF CYTOKINES IN NORMAL AND PATHOLOGICAL SITUATIONS

Marc Feldmann, Steve Dower and Fionula M. Brennan

INTRODUCTION

Cytokines are proteins or glycoproteins, which act as local messengers produced by cells of any type, but most frequently by leucocytes. This definition excludes the hormones, which are produced by specialized cells in endocrine glands, and are transmitted to distant sites by the blood. Some hormones, for example erythropoietin (Epo) which regulates red cells, are clearly related in function to the cytokines and the Epo receptor is part of the 'cytokine' receptor family. Unlike hormones, in most cases cytokines are not produced constitutively, but transiently after stimulation, usually in small quantities.

The term *cytokines* is the current nomenclature for these molecules which encompasses proteins also described in the literature as *interleukins* (1-15 at present), *interferons* (α, β, γ, ω), *growth factors, tumor necrosis factors* and *chemotactic cytokines (chemokines)*. These proteins are essential components of most important biological processes, including cell growth, development, repair, fibrosis, immunity and inflammation.

Most cytokines, unlike hormones, are not found in bioactive forms in plasma or serum, but there are exceptions. Interleukin (IL)-6 is frequently found in the serum in a bioactive form, as is the active form of macrophage colony stimulating factor (M-CSF).

A problem which has bedeviled the field over the years is nomenclature. In many cases the same protein has been described by different groups using different assays and are thus given different names, thus Carswell and colleagues[1] described tumor necrosis factor, whereas

Cytokines in Autoimmunity, edited by Fionula M. Brennan and Marc Feldmann.
© 1996 R.G. Landes Company.

Cerami et al described the same protein as 'cachectin'.[2] As in the case of TNF, the name which is most commonly used often is a very partial reflection of the actions of this protein.

One of the key problems in the field in the past has been to identify and characterize cytokines. This is because they act typically as signaling molecules, working at low concentrations, usually 10^{-10} to 10^{-13} mol/liter, or roughly 1 ng to 1 pg/ml. Their potency is due to the high affinity of their receptors, in the range of 10^{-9} to 10^{-12} mol/liter, and the low receptor occupancy needed for cell activation. Even though more than 80 cytokines have been identified to date it is certain that there are many more, although only pessimists expect this number to approach 1000.

Every cell type expresses multiple cytokine receptors, with some receptors being virtually ubiquitous (e.g., IL-1, IL-6, TNF, IFN). However the effects of a single cytokine on different cell types varies, with this property being known as 'pleiotropy.' There are often several cytokines which can direct the same action. Thus IL-1 and TNFα can both upregulate adhesion molecules in endothelium, and IL-6 and LIF can induce hepatocytes to produce acute phase response proteins such as C reactive protein. This property of overlapping biological effects is known as cytokine 'redundancy'. In some instances the mechanism of 'redundancy' has become known. It can be due to the sharing of signal-transmitting components of the cytokine receptors. Thus both IL-6 and LIF receptors include the gp130 signaling chain, and receptors for IL-2, IL-4, IL-7, IL-9 and IL-15, all T cell growth factors, share what was initially called the IL-2Rγ chain, now just the γc (common). However, there are also differences between the actions of the above cluster of cytokines, dependent on distinct receptor chains and signaling pathways. The properties of cytokines in general are reviewed in references 3-6 and individual cytokines in references 2, 7-16.

CYTOKINE NETWORKS

A common property of cytokines is that they can induce the production of other cytokines.[17] Thus the cytokine products of one cell, for example an antigen presenting cell (APC), including IL-1 and IL-6, can signal to another cell, e.g., a T cell to help it produce IL-2, which may then act on both itself, a process termed 'autocrine' stimulation, or neighboring T cells, termed 'paracrine' stimulation to help produce yet other cytokines, such as IFNγ and GM-CSF. These latter proteins may then feedback to upregulate the activities of the APC, thus illustrating how cytokines can act in networks as signaling molecules, in concert with other signals (e.g., via the T cell receptor for antigen).

There are many other examples of cytokine networks. A prime example is the capacity of TNFα to induce IL-1,[17,18] both of which induce IL-6 and GM-CSF. This network is seen in inflammation in mice, monkey and humans, and has been described in the response to

LPS in animals[19] and in rheumatoid arthritis synovium, both in vitro[18] and in vivo (see chapter 2).

PROPERTIES OF CYTOKINES

CYTOKINE FAMILIES

With developments in molecular and structural biology, it has become apparent that many cytokines belong to 'families', which are related in structure, to some extent in sequence (rarely more than 30% or so) but much more so in 3-D structure. The clearest definition of cytokine families is by binding with similar affinities to the same receptor, e.g., IL-1α and β to the type I and II IL-1 receptors, TNFα and lymphotoxin (LT) to p55 and p75 TNF receptors.

X-ray diffraction and nuclear magnetic resonance analysis of cytokine molecules have identified the 3D structures of cytokines. Many consist of four α helices[20] (hemopoietin family), while others have β sheets, and the members of the TNF family have a jelly roll motif[21] (see Table 1.1). The largest families of cytokines include the chemokines and the interferon α/β family. The structure of several cytokines is represented in the figures: IL-4, a hemopoietin, and IL-8, a chemokine, are shown in Figure 1.1; TNF is illustrated in Figure 1.2.

While cytokines were originally considered to be secretory molecules, studied in the supernatants of activated cells, there is increasing evidence that many cytokines also exist as cell surface bound forms. This has been clearly documented for TNFα, LTβ, IL-1α, TGFα, M-CSF and stem cell factor (SCF). The cell surface forms of these proteins are capable of signaling. This is potentially of importance as during cell-cell contact, high local concentrations of cytokines may be present at the cell surface.

While most cytokines are synthesized with signal sequences encoding a leader peptide and are exported in the normal manner upon cell activation, some cytokines lack signal sequences and have unusual or as yet unknown routes of cell exit. For example IL-1β depends on IL-1 converting enzyme[22] ('ICE') to cleave the 33 kd propeptide found in the cell to yield the 17 kd peptide found outside the cell; however, its route of exit needs further clarification. For FGF and IL-1α the mode of exit is unclear, and it has been proposed that IL-1α is only released after cell death.

Most cytokines are single chain proteins, but some are homodimers (IFNγ, IL-10, TGFβ) or homotrimers (TNFα, LT and members of TNF family, Fig. 1.2). Only IL-12 is a heterodimer. One chain of IL-12, p40, resembles a hemopoietin (or cytokine) soluble receptor chain. While most cytokines are released from cells in a bioactive form, this is not the case for TGFβ,[23] which needs to be activated by acid or enzymes before it is biologically active. Many cytokines bind to glycosaminoglycans such as heparin, biglycan, decorin or the hyaluronic

Table 1.1. Cytokine families: Grouped by structural similarity

Hematopoetins		TNF Family		Chemokines		PDGF Family	
				α (C-X-C) family			
IL-2	(interleukin-2)	TNFα	(tumor necrosis factor α)	IL-8	(interleukin-8)	PDGF A	(platelet derived growth factor)
IL-3	(interleukin-3)	LTα	(lymphotoxin α)	gro α/β/γ	(melanocyte grown stimulating factor)	PDGF B	(platelet derived growth factor)
IL-4	(interleukin-4)	LT β	(lymphotoxin β)	NAP-2	(neutrophil activating protein)	CSF-1	(colony stimulating factor-1)
IL-5	(interleukin-5)	CD40L	(CD40 ligand)	ENA 78	(epithelial neutrophil activating peptide)	Steel Factor	
IL-6	(interleukin-6)	CD30L	(CD30 ligand)	GCP-2	(granulocyte chemotactic protein)		
IL-7	(interleukin-7)	CD27L	(CD27 ligand)	PF4	(platelet factor 4)		
IL-9	(interleukin-9)	4-1BBL		CTAP-3	(connective tissue activating peptide 3)		
IL-11	(interleukin-11)	FasL	(Fas ligand)	Mig	(monokine induced by IFNγ)		
IL-12	(interleukin-12)			γIP-10	(γ interferon inducible protein 10)		
EPO	(erythropoietin)						
LIF	(leukemia inhibitor factor)						
GM-CSF	(granulocyte-macrophage colony stimulating factor)						
G-CSF	(granulocyte colony stimulating factor)						
Onco M	(oncostatin M)						
CNTF	(ciliary neurotrophic factor)						
GH	(growth hormone)						
	(prolactin)						
tpo	(thrombopoetin)						
		IL-1 family		**β (C-C) family**			
		IL-1α	(interleukin-1)	MCP-1	(monocyte chemoattractant protein 1)		
		IL-1β	(interleukin-1β)	MCP-2	(monocyte chemoattractant protein 2)		
		IL-1ra	(interleukin-1 receptor antagonist)	MCP-3	(monocyte chemoattractant protein 3)		
		bFGF	(basic fibroblast growth factor)	MIP-1β	(macrophage inflammatory protein 1β)		
		aFGF	(acidic fibroblast growth factor)	MIP-1α	(macrophage inflammatory protein 1α)		
		ECGF	(endothelial cell growth factor)	RANTES	(regulated upon activation normal T cell expressed and secreted)		
						TGFβ Family	
						TGFβ	1,2,3,4,5 (transforming growth factor)
						(inhibin β 2A, 2B)	
						(activin 1, 2A, 2b, 4)	
						BMP 1,2A,2B 4 (bone morphogenetic protein)	

acid receptor CD44,[24] and are thus sequestered in the extracellular matrix of the connective tissues of skin and bone. Such cytokines include TGFβ, FGF and LIF and many of the chemokine family such as MIP-1α and IL-8. For chemokines, binding to tissue constituents helps to build up the chemotactic gradients which are essential for allowing extavazation of leucocytes into sites of inflammation.

There is now considerable evidence that a cell's response to a cytokine can be augmented or inhibited by other cytokines. For example, IFNγ synergises with TNF to induce IL-1, a mechanism involving upregulation of TNF receptors.[25] In other instances, there is antagonism, for example

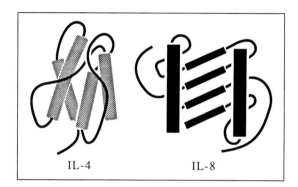

Fig. 1.1. Diagrammatic illustration of the structure of the cytokines IL-4 and IL-8.

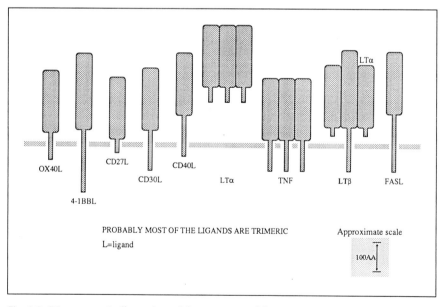

Fig. 1.2. Diagrammatic illustration of the structure of the TNF family of molecules. Most of these molecules are membrane bound with the exception of LTα which is secreted and TNFα which can exist both as a membrane bound pro-TNFα and as a secreted molecule.

IFNγ interferes with the fibroblast growth and fibrosis induced by platelet derived growth factor (PDGF) and antagonizes IL-4 induced IgE production.[26]

IL-10 is often antagonistic to the proinflammatory cytokines. It does this in many different ways: by diminishing the synthesis of monocyte cytokines (IL-1, TNF, IL-6), but also by diminishing T cell activity. Most of the latter action is indirect, by downregulating antigen-presenting function, but there are also direct antagonistic effects on IL-2 production. The properties of proinflammatory cytokines are summarized in Table 1.2. The properties of anti-inflammatory cytokines are summarized in Table 1.3. Properties of chemotactic cytokines are summarized in Table 1.4 (a and b).

CYTOKINE RECEPTORS

Although cytokine receptors vary in abundance, their expression levels are usually low, from 10 to 10,000 sites/cell, usually of high affinity. Sometimes receptors are of dual affinity. It is common for several cytokines to share a receptor (R), e.g., IL-1α, β and the IL-1 receptor antagonist (IL-1ra) share the IL-1R type I and II, TNF and LT share the p55 and p75 TNF-R,[27] acidic and basic FGF share receptors, as do EGF and TGFα, IFNα and β.[28] While most cytokine receptor chains are of the single transmembrane type, the chemokine receptors (including IL-8) have the seven transmembrane segments common to the rhodopsin receptor family, also often referred to as the 'serpentine' receptor family or 'seven spanners'. A pictorial representation of the cytokine receptor families are illustrated in Figure 1.3.

It is now becoming evident that in most instances cytokine receptors (a receptor being defined as a ligand binding and signaling complex) are not single peptide chains. The IL-2 receptor, among the first to be studied, is comprised of three chains α, β and γ,[29] the IL-6 receptor has two types of chains, the IL-6R and the gp130 chain.[30] In many instances there are chains common to several receptors, and in such cases the common chains are involved in signaling. Thus the IL-2Rγ chain (γc) also associates with the IL-4, IL-7, IL-9 and IL-15 receptors, the gp130 chain with IL-6, CNTF, oncostatin M, LIF, IL-11 and cardiotropin-1 receptors. A common β chain associates with IL-3, GM-CSF and IL-5 receptors. In other instances, there are associations of multiple copies of the same chain, e.g., three in the TNF-R p55 or p75, two in the PDGF-R. Current concepts of receptor complexes and chain sharing are illustrated in Figures 1.4, 1.5 and 1.6, although the exact stoichiometry is not yet certain. Thus there is data suggesting that two IL-6 molecules interact with two IL-6R and two gp130 molecules.

In addition to shared receptor chains, there are also examples of dual receptors for the same ligand. Thus IL-1β (and α) bind to both the type I and type II IL-1R. In this case however it has been deter-

The Role of Cytokines in Normal and Pathological Situations

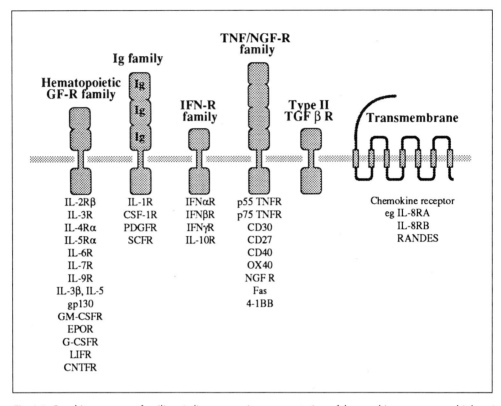

Fig. 1.3. Cytokine receptor families. A diagrammatic representation of the cytokine receptors which are grouped broadly into six categories based on their molecular structure.

mined that all the signaling involves the IL-1 type I receptor,[31] while the type II receptor is a decoy, and when cleared acts as a soluble inhibitor.

There are several major families of cytokine receptors (Fig. 1.3). The largest is the hemopoietin or cytokine receptor family which is characterized by an extracellular region composed of one or more domains containing four conserved cysteines and a tryptophan-serine-X-tryptophan-serine amino acid motif in the membrane proximal domain (Fig. 1.7). Other receptors, such as IL-1R, PDGF-R and M-CSFR, have Ig-like external domains. The latter two have tyrosine kinase intracytoplasmic domains (Fig. 1.8). The IFN receptors form a family which also includes the IL-10 receptor, and is homologous to tissue factor. There is also a large family of proteins which resemble the TNF receptor. These include the low affinity nerve growth factor receptor, and a cluster of proteins involved in immune activation (CD30, CD27, CD40, 41BB and OX40). Their structure is illustrated in Figure 1.9.

Table 1.2. Properties of proinflammatory cytokines

Cytokine	MW (kDa)	Sources	Inducers	Effects	Production Inhibited By
IL-1α	33 membrane 17 soluble	Most cells, especially Mφ, KC, EC membrane associated	LPS, other microbial injurious agents, cytokines: TNF, GM-CSF IL-1, Subs P, IFNγ as costimulation, IL-2	Induces inflammation in most cells, e.g., prostaglandin production, metalloproteinases etc. upregulates adhesion molecules (ICAM-1, VCAM-1 E selection) upregulates other cytokines (IL-2, IFN, CSF TNF, IL-6, IL-8 etc.) upregulates acute phase proteins upregulates T and B cell activation (costimulus) 'Endogenous Pyrogen', stimulates Hypothalamic Pituitary - Adrenal axis	IL-4, IL-13 IL-10 TGFβ
IL-1β	33 → 17 Converted by IL-1 converting enzyme (ICE)	Mφ, neutrophils, astrocytes	As above	As above	As above

Cytokine	Size	Source cells	Inducers	Main actions	Inhibitors
TNFα	17Kd trimeric	M, neutrophils astrocytes	Depends on cell type Mostly as for IL-1	Induces inflammation, e.g., prostaglandins, leukotrienes Upregulates adhesion molecules Upregulates other cytokine (IL-1, IFN, CSF, IL-6, IL-8 etc.) Upregulates acute phase Proteins Upregulates T and B cell activation Upregulates macrophage and neutrophil activation Suppress, e.g., bone marrow, upregulates HLA class I expression Tumor cell cytotoxicity Endogenous pyrogen	IL-4, 13, IL-10 TGFβ
LT	25 Kd trimeric	T and B lymphocytes LGL (NK)	Antigens mitogens	As above for TNFα.	IL-10, IL-4 IL-13, LT
IL-6	20	M, fibroblasts, B, T lymphocytes	Like IL-1 and TNF	B cell growth, Ig production, induces acute phase response, stem cell activation, NK activation, Platelet production, noninflammatory mesangial cell proliferation, activates osteolysis, induces IFN	As above
IFNγ	20-25 dimer	CD4 and CD8 T cells CD4Th1' cells NK (LGL)	T cell activation IL-12, IL-2	Induces class II and class I. Strongest activator of monocytes, augmenting cell surface receptors and priming for cytokine production. Involved in differentiation of CTL, blocks Th$_2$ activity (production IL-4 and IL-5) promotes DTH. Inhibits B cell proliferation and IgE production. Activates neutrophils and NK cells.	IL-10, TGFβ

M, macrophages; KC, keratinocytes; EC, endothelial cell; ICAM, inducible cell adhesion molecule; VCAM, vascular cell adhesion molecule; LGL, large granular lymphocyte; NK, natural killer cell; DTH, Delayed type IV hypersensitivity; CTL, cytotoxic T lymphocyte; Ig, immunoglobulin

Table 1.3. Properties of anti-inflammatory cytokines

Cytokine	MW	Sources	Stimuli	Effects
IL-10	18K, dimer	M, T cell, B cell, KC	LPS for M ? others T cell activation	Inhibits M cytokine production (e.g. IL-1, IL-6, TNFα, GM-CSF, IL-12) Inhibits antigen presentation (class II, B7) Upregulates cytokine inhibitor (sTNF-R, IL-1ra) Downregulates cytokine receptor expression Strong B cell activation, Ig production Induces MMP expression
TGFβ	25 kD, dimer	most cells	depends on cell type	activation of connective tissue growth and synthesis of extracellular matrix inhibitor or hemopoiesis, immune cell activity and inflammation.
IL-4	20K	T cells mast cells	T cell activation IgE activation	T cell growth factor, inducer of Th$_2$ cells Co-activator of B cell growth and Ig secretion (IgE and IgG1 especially) upregulates class II on B cells, activator of most cells and basophils Inhibitor of macrophage proinflammatory cytokine synthesis (IL-1, TNF, IL-6 etc.).
IL-13		T cells mast cells	T cell activation IgE activation	Co-activator of B cell growth and Ig secretion (IgE and IgG1 especially) upregulates class II on B cells, activator of most cells and basophils Inhibitor of macrophage proinflammatory cytokine synthesis (IL-1, TNF, IL-6 etc.).

M = macrophages; KC = keratinocytes; MMP = matrix metalloproteinase.

Table 1.4a. Properties of chemotactic cytokine (chemokines). α (C-X-C) chemokines mostly act on neutrophils

	Sources	Inducers	Actions	Receptor
IL-8	Almost all cells especially macrophages, also neutrophils	Depends on cell type LPS, proinflammatory cytokines	Attracts neutrophils, basophils, eosinophils, T cells. Keratinocyte proliferation, activates neutrophils (degranulation, enzyme release, respiratory burst)	IL-8RA IL-8RB
MGSA/GROα β γ	Almost all cells	IL-1, TNF, LPS etc.	Neutrophil chemotaxis and activation, respiratory burst and enzyme release, melanoma cell proliferation, fibroblast proliferation, neutrophils. attract basophils	IL-8RB ? ?
ENA 78	Epithelial cells	IL-1, TNF etc.	Acts as neutrophils	IL-8RB
PF4	Platelet granules	Platelet activators - immune complexes, thrombin, collagen, adrenaline	Fibroblast activation and chemotaxis inhibits angiogenesis, stimulates ICAM-1 expression.	
CTAP/BT6	Platelet granules	Platelet activators - immune complexes, thrombin, collagen, adrenaline	Fibroblast activation, growth, chemotaxis	
NAP-2	Cleavage BTG	Sites platelet aggregation	Neutrophil chemoattractant and activation	
IP-10	Most cells	LPS, IL-1, TNF	Chemoattractant monocytes and T cells	

Others: Mig, GCP-2, less well defined. Genes for α chemokines are on human chromosome 4.

Table 1.4b. Properties of chemotactic cytokine (chemokines). β (C-C) chemokines: Mostly act on monocytes and lymphocytes

	Sources	Inducers	Actions	Receptor
MCP-1	Monocytes, fibroblasts	LPS, IL-1, TNF	Monocyte and basophil chemotaxis and activation	MCP-1R
MCP-2	Keratinocytes, endothelium		Monocyte and basophil chemotaxis and degranulation	
MCP-3			Monocytes, basophils, eosinophils	
MIP-1α	Monocytes, lymphocytes	LPS, IL-1, TNF, T cell activators	Monocyte chemotaxis T cells (CD8$^+$ especially), B	MIP1α/RANTES
MIP-1β	Monocytes, lymphocytes	LPS, IL-1, TNF, T cell activators	Monocyte chemotaxis T cells (CD4 especially)	
RANTES	T lymphocytes, monocytes endothelium	T cell activators macrophage action	Monocyte chemotaxis T cells (CD4$^+$ CD45 RO$^+$) eosinophils, basophil chemotaxis and activation	MIPα /RANTES
1-309	Lymphocytes	T cell activators	Monocyte chemotaxis	

Genes for β chemokines are on human chromosome 17.

The Role of Cytokines in Normal and Pathological Situations

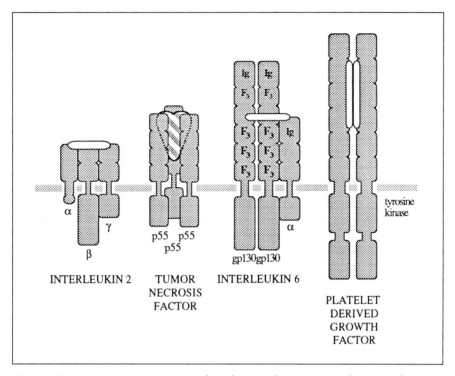

Fig. 1.4. Diagrammatic representation of cytokine-cytokine receptor chain complexes.

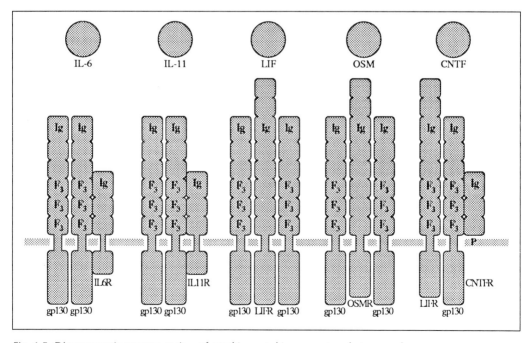

Fig. 1.5. Diagrammatic representation of cytokine-cytokine receptor chain complexes.

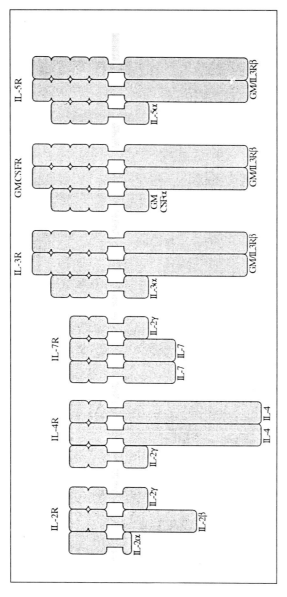

Fig. 1.6. Diagrammatic representation of cytokine-cytokine receptor chain complexes.

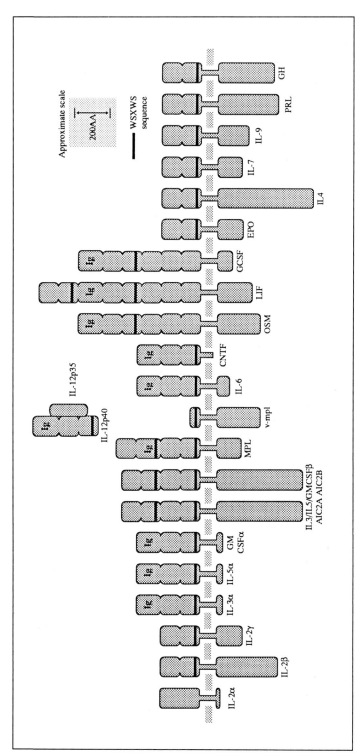

Fig. 1.7. Diagrammatic representation of the hemopoietin cytokine receptor family.

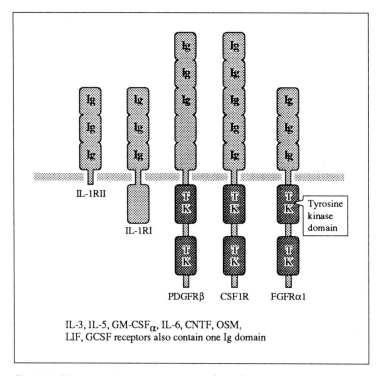

Fig. 1.8. Diagrammatic representation of cytokine receptors containing immunoglobulin-like external domains.

The mechanisms by which cytokine receptors signal are beyond the scope of this chapter, but have been reviewed recently.[32,33]

SOLUBLE CYTOKINE RECEPTORS

Soluble cytokine receptors are found in normal and pathological body fluids.[34,35] These represent the ligand binding extracellular domains of the single transmembrane cytokine receptors. Usually multi-nanogram/ml levels have been detected in body fluids such as serum and urine.[35] In fact it is now known that many other cell membrane receptors also exist in soluble form, e.g., hormone receptors, adhesion molecules and low density lipoprotein receptors. While many of these soluble receptors bind to the ligand with appreciable affinity and can thus act as inhibitors[35,36] (e.g., of TNF, IL-1, IFNγ), this is not the case for all the soluble receptors. The one derived from the IL-6R is strikingly different, as it acts as an agonist. The concept of soluble receptors is illustrated in Figure 1.10.

The cytokine field has now progressed to the state where it is possible to quantitate the expression of the agonist (cytokine), its cell surface receptor, and its inhibitor which most commonly is the soluble receptor. In one instance, the inhibitor is not a soluble receptor, but is a

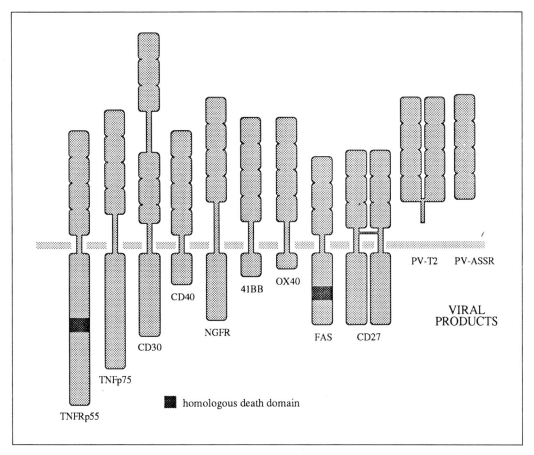

Fig. 1.9. Diagrammatic representation of the TNF receptor family.

receptor antagonist,[37] of the IL-1 receptor. Three forms of this protein exist homologous to IL-1β and members of the IL-1 family. There is a secreted form produced mostly by macrophages, and two intracytoplasmic forms, mostly produced in keratinocytes and epithelial cells. The IL-1 receptor antagonist, abbreviated IL-1ra, has a higher affinity for the IL-1R than IL-1α and IL-1β but does not signal. Due to the low receptor occupancy needed for IL-1 to signal, considerable (~100 fold) molar excess is needed for IL-1ra to fully inhibit IL-1.

CYTOKINE PRODUCTION BY CELLS IN INFLAMMATION AND IMMUNITY

Activation of cells of the macrophage lineage by bacterial toxins such as LPS rapidly induces a group of proinflammatory cytokines. TNFα is produced first, then IL-1α and β, followed by IL-6 and GM-CSF. The relative kinetics of products of the first three cytokines are reproducible in vitro and in vivo, in several species. This group of

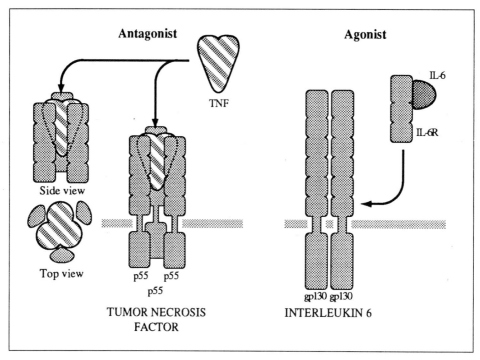

Fig. 1.10. Concept of soluble cytokine receptor interactions with ligand.

cytokines initiate an inflammatory response which involves the upregulation of adhesion molecules on endothelium, and, as activated macrophages cells also produce multiple chemokines, there is a rapid recruitment of other cells to the inflamed site. This consists first of neutrophils, followed by monocytes and T cells; the activation of the cells adds to the inflammatory mediators produced locally. Under normal circumstances cytokine production induced by LPS rapidly switches off, and it is known that these cells are subsequently refractory to further stimuli with LPS.

The production of cytokines from T cells during immune induction is similarly brief. IL-2 and IFNγ are the cytokines most frequently produced, but their production only lasts about 48 hours after initial stimulation.[9] One of the most interesting aspects of T cell function is their segregated production of cytokines. This was first discovered in the mouse for CD4+ cells by Mosmann and Coffman.[38] They found that certain CD4+ T cell clones made IL-2, IFNγ and TNFα and were termed 'Th$_1$', while others made IL-4, IL-5, IL-6, IL-10 and IL-13 and were termed 'Th$_2$'. The Th$_1$ cells were involved in delayed type hypersensitivity responses and some antibody responses, and are considered proinflammatory. The Th$_2$ cells were involved in antibody responses, especially IgA, IgG1 and IgE responses. Of interest is that products of Th$_1$ cells, e.g., IFNγ downregulate Th$_2$ cells, and Th$_2$ products, e.g., IL-4 and IL-10 diminish Th_1 responses, mostly by effects on antigen presenting cells. In humans, most T cells do not segregate as clearly, and are often termed Th_0, producing both IFNγ and IL-4. The development of naive T cells into Th_2 cells depends on IL-4, whereas the development into Th_1 cells depends on IL-12. Thus cytokines themselves can alter the subsequent cytokine profile produced by T cells. A summary of the properties of Th_1 and Th_2 cells is in Table 1.5.

There is now considerable interest in evaluating whether disease states are due to abnormalities of the Th_1/Th_2 balance, and in most autoimmune disease models, such as experimental allergic encephalomyelitis (EAE), it is considered that Th_1 levels are excessive, and Th_2 cells protective. However the reverse is likely to be the case in systemic lupus erythematosus (SLE). There is also evidence that high Th_2 levels are involved in allergic diseases. The cytokine profile produced is of clinical importance in allergy, autoimmunity and infection. For example the latter is clearly demonstrable in mice infected with Leishmania. Genetically susceptible BALB/c mice can be rendered resistant by injection with a neutralizing antibody to IL-4.[39] Other examples are discussed in the following chapters.

REGULATION OF CYTOKINE ACTION

Cytokine action can in principle be regulated at many steps. One of the most critical is production of the ligand, the cytokine, which is usually transient, and rate limiting.[9] There is also regulation at the receptor level, with cytokine and other signals inducing up and down regulation of receptor expression.[29-31] Most importantly, it has been found that single transmembrane receptors are cleaved to release the extracellular domain, which acts as a soluble inhibitor.[35,36] This process is regulated, and the main role of this process may be to prevent signaling. There are natural antibodies to IL-1α, IL-6 and IL-8,[40] in many but not all individuals. Cytokine signaling may also be downregulated intracellularly by receptor desensitization and by competition for common signaling components. Aspects of cytokine regulation are illustrated in Figure 1.11.

WHAT HAPPENS TO CYTOKINES IN DISEASE PROCESSES?

In autoimmune diseases, there is often a persistent immune and inflammatory response, with subsequent repair and fibrosis. It is evident from our current understanding that there must be abnormal cytokine and cytokine receptor expression. What needs to be established is which cytokines have the most influence on major mechanisms of importance in the disease process. This information is not easy to obtain, as the importance of a cytokine in pathogenesis does not correlate with its abundance. For assaying importance, the assays which are most informative in this context are functional, for example what happens if a certain cytokine is neutralized by an antibody. This approach is more helpful than asking what happens with excess cytokine. The neutralization approach has the advantage that it is widely applicable, as neutralizing antibodies to any cytokine (or receptor) can be produced, and the same approach works not only in vitro, but also in animal models and in clinical trials. We have successfully used this

Table 1.5. Functional properties of human T helper subsets

Subset	Cytokine Produced	Main Functions of Cytokine
Th1 Subset	IL-2	T cell growth factor
	IFNγ	Stimulates macrophage activity, cytolytic activity of NK cells Activates neutrophils and vascular endothelial cells Required for maturation of CD8+ CTLs Promotes differentiation to Th1 cells, inhibits proliferation of Th2 cells Stimulates switching of B cells to IgG2a and IgG3 production
	LT	Initiates a cascade of cytokines and other factors associated with the inflammatory response
Th0 Subset	IL-3	Promotes growth and differentiation of multipotential progenitor cells
	IL-6	Induces growth of T cells and B cells
	IL-9	Putative survival factor for T cells Supports growth of mast cell progenitors Potentiates the effects of IL-4 on stimulation of IgG, IgE and IgM production by B cells
	IL-10	Potent immunosuppressant of macrophage function Suppresses production of proinflammatory cytokines Enhances B cell proliferation and Ig secretion, switch factor for IgG4 Inhibitor of T cell growth
	IL-13	Similar effects to IL-4 but no effects on T cells
	GM-CSF	Promotes growth
Th2 Subset	IL-4	Growth factor for Th2 cells, promotes differentiation of naive cells to Th2 phenotype Growth factor for mast cells Induces proliferation and differentiation of B cells Stimulates switching of B cells to IgG4 and IgE production Inhibits monocyte/macrophage activation
	IL-5	Stimulates growth and differentiation of eosinophils Acts on mature B cells to increase Ig synthesis, especially IgA

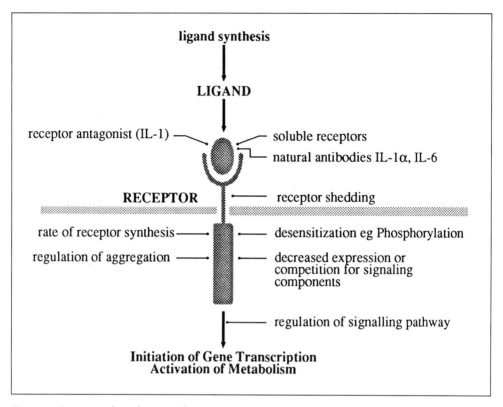

Fig. 1.11. Concept of cytokine regulation.

approach in the analysis of cytokine regulation in rheumatoid arthritis, as described in chapter 2.

ACKNOWLEDGMENTS

We thank Louise Webb for producing Table 1.5 and constructive comments.

REFERENCES

1. Carswell EA, Old LJ, Kassel RL et al. An endotoxin-induced serum factor that causes necrosis of tumors. Proc Natl Acad Sci 1975; 72:3666-3670.
2. Beutler B, Cerami A. The biology of cachectin/TNF—a primary mediator of the host response. Ann Rev Immunol 1989; 7:625-655.
3. Oppenheim JJ, Saklatvala J. Cytokines and their receptors. In: Oppenheim JJ, Rossio JL, Gearing AJH, eds. Clinical applications of cytokines. Role in pathogenesis, diagnosis and therapy. Oxford: Oxford University Press, 1993:3-15.
4. Aggarwal BB, Puri RK. Common and uncommon features of cytokines and cytokine receptors: an overview. Aggarwal BB, Puri RK, eds. In: Human

cytokines: their role in disease and therapy. Blackwell Science, 1995:4-24.
5. Callard RE, Gearing AJH. The Cytokine Facts Book. Academic Press, 1994:2-6.
6. Paul WE. Pleiotropy and redundancy of T cell derived lymphokines in the immune responses. Cell 1989; 57:521-524.
7. Oppenheim JJ, Zachariae COC, Mukaida N et al. Properties of the novel proinflammatory supergene "intercrine" cytokine family. Ann Rev Immunol 1991; 9:617.
8. Moore KW, O'Garra A, de Waal-Malefyt R et al. Interleukin-10. Ann Rev Immunol 1993; 11:165-190.
9. Smith KA. Interleukin-2: inception, impact and implications. Science 1988; 240:1169-1176.
10. Metcalf D. Hematopoietic regulators : redundancy or subtlety? Blood 1993; 82:3515-3523.
11. Kishimoto T, Akira S, Taga T. Interleukin-6 and its receptor: a paradigm for cytokines. Science 1992; 258:22-26.
12. Dinarello CA. The interleukin-1 family: 10 years of discovery. FASEB J 1994; 8:1314-1325.
13. Paul WE. Interleukin-4: a prototypic immunoregulatory lymphokine. Blood 1991; 77:1859-1870.
14. Trinchieri G. Interleukin-12: A proinflammatory cytokine with immunoregulatory functions that bridge innate resistance and antigen-specific adaptive immunity. Ann Rev Immunol 1995; 13:251-276.
15. Henney CS. Interleukin 7: effects on early events in lymphopoiesis. Immunol Today 1989; 10:170-173.
16. Farrar MA, Schreiber RD. The molecular cell biology of interferon γ and its receptor. Ann Rev Immunol 1993; 11:571-611.
17. Dinarello CA, Cannon JG, Wolff SM et al. Tumor necrosis factor (cachectin) is an endogenous pyrogen and induces production of interleukin 1. J Exp Med 1986; 163:1433-1450.
18. Brennan FM, Chantry D, Jackson A et al. Inhibitory effect of TNFα antibodies on synovial cell interleukin-1 production in rheumatoid arthritis. Lancet 1989; 2:244-247.
19. Fong Y, Tracey KJ, Moldawer LL et al. Antibodies to cachectin/tumor necrosis factor reduce interleukin 1β and interleukin 6 appearance during lethal bacteremia. J Exp Med 1989; 170:1627-1633.
20. Boulay JL, Paul WE. Hematopoietin sub-family classification based on size, gene organization and sequence homology. Curr Biol 1993; 3:573-581.
21. Jones EY, Stuart DI, Walker NPC. Structure of tumour necrosis factor. Nature 1989; 338:225-228.
22. Cerretti DP, Kozlosky CJ, Mosley B et al. Molecular cloning of the interleukin-1β converting enzyme. Science 1992; 256:97-100.
23. Roberts AB, Sporn MB. The transforming growth factors-beta. In: Sporn MB, Roberts AB, eds. Handbook of Experimental Pharmacology. Heidelberg: Springer Verlag, 1990:419-472.

24. Noble NA. In vivo interactions of TGF-beta and extracellular matrix. Prog Growth Factor Res 1992; 4:369-382.
25. Aggarwal BB, Eessalu TE, Hass PE. Characterization of receptors for human tumour necrosis factor and their regulation by gamma-interferon. Nature 1985; 318:665-667.
26. Coffman RL, Carty J. A T cell activity that enhances polyclonal IgE production and its inhibition by interferon-γ. J Immunol 1986; 136:949.
27. Gray PW, Barrett K, Chantry D et al. Cloning of human tumor necrosis factor (TNF) receptor cDNA and expression of recombinant soluble TNF-binding protein. Proc Natl Acad Sci USA 1990; 87:7380-7384.
28. Novick D, Cohen B, Rubinstein M. The human interferon α/β receptor: characterization and molecular cloning. Cell 1994; 77:391-400.
29. Taniguchi T, Minami Y. The IL-2/IL-2 receptor system: A current overview. Cell 1993; 73:5-8.
30. Hibi M, Murakami M, Saito M et al. Molecular cloning and expression of an IL-6 signal transducer, gp130. Cell 1990; 63:1149-1157.
31. Sims JE, Gayle MA, Slack JL et al. Interleukin 1 signalling occurs exclusively via the type 1 receptor. Proc Natl Acad Sci 1993; 90:6155-6159.
32. Marshall CJ. Specificity of receptor tyrosine kinase signaling: Transient versus sustained extracellular signal-regulated kinase activation. Cell 1995; 80:179-278.
33. Taniguchi T. Cytokine signaling through nonreceptor protein tyrosine kinases. Science 1995; 268:251-255.
34. Fernandez-Botran R. Soluble cytokine receptors: their role in immunoregulation. FASEB J 1991; 5:2567-2574.
35. Novick D, Englemann H, Wallach D et al. Soluble cytokine receptors are present in normal human murine. J Exp Med 1989; 170:1409-1414.
36. Engelmann H, Aderka D, Rubinstein M et al. A tumor necrosis factor-binding protein purified to homogeneity from human murine protects cells from tumor necrosis factor toxicity. J Biol Chem 1989; 264:11974-11980.
37. Arend WP. Interleukin-1 receptor antagonist. Adv Immunol 1993; 54:167-227.
38. Mosmann TR, Coffman RL. Th$_1$ and Th$_2$ cells: Different patterns of lymphokine secretion lead to different functional properties. Ann Rev Immunol 1989; 7:145-173.
39. Sadick MD, Heinzel FP, Holaday BJ et al. Cure of murine leishmaniasis with anti-interleukin 4 monoclonal antibody. J Exp Med 1990; 171:115-127.
40. Bendtzen K, Svenson M, Jonsson V et al. Autoantibodies to cytokines-friends or foes? Immunol Today 1990; 11:167-169.

CHAPTER 2

CYTOKINES IN RHEUMATOID ARTHRITIS

Fionula M. Brennan, Ravinder N. Maini and
Marc Feldmann

ABSTRACT

Rheumatoid arthritis (RA) is an autoimmune disease with inflammatory manifestations in the peripheral synovial joints, which are infiltrated by blood-borne cells, chiefly T cells, macrophages and plasma cells. We have investigated the role of cytokines in RA and from this analysis have proposed that tumor necrosis factor α (TNFα) has a pivotal role in the pathogenesis of this disease.

In this chapter, we review the role of many cytokines in the pathogenesis of this disease, and in particular, observations which indicate that TNFα plays a pivotal role in this process. These findings have led to the development of therapeutic strategies and clinical trials to block this proinflammatory cytokine in RA (as discussed in detail in chapter 12 of this book). In addition to proinflammatory cytokine production at sites of inflammation such as the RA synovial joint, there is also much evidence for homeostatic immunoregulatory mechanisms which include the production of cytokine inhibitors such as soluble TNF-R and the IL-1 receptor antagonist, and cytokines with immunoregulatory properties like IL-10 and TGFβ. These findings indicate that in the RA joint an attempt at immune regulation is occurring. Such observations may well lead to the development of alternative approaches for therapeutic manipulation in this disease, by upregulating the endogenous inhibitory mechanisms.

INTRODUCTION

Rheumatoid arthritis (RA) is a chronic inflammatory autoimmune disease, in which the peripheral synovial joints become swollen and

Cytokines in Autoimmunity, edited by Fionula M. Brennan and Marc Feldmann.
© 1996 R.G. Landes Company.

inflamed, leading eventually to joint failure as a result of the destruction of articular cartilage and subchondral bone. The pathogenic mechanisms which underlie this disease are thought to be due to a complex interplay of genetic and environmental factors.[1] The importance of the genetic factors are not however understood, as the concordance for disease in identical twins is low (15-30%).[2] The largest contribution to this genetic susceptibility is thought to be contained within the HLA genetic component, with the large majority of RA patients being DR4 and/or DR1. Interestingly, similar amino acids exist in position 67-74 of the peptide binding groove on the HLA-DR β chain of DR1 and DR4 (w4, 14 and 15), which has led to the emergence of the 'shared epitope' hypothesis, suggesting that at some stage of the pathogenesis, T cells which recognize DR1 or DR4 must be involved.[3] Cytokine and cytokine receptor genes (some of which are encoded within the MHC loci), and T cell receptors may also be of importance in genetic susceptibility.

In contrast to normal joint synovium, which has few cells, the rheumatoid synovium is infiltrated with cells derived from blood. The lining layer becomes thicker, and perivascular follicles of cells emerge in the deeper layer. The most abundant cells are T lymphocytes and macrophages; but plasma cells, dendritic cells, activated fibroblasts, and endothelial cells are also abundant. In addition there is upregulation of HLA class II and other adhesion molecules of relevance in antigen presentation.[4] Occasionally autoantigen reactive T cells such as those specific for collagen type II[5] can be detected in RA joints. However, in most active RA patients autoantigen reactive T cells cannot be isolated, there is a diminished immune response with reduced T cell proliferation; delayed hypersensitivity skin test responses are also low.[6] These results suggest that there are mechanisms downregulating T cell function in RA patients with active disease. Although the etiology of the disease is unknown, and the specific contribution of autoreactive T cells to the pathogenesis of different stages of the disease is disputed, it is now generally well accepted that the eventual destruction of the articular cartilage and the subchondral bone is brought about by activated cells within the synovium, cartilage and adjacent bone, and, in particular, the cytokine and enzyme products which they release.

CYTOKINE ANALYSIS

Measurement of cytokine levels in blood is of limited value because cytokines in such samples are evaluated at a site distant from the site of inflammation and are invariably biologically inactive, being present in an excess of cytokine inhibitors. In a chronic inflammatory disease like RA, in which the local sites (synovial joints) display the most marked pathology, it seems logical to document cytokines produced at this site, as they are most relevant to the disease process. It is for this reason that we have chiefly studied synovial cytokine expression and that we developed an in vitro culture system using synovial membrane mononuclear cells (MNC) isolated from synovium obtained during joint replacement surgery. Cytokine secretion in synovial fluids was not studied, as the presence of enzymes, rheumatoid factors, and high concentrations of hyaluronan, in addition to specific cytokine inhibitors, can all inhibit the detection of cytokine bioactivity and also, to a lesser extent, interfere with their detection in immunoassays. Thus mononuclear cells within the synovium were separated from the extracellular matrix by enzyme digestion, and were cultured for up to 5-6 days without exogenous stimulation. Initially mRNA was assayed as an index of local synthesis, and subsequently the production of cytokine protein in the supernatants of these short term cultures was determined. These in vitro studies were subsequently supplemented with immunohistological analysis of both cytokines and their respective receptors in synovial membrane sections. As a comparison we performed parallel experiments upon tissues from joints with a degenerative disease, osteoarthritis, which in its late stage also destroys connective tissue and leads to joint replacement.

CYTOKINE EXPRESSION IN RHEUMATOID SYNOVIAL TISSUE

Using isolated cells from RA synovial membranes, we demonstrated initially that mRNA for both T cell (IFNγ, IL-2, LT)[7] and macrophage derived (IL-1, TNFα, IL-6)[8,9] cytokines were reproducibly found in all samples, although varying in their abundance (Table 2.1). This was true regardless of the duration of the disease or existing drug therapy, including agents such as corticosteroids which have been reported to downregulate proinflammatory cytokine synthesis. The results suggested that cells at this disease site were producing cytokines chronically, unlike the regulated transient production observed in peripheral blood mononuclear cells (PBMC) activated by mitogen. This hypothesis was tested by placing the dissociated synovial cells in tissue culture, in the absence of extrinsic stimulation. Over a 6-7 day culture period the cell mixture consisting of activated T lymphocytes, macrophages, fibroblasts and endothelial cells remained relatively stable, before fibroblast outgrowth occurred. During this period the production of a number of cytokines was found to persist in vitro including IL-1,[8] TNFα,[8,9] IL-6,[9] IL-8,[10] TGFβ,[11] GM-CSF,[12,13] and as shown more recently, IL-10.[14] However, in contrast to cytokine proteins principally derived from macrophages such as IL-6, IL-1, TNFα, it was more difficult to demonstrate the 'expected' levels of the soluble cytokine products of T cells such as IL-2, IFNγ and LT despite the presence of activated T cells as judged by cell surface marker analysis.[15,16] This, together with the observation that T cells from RA synovial tissue proliferate suboptimally if stimulated with recall antigens or mitogens, has led to the speculation that T cells in RA may be downregulated in some way, or may conceivably be of minimal relevance in late disease.[17] The physiology of T cells, however, is unlike that of macrophages, in that they migrate to sites of inflammation in which they often adhere directly to their target cells. Thus T cells do not need to secrete abundant quantities of cytokines to transmit effective signals. Furthermore, the recent observations that some cytokines such as LT (LTα) can be anchored in the cell membrane by binding to the membrane form of LT (LTβ)[18] indicates that some T cell cytokines may function as membrane-bound molecules, which would not be detected in supernatants.

Therefore, the mere presence of cytokines does not tell us about their relevance (if any) in the pathogenesis of the disease and neither

Table 2.1. Cytokine expression in RA synovial tissue

Cytokine		mRNA	Protein
IL-1α & β	(interleukin 1)	Yes	Yes
TNFα	(tumor necrosis factor α)	Yes	Yes
LT	(lymphotoxin)	Yes	+/−
GM-CSF	(granulocyte macrophage colony stimulating factor)	Yes	Yes
M-CSF	(macrophage colony stimulating factor)	Yes	Yes
IL-6	(interleukin 6)	Yes	Yes
LIF	(leucocyte inhibitory factor)	Yes	Yes
IL-11	(interleukin 11)	?	?
Onco M	(Oncostatin M)	?	?
IL-2	(interleukin 2)	Yes	+/−
IL-3	(interleukin 3)	No	No
IL-7	(interleukin 7)	?	?
IL-9	(interleukin 9)	?	?
IL-15	(interleukin 15)	Yes	Yes
IFNα	(interferon α)	Yes	Yes
IFNβ	(interferon β)	?	?
IFNγ	(interferon γ)	Yes	+/−
IL-12	(interleukin 12)	Yes	Yes
IL-4	(interleukin 4)	?	No
IL-10	(interleukin 10)	Yes	Yes
IL-13	(interleukin 13)	Yes	Yes
TGFβ	(transforming growth factor β)	Yes	Yes
IL-8	(interleukin 8)	Yes	Yes
Gro α	(melanoma growth stimulating activity)	Yes	Yes
MIP-1α	(macrophage inflammatory protein 1 α)	Yes	Yes
MIP-1β	(macrophage inflammatory protein 1 β)	Yes	Yes
MCP-1	(monocyte chemoattractant protein 1)	Yes	Yes
ENA-78	(epithelial neutrophil activating peptide 78)	Yes	Yes
RANTES	(regulated upon activation T cell expressed & secreted)	Yes	Yes
FGF	(fibroblast growth factor)	Yes	Yes
PDGF	(platelet-derived growth factor)	Yes	Yes

do the quantities of cytokines detected reflect their importance. Much greater insight is obtained by investigating cellular interactions in the synovial cultures by using neutralizing antibodies to individual cytokines. We focused predominantly on TNFα and IL-1, as both these cytokines were reported to induce PGE2 production, cartilage destruction[19,20] and bone resorption[21,22] in vitro. Furthermore, if injected intra-articularly into the knee joints of rabbits, IL-1 induces a transient synovitis and proteoglycan loss from articular cartilage.[23] More recently it was shown that administration of IL-1 and TNFα accelerates the development of arthritis in rodents susceptible to the development of collagen induced arthritis (reviewed by Brennan[24]).

In the RA MNC culture system we had noted that there was an unusually large proportion of IL-1α mRNA and protein compared with the usually dominant form of IL-1 (IL-1β).[8] These results suggested that the normal balance of the two cytokines, or their regulation, may be disturbed. Further, IL-1 was produced continuously for the entire period of the cultures, indicating that the factor(s) or signals responsible for chronic production of IL-1 were contained within the RA suspension culture. Likely candidates were cytokine molecules themselves, which can regulate their own expression and that of other cytokine molecules by autocrine and paracrine pathways. We and others had observed that TNFα strongly induces IL-1 activity in monocytes, at a level comparable to lipopolysaccharide (LPS).[25] Thus we determined the effect of neutralizing TNFα on IL-1 production in the RA MNC cultures. Surprisingly, in all RA cultures tested, IL-1 bioactivity was markedly inhibited within 3 days in the presence of anti-TNF antibodies.[26] This implied that an important signal for IL-1 production in the RA synovial tissue was TNFα, and that by blocking one proinflammatory cytokine (TNFα) the production of another equally proinflammatory protein, namely IL-1, could also be blocked.

These results gave the first indication of the importance of TNFα in the pathogenesis of RA and prompted us to investigate whether other cytokines in the RA MNC cultures were also regulated by TNFα. This indeed proved to be the case, as it was found that anti-TNFα antibodies also inhibited the production of another proinflammatory cytokine, granulocyte monocyte colony stimulating factor (GM-CSF).[12,27] GM-CSF in addition to being a growth factor for monocytes in hemopoiesis, also activates granulocytes, mature monocytes and macrophages. It has been implicated in contributing to the pathogenesis of RA, based on the observation that it can induce and maintain HLA class II expression on monocytes.[13] It may also affect other cell types in RA tissue, as it can also augment neutrophil mediated cartilage degradation and adherence.[28]

In more recent studies we have observed diminution in IL-6 and IL-8 production in RA synovial cell cultures incubated with either a neutralizing monoclonal anti-TNFα antibody or the IL-1 receptor antagonist, (IL-1ra)[29] (Fig. 2.1). IL-6 and IL-8 are both found in large (ng) quantities in RA culture supernatants. Although IL-6 does not directly exhibit the proinflammatory properties of TNFα and IL-1, it is a potent B cell growth and differentiation factor, induces acute phase proteins and is involved in bone erosion.[30] Thus, through augmentation of rheumatoid factor and other autoantibodies in the synovium, it could indirectly exacerbate inflammation. IL-8 belongs to the newly designated 'chemokine' family which is an abbreviation for chemotactic cytokine.[31] It is produced by a wide range of cell types in the joints, and functions as a potent neutrophil chemoattractant and activation factor. The presence of other members of the chemokine family in RA synovial tissue has been investigated. One interesting member molecule of this family is RANTES (Regulated upon Activation, T Cell Expressed and Secreted) which is chemotactic for memory CD4 cells (CD45RO) and monocytes. In a recent paper the presence of this

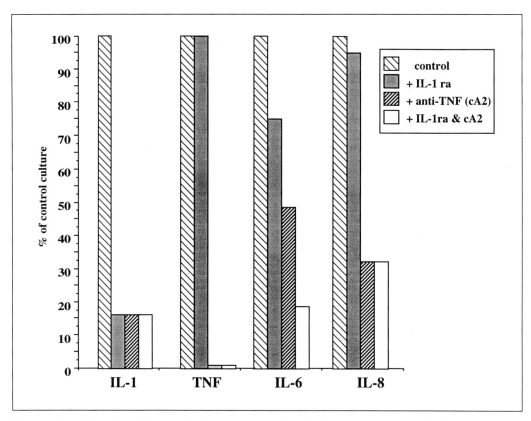

Fig. 2.1. Regulation of cytokine production in RA synovial cell cultures. Dissociated cells from RA synovial membranes were cultured for 2 days with medium alone or in the presence of anti-TNFα mab, cA2, (2.5 μg/ml) and/or IL-1ra (100 ng/ml). TNF and IL-1 levels were measured by bioassay and IL-6 and IL-8 levels (ng/ml) were measured by ELISA.

chemokine in RA tissue was described, and it was suggested that it may be responsible, in part, for the selective migration of CD45RO memory cells to this site. Other chemokines of interest include MCP-1 (monocyte chemoattractant protein-1), which is also produced by activated macrophages in RA synovium.[32] More recently, macrophage inflammatory protein 1α[33] and epithelial neutrophil activating peptide 78 (abbreviated ENA78),[34] cytokines chemotactic for macrophages and neutrophils have also been described to be produced spontaneously by RA synovial cells in culture. The involvement of TNFα in inducing RANTES or other chemokines such as MCP or MIP-1α has yet to be investigated.

IL-1 and TNFα also both induce the expression of adhesion molecules such as ICAM-1, E-Selectin and V-CAM1 on endothelium and other cell types, reviewed.[35] Thus it was of interest to observe that in the RA MNC cultures treated with anti-TNFα antibody, the cells were less tightly aggregated, and HLA class II antigens were also down modulated (Brennan et al, unpublished). The multi-functional effects of TNFα in RA synovial tissue are illustrated in Figure 2.2. From these studies we have postulated that TNFα has a pivotal role in the cytokine interactivities and that the cytokine 'cascade' is unidirectional, in that TNFα induces IL-1 but not visa versa, but that

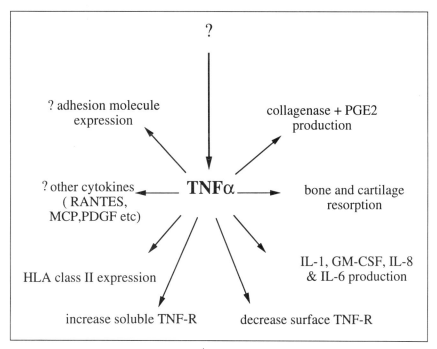

Fig. 2.2. Effects mediated by TNFα in rheumatoid arthritis. Modified from Br J Rheumatol, 1992, 31:293, and reproduced with permission from Oxford University Press.

cytokines further 'downstream' can be modulated by both TNF or IL-1.[29] This concept is illustrated in Figure 2.3, and indicates that the interactions between cytokines in an inflammatory tissue such as rheumatoid synovium do not necessarily reflect their potential pleiotropism as identified in vitro on transformed and normal cell lines. In contrast, in an inflamed tissue in vivo, it matters where cytokines are produced, how much are made and where their receptors are expressed.

Using immunohistological techniques the presence of TNFα in RA synovium was confirmed to be mostly in the CD68 positive macrophages in the synovial lining layer, and in the cartilage pannus junction.[36] As these cells also express augmented TNF receptor (p55 and p75) this indicates the potential for further TNF signal transduction in these cells. Lesser amounts of TNFα were also detected in some T cells, and interestingly, in endothelial cells.[37]

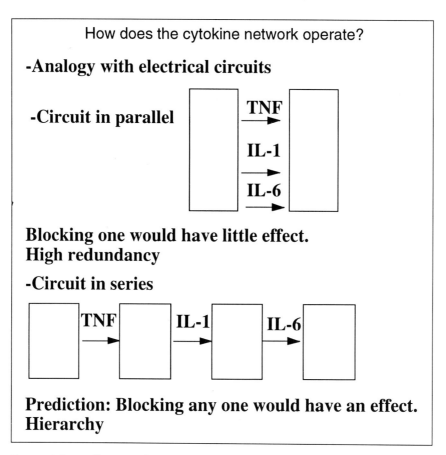

Fig. 2.3. Scheme illustrating the cytokine network. Studies on RA synovial tissue suggest a 'circuit in series' network. Reprinted with permission from BB Aggarwal and RK Puri, eds; Human Cytokines: Their Role in Disease and Therapy, Blackwell Sciences.

STUDIES IN ANIMAL MODELS

Much supportive evidence concerning the importance if cytokines in arthritis, and especially the major role of TNFα, has come from animal studies, including those in transgenic mice. The DBA/1 mouse occasionally develops arthritis spontaneously later in life, and does so regularly after injection intradermally of collagen type II in complete Freund's adjuvant. The arthritis resembles RA, particularly in the erosion of cartilage and bone, and has provided a useful method to evaluate the effect of blocking TNF on the disease process. A hamster monoclonal anti-mouse TNF antibody (TN3.19.2) was injected *after* the onset of arthritis, thus potentially mimicking the clinical therapeutic situation, and was found to ameliorate the disease process, as judged by all the three aspects measured: (i) degree of footpad swelling, a measure of inflammation; (ii) recruitment of new diseased limbs, a measure of disease progression; and (iii) most importantly, by histological analysis of erosions and cell infiltrate.[38] Similar results have been reported by others in this animal model.[39,40]

Perhaps one of the clearest definitions of the pathogenic role of TNFα in arthritis has come from is the work of George Kollias and his colleagues[41] who have generated transgenic mice expressing human TNFα, from a transgene modified, in the 3' untranslated AU rich region (which yields unstable mRNA), by replacement with the β-globin 3' UTR. These mice develop a rheumatoid-like arthritis from 4 weeks of age, preventable by treatment with anti-human TNFα antibodies. It is not clear why the mice develop arthritis only, as the disregulated TNF expression should be widespread in the tissues. This result suggest that the joint tissue is particularly sensitive to the proinflammatory effects of TNFα or that TNFα is most readily inducible in joints. It appears that secreted TNFα is not obligatory in this model, as mice which express disregulated human TNFα under the strong T cell promoter CD2, in which the human TNFα transgene lacks the 12 amino acid sequence essential for cleavage of membrane bound 26 kD TNFα, also develop arthritis (Kollias, unpublished observation, reported at TNF Congress, Monterey, CA, 1994, also see chapter 11).

REGULATION OF CYTOKINE RESPONSES IN RHEUMATOID ARTHRITIS

Despite the chronic inflammation in RA often lasting many years, the disease is also characterized by periods of relative quiescence, indicating that homeostatic immunoregulatory mechanisms are operational. This is often the case during pregnancy. From our in vitro studies we have observed that in many cases these homeostatic immunoregulatory mechanisms are upregulated, albeit insufficiently, in an 'attempt' to combat the inflammatory processes. This is particularly well illustrated with respect to cytokine expression, both by an increase in the expression of inhibitors of cytokines, and also by an increase in the production of cytokines with anti-inflammatory and/or immunoregulatory properties.

CYTOKINE INHIBITORS

An important step in understanding cytokine regulation has come from the elucidation and study of specific cytokine inhibitors, of which there are two groups. The major group consists of soluble cytokine receptors (reviewed in ref. 42), and are derived from the extracellular domain of most of the cytokine receptors already characterized, with the exception of the G-protein coupled chemokine receptors. The second group of receptor antagonists is represented solely by the IL-1 receptor antagonist (IL-1ra), a member of the IL-1 family with 25% homology to IL-1α which binds to the same receptors but is not capable of signalling.[43]

The best studied example of soluble receptors are the soluble TNF receptors. These were originally described in the late 80s independently by three groups, those of Dayer,[86] Wallach,[87] and Olsson,[88] in the urine of febrile patients. Both p55 and p75 TNF-R were subsequently found in biological fluids of normal individuals including plasma and urine. We have found that both p55 and p75 TNF-R are elevated in the plasma of RA patients,[44] and that these levels are even more augmented in synovial fluid. This suggests that the source of these molecules in RA serum is the synovial membrane. Surface TNF receptor expression is increased in RA synovial tissue, both at mRNA level and on the surface of cells.[37,45] Immunohistological studies indicated that the macrophages in the lining layer and at the cartilage pannus junction express increased levels of both receptors, whilst the T lymphocytes express elevated levels of the p75 TNF-R. In RA MNC cultures, soluble p75 and p55 TNF-R are released spontaneously with the former more abundantly. This is also reflected in both synovial fluid exudate and in plasma, where soluble p75 TNF-R is more abundant than p55 TNF-R. This does not necessarily indicate that this TNF-R is more abundant on the surface of all cells, but appears to be the principle soluble TNF-R released from cells upon activation. Both these soluble TNF-R function as TNF blockers, as the TNF inhibitory activity detected both in synovial fluid[44] and synovial cell culture supernatants[46] is reversed with antibodies directed against both these receptors (Fig. 2.4). However, despite the elevated levels of these molecules, this regulatory mechanism is clearly insufficient as we have found bioactive TNF is still detectable in all RA synovial joint cell cultures. This imbalance between production of TNF, surface and soluble TNF-R in health and disease is summarized in Figure 2.5.

IL-1ra was originally described by Dayer in the urine of febrile individuals.[47] This protein shares a high degree of homology with IL-1α and IL-1β, binds both IL-1 receptors in man, but does not transduce detectable signals in any known circumstance. Since low IL-1 receptor occupancy is sufficient to trigger, in order to effectively block IL-1 it must occupy >98% IL-1 receptors on the cell surface, and thus must be present in a large excess over the ligand. The presence of IL-1ra in synovial fluid mononuclear cells and synovial fluid has been demonstrated[48] and it has been immunolocalised (to macrophages) in RA and OA synovial tissue.[49,50] A second IL-1 inhibitor was also detected in synovial fluid, and was found to be the soluble type II IL-1 receptor.[51] This shed receptor, unlike its membrane bound counterpart binds IL-1β, but not the IL-1ra. The presence of both IL-1ra and soluble

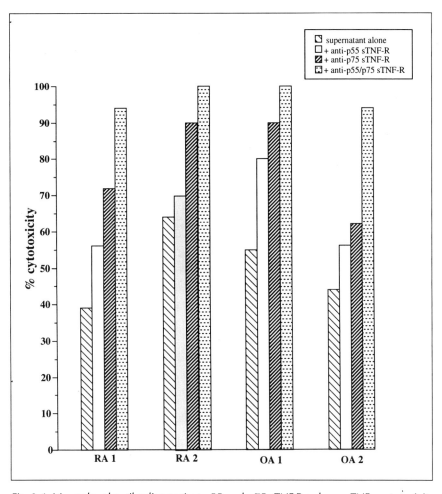

Fig. 2.4. Monoclonal antibodies against p55 and p75 sTNF-R enhance TNFα cytotoxicity in synovial joint cell culture supernatants. RA (n = 2) and OA (n = 2) supernatants were preincubated with medium alone, monoclonal anti-p55, anti-p75 antibody or both antibodies together as described above, before assessing TNFα bioactivity. Results are expressed as percentage cytotoxicity of culture supernatant as determined in the TNF bioassay. Reprinted with permission from Scandinavian University Press, Scan J Immunology 1995; 42:158.

IL-1R could enable IL-1 bioactivity to be countered more effectively both by blocking the receptor and by neutralizing the ligand. However, despite their increased levels in synovial tissue this homeostatic mechanism is obviously insufficient, as IL-1 bioactivity is still detected in RA joint cell cultures.[26]

REGULATION OF CYTOKINE INHIBITOR PRODUCTION

The observation that cytokine inhibitor production is augmented, although insufficiently to neutralize all TNFα in RA synovium, has led us to investigate the mechanisms of sTNF-R release from mono-

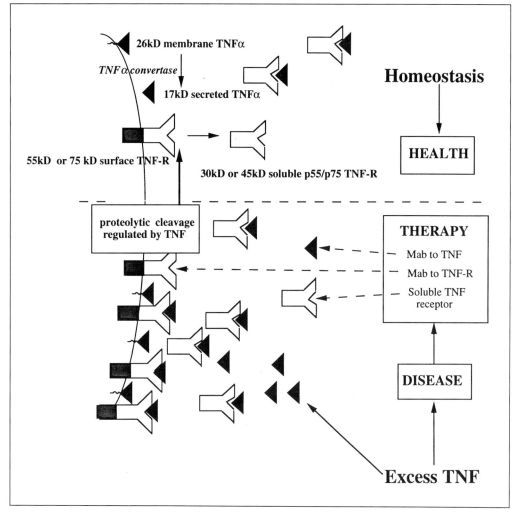

Fig. 2.5. Interaction between TNFα, surface TNF receptor and soluble TNF receptor in health and disease. Modified from JJ Oppenheim et al, Clinical applications of cytokines: role in pathogenesis, diagnosis and therapy, reprinted with permission from Oxford University Press.

cytes and their regulation. These studies have confirmed that activators of monocytes including LPS, IL-1 and TNFα itself[52] can cause down regulation of surface TNF receptor expression, whilst upregulating sTNF-R levels in the culture supernatants. However, the net level of surface TNF receptor in joints is higher than on resting cells, indicating that receptor expression is a very dynamic equilibrium.

We were particularly interested in investigating to what extent immunoregulatory cytokines such as TGFβ, IL-4 and IL-10 modulate TNF receptor expression. All three cytokines inhibit TNFα and IL-1 production in monocytes[53-55] and all stimulate the secretion of the IL-1ra.[55-57] We confirmed that exposure of monocytes to IL-1α in the presence of TGFβ, IL-4 or IL-10 inhibited TNFα production, and all three cytokines induced down regulation of surface TNF receptor expression. IL-4 and TGFβ suppressed the release of soluble TNF-R,[52] but in contrast IL-10 augmented p55 and p75 sTNF-R release in a dose dependent manner, and induced TNF-R mRNA expression (Fig. 2.6). These results indicate that IL-10 reduces the proinflammatory potential of

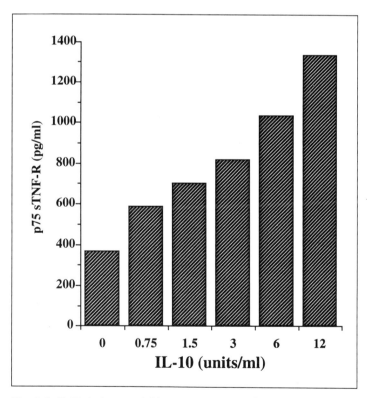

Fig. 2.6. IL-10 induces soluble p75 TNF-R production in monocyte cultures. Soluble p75 TNF-R production measured in the supernatant by a specific ELISA.

TNF in at least three ways: by down regulating surface TNF-R expression, increasing production of soluble TNF-R, and inhibiting the production and hence release of the ligand.

IMMUNOREGULATORY CYTOKINES

The data described in the preceding sections indicate that homeostatic, immunoregulatory mechanisms occur in the joint. In addition to specific inhibitors of cytokines, some cytokines themselves have immunosuppressive function. It has therefore been of interest to evaluate which of these molecules are present in RA synovial tissue, and to what degree they regulate the inflammatory responses.

TRANSFORMING GROWTH FACTOR β

Transforming growth factor β (TGFβ) is a small family of multifunctional cytokines (TGFβ1, 2 and 3) which displays both growth promoting and growth inhibitory properties on a wide range of cell types.[58] In addition TGFβ exhibits immunosuppressive effects on cells of the immune system. Thus it inhibits T lymphocyte proliferation and cytokine release.[59,60] It also inhibits the proliferation and immunoglobulin secretion of many isotypes in B cells whilst inducing IgA and IgG2 release.[61] On monocytes it also inhibits cytokine production, HLA class II antigen and adhesion molecule expression.[53] Thus it was of interest that we detected significant quantities of TGFβ in RA cultures at the mRNA level and in both RA MNC culture supernatants and in synovial fluid at the protein levels by both immunoassay and bioassay.[11] However despite its abundance, proinflammatory cytokine production in RA synovial tissue continues. Experiments were performed to evaluate the effect of additional (exogenous) TGFβ on RA joint cell cultures. However, these did not demonstrate any reduction in cytokine (IL-1α) synthesis, in keeping with the concept that either the receptors were maximally saturated or that TGFβ was ineffective, as the cells were already previously activated.[11]

Investigations to assess the immunosuppressive potential of TGFβ in vivo have also yielded conflicting results. For example, if injected locally into the joints of normal rats, TGFβ resulted in a rapid leucocyte infiltration with synovial hyperplasia leading to synovitis,[62,63] whereas if injected systemically into rats 'susceptible' to arthritis it inhibited the development of polyarthritis.[64,65] Furthermore, it was recently reported that anti TGFβ antibody, if injected locally into the joint of rats with arthritis, diminished the on going inflammation.[66] These studies illustrate the multipotential properties of TGFβ, and its differential effects if injected systemically or locally into the joint. Moreover, in addition to possessing immunoregulatory properties on cytokine production, TGFβ clearly has other proinflammatory effects, such as acting as a chemotactic factor for monocytes. Furthermore, TGFβ is likely to be a key cytokine involved in repair and fibrosis in the joints. For example, whilst inhibiting production of metalloproteinases such as collagenase,[67] it stimulates the production of type I and type XI collagen.[68] Thus locally TGFβ may promote scarring and tissue repair, and promote reparative processes in arthritic synovial connective tissue by inhibiting cartilage and bone destruction. However, in chronic lesions where there is overproduction of TGFβ this can contribute to the 'ongoing' damage by recruiting inflammatory macrophages and fibroblasts with the potential for tissue destruction.

INTERLEUKIN 4

IL-4 is produced by activated T cells and mast cells and in common with other T cell cytokines is not found at significant levels in RA synovium (Table 2.1). There is more IL-4 in reactive arthritis, which is a self limiting disease, suggesting that perhaps a deficiency of IL-4 is important in promoting chronic disease. Because of its properties, interest has been directed towards the use of IL-4 as an immunomodulatory cytokine in RA. This is based on the observations that IL-4 inhibits LPS-induced IL-1, TNFα, IL-6 and PGE2 production in monocytes. In addition it inhibits metalloproteinase biosynthesis in human alveolar macrophages,[69] but unlike IL-10 does not induce the tissue inhibitor of metalloproteinases (TIMP), (J.M. Dayer, personal communication). In one report using RA synovial explant cultures, IL-4 was shown to inhibit IL-1β, TNFα and IL-6 production.[70] Using our RA MNC suspension culture we were unable to show significant inhibition of TNF bioactivity by IL-4.[71] Suppression of LPS-induced PBMC monokine production by IL-4 can be demonstrated and depends on pretreatment of these cells with IL-4. Thus the inability of IL-4 to inhibit monokine production in our rheumatoid joint cell culture system may be simply due to the chronic activation state of the macrophages. Furthermore we observed that addition of IL-4 to RA MNC cultures enhanced p55 and p75 surface TNF-R expression.[71] Thus, in inflammatory sites, although IL-4 may reduce TNF bioactivity, it could enhance TNF signal transduction by increasing TNF-R surface expression. Clearly the overall effect of IL-4 in an inflammatory tissue will depend on the target cells, differentiation status and the influence of other cytokines in the environment. Although the use of IL-4 as a therapeutic agent in RA has been proposed, this would have to be balanced in light of its T and B cell activation properties,[72,73] and its effect on HLA class II expression.[74,75] These effects aside, it is interesting to note that IL-4 production in RA joints is low, and the incidence of allergies appear lower in RA patients.[76] The outcome of projected clinical trials is awaited with great interest.

INTERLEUKIN 10

In the past year we have documented that IL-10, previously known as 'cytokine synthesis inhibitory factor'[77] is highly expressed in RA joints, and has an important immunoregulatory role.[14] Other workers have recently found that IL-10 is spontaneously produced by RA blood cells.[78]

The evidence for IL-10 expression in joints in vivo is derived from mRNA detection by RT-PCR immunohistology, and immunoassays of 24 hour, RA synovial joint cell culture supernatants. Furthermore, upon addition of neutralizing anti-IL-10 antibodies to these cultures there followed within 24 hours a 2- to 3-fold augmentation in the spontaneous release of TNF and IL-1. As IL-10 was initially described by its inhibition of IFNγ synthesis, it was of interest to determine what the effect of neutralizing IL-10 was on IFNγ production in the RA synovial cell cultures. In 2 out of the 7 cultures, there was an elevation from undetectable (<50 pg/ml) to 1100 and 600 pg/ml within 24 hours. This observation needs to be extended with more samples and assays of later time points, but it is conceivable that IL-10 is the major regulator of T cell derived cytokine production. Furthermore, addition of exogenous IL-10 to these cultures reduced IL-1 and TNFα production by 2 to 3-fold indicating that IL-10 receptors are not saturated by the endogenous IL-10, and that regulation of proinflammatory cytokines might be achieved by further addition of IL-10. This possibility is further strengthened by our observation, discussed earlier in this chapter[52] that IL-10 induces the production of the native TNF inhibitor, sTNF-R. However, although IL-10 has some modulatory effects on the production of proinflammatory cytokines such as TNFα, clearly its endogenous production is insufficient to control the disease process. It is not clear to what degree IL-10 given as a therapeutic modality may be of benefit in inflammatory diseases long term. This is because although IL-10 has predominant inhibitory effects, it is also a chemotactic factor for CD8 T cells,[79] and most importantly it is a powerful growth factor, and activator of B cells,[79] and enhances antibody-dependent cellular cytotoxicity.[80] In IL-10 transgenic mice, diabetes mellitus is precipitated if crossed with NOD mice. However, studies in the DBA/1 collagen type II mouse model of arthritis have established that IL-10 treatment in vivo may downregulate arthritis. The effect is noted upon treatment after disease onset, and both inflammation (e.g., paw swelling) and tissue destruction (histology) are considerably reduced.[81] Clinical trials of IL-10 in RA patients using the above data as the rationale are in progress.

Chronic Exposure of T Cells to TNF

The studies described above indicate that in the RA synovium, the production of proinflammatory cytokines (and their inhibitors) is upregulated in an environment in which the specific cytokine receptors are also increased on cells. One particularly interesting observation is that the T lymphocytes in the joint express abundant surface p75 TNF-R. We therefore investigated whether chronic exposure of activated T lymphocytes to TNFα alters their function. Pretreatment of tetanus toxoid specific T cell clones with TNF for 14 days resulted in an impaired response to tetanus toxoid, but not to IL-2 or PHA.[82] Furthermore, chronic exposure to TNF resulted in impaired cytokine production in these T cell clones. The immunosuppressive effect of TNFα on T cells in vivo was further studied using PBM from RA patients, before and after treatment with a chimeric anti-TNFα antibody cA2, as part of a clinical trial. Treatment with anti-TNFα restored the diminished proliferative response of these cells to both recall antigens and mitogens[82] indicating that persistent expression of TNF in vitro and in vivo paradoxically impairs cell mediated immune responses.

CONCLUDING REMARKS

This chapter has summarized our work and that of other groups over the last 8 years investigating to what extent cytokines contribute to the pathogenesis of RA. A more detailed discussion of cytokines in rheumatoid arthritis may be found in Annual Reviews in Immunology, 1996.[83] Our identification of TNFα as a pivotal molecule in the rheumatoid process was an important observation in leading research from the laboratory towards the clinic, and the gradual unraveling of the inhibitory mechanisms which are naturally present. It has thus helped us to understand the mechanisms which combat inflammation. What is not clear from these studies is to what degree the balance between pro- versus anti-inflammatory cytokines modulates disease activity. In RA, like many other autoimmune diseases, the disease manifestations 'wax and wane' over a period of many years. It is tempting to speculate that remission may be associated with an overall increase in cytokine inhibitory mechanisms which, albeit temporarily, inhibit inflammation. Despite the chronicity—or indeed the treatment of these patients with a wide range of disease modifying drugs—the disease itself continues to progress. Further studies to learn how the production of immunosuppressive cytokines could be upregulated 'long term' at sites of inflammation is now a major goal.

From the study of cytokine expression in RA joints, a number of other therapeutic possibilities have emerged, for example, the immunosuppressive cytokines IL-10, IL-4 or conceivably TGFβ. Blocking other proinflammatory cytokines such as IL-1 and IL-6 are possibilities which are under discussion. The success of TNFα blockade in the clinic[84,85] (chapter 12) has demonstrated that understanding cytokine interactions in disease processes can lead to therapeutic advances.

Acknowledgment

The Kennedy Institute is supported by the Arthritis and Rheumatism Council of Great Britain.

REFERENCES

1. Feldmann M. Molecular mechanisms involved in human autoimmune diseases: relevance of chronic antigen presentation, class II expression and cytokine production. Immunology 1989; Supplement 2:66-71.
2. Silman AJ, MacGregor AJ, Thomson W et al. Twin concordance rates for rheumatoid arthritis: Results from a nationwide study. Br J Rheumatol 1993; 32:903.
3. Gregersen PK, Silver J, Winchester RJ. The shared epitope hypothesis. An approach to understanding the molecular genetics of susceptibility to rheumatoid arthritis. Arthritis and Rheumatism 1987; 30:1205-1213.
4. Klareskog L, Forsum U, Scheynius A et al. Evidence in support of a self perpetuating HLA-DR dependent delayed type cell reaction in rheumatoid arthritis. Proc Natl Acad Sci USA 1982; 72:3632-3636.
5. Londei M, Savill CM, Verhoef A et al. Persistence of collagen type II-specific T-cell clones in the synovial membrane of a patient with rheumatoid arthritis. Proc Nat Acad Sci U S A 1989; 86:636-640.
6. Silverman HA, Johnson JS, Vaughan JH et al. Altered lymphocyte reactivity in rheumatoid arthritis. Arthritis Rheum 1976; 19:509-515.
7. Buchan G, Barrett K, Fujita T et al. Detection of activated T cell products in the rheumatoid joint using cDNA probes to Interleukin-2 (IL-2) IL-2 receptor and IFNγ. Clin Exp Immunol 1988a; 71:295-301.
8. Buchan G, Barrett K, Turner M et al. Interleukin-1 and tumour necrosis factor mRNA expression in rheumatoid arthritis: prolonged production of IL-1α. Clin Exp Immunol 1988b; 73:449-455.
9. Hirano T, Matsuda T, Turner M et al. Excessive production of interleukin 6/B cell stimulatory factor-2 in rheumatoid arthritis. Eur J Immunol 1988; 18:1797-1801.
10. Brennan FM, Zachariae CO, Chantry D et al. Detection of interleukin 8 biological activity in synovial fluids from patients with rheumatoid arthritis and production of interleukin 8 mRNA by isolated synovial cells. Eur J Immunol 1990a; 20:2141-2144.
11. Brennan FM, Chantry D, Turner M et al. Detection of transforming growth factor-β in rheumatoid arthritis synovial tissue: lack of effect on spontaneous cytokine production in joint cell cultures. Clin Exp Immunol 1990b; 81:278-285.
12. Haworth C, Brennan FM, Chantry D et al. Expression of granulocyte-macrophage colony-stimulating factor in rheumatoid arthritis: regulation by tumor necrosis factor-α. Eur J Immunol 1991; 21:2575-2579.
13. Alvaro-Garcia JM, Zvaifler NJ, Firestein GS. Cytokines in chronic inflammatory arthritis. IV. GM-CSF mediated induction of class II MHC antigen on human monocytes: a possible role in RA. J Exp Med 1989; 146:865-875.
14. Katsikis P, Chu CQ, Brennan FM et al. Immunoregulatory role of interleukin 10 (IL-10) in rheumatoid arthritis. J Exp Med 1994; 179:1517-1527.

15. Firestein GS, Xu W-D, Townsend K et al. Cytokines in chronic inflammatory arthritis. I. Failure to detect T cell lymphokines (interleukin 2 and interleukin 3) and presence of macrophage colony-stimulating factor (CSF-1) and a novel mast cell growth factor in rheumatoid synovitis. J Exp Med 1988; 168:1573-1586.
16. Brennan FM, Chantry D, Jackson AM et al. Cytokine production in culture by cells isolated from the synovial membrane. J Autoimmun 1989a; 2 (Suppl):177-186.
17. Firestein GS. How important are T cells in chronic rheumatoid synovitis? Arthritis Rheum 1990; 33:768-773.
18. Browning JL, Ngam-ek A, Lawton P et al. Lymphotoxin β, a novel member of the TNF family that forms a heteromeric complex with lymphotoxin on the cell surface. Cell 1993; 72:847-856.
19. Dayer JM, Beutler B, Cerami A. Cachectin/tumor necrosis factor stimulates collagenase and prostaglandin E2 production by human synovial cells and dermal fibroblasts. J Exp Med 1985; 162:2163-2168.
20. Saklatavala J. TNFα stimulates resportion and inhibits synthesis of proteoglycan in cartilage. Nature 1985; 322:547-549.
21. Gowen M, Wood DD, Ihrie EJ et al. An interleukin-1 like factor stimulates bone resorption in vitro. Nature 1983; 306:378-380.
22. Thomas BM, Mundy GR, Chambers TJ. Tumour necrosis factor α and β induce osteoblastic cells to stimulate osteoclast bone resorption. J Immunol 1987; 138:775-780.
23. Pettipher ER, Higgs GA, Henderson B. Interleukin 1 induces leukocyte infiltration and cartilage proteoglycan degradation in the synovial joint. Proc Natl Acad Sci USA 1986; 83:8749-8753.
24. Brennan FM. Role of cytokines in experimental arthritis. Clin Exp Immunol 1994; 97:1-3.
25. Portillo G, Turner M, Chantry D et al. Effect of cytokines on HLA-DR and IL-1 production by a monocyte tumour, THP-1. Immunology 1989; 66:170-175.
26 Brennan FM, Chantry D, Jackson A et al. Inhibitory effect of TNF α antibodies on synovial cell interleukin-1 production in rheumatoid arthritis. Lancet 1989b; 2:244-247.
27. Alvaro-Garcia JM, Zvaifler NJ, Brown CB et al. Cytokines in chronic inflammatory arthritis. VI. Analysis of the synovial cells involved in granulocyte-macrophage colony stimulating factor production and gene expression in rheumatoid arthritis and its regulation by IL-1 and TNF-α. J Immunol 1991; 146:3365-3371.
28. Kowanko IC, A. F. Granulocyte macrophage colony-stimulating factor augments neutrophil-mediated cartilage degradation and neutrophil adherence. Arthritis Rheum 1991; 11:1452-1460.
29. Butler D, Maini RN, Feldmann M et al. Modulation of proinflammatory cytokine release in rheumatoid synovial membrane cell cultures with an anti TNFα monoclonal: comparison with blockade of IL-1 using the recombinant IL-1 receptor antagonist. J Exp Med 1995.

30. Hirano T, Akira S, Taga T et al. Biological and clinical aspets of interleukin 6. Immunol Today 1990; 11:443-449.
31. Taub DD, Oppenheim JJ. Review of the chemokine meeting the third international symposium of chemotactic cytokines. Cytokine 1993; 5:175-179.
32. Koch AE, Kunkel SL, Harlow LA et al. Enhanced production of monocyte chemoattractant protein-1 in rheumatoid arthritis. J Clin Invest 1992; 90:772-9.
33. Koch AE, Kunkel SL, Harlow LA et al. Macrophage inflammatory protein-1 α. A novel chemotactic cytokine for macrophages in rheumatoid arthritis. J Clin Invest 1994; 93:921-8.
34. Koch AE, Kunkel SL, Harlow LA et al. Epithelial neutrophil activating peptide-78: a novel chemotactic cytokine for neutrophils in arthritis. J Clin Invest 1994; 94:1012-1018.
35. Springer TA. Traffic signals for lymphocyte recirculation and leukocyte emigration: The multistep paradigm. Cell 1994; 76:301-314.
36. Chu CQ, Field M, Feldmann M et al. Localization of tumor necrosis factor α in synovial tissues and at the cartilage-pannus junction in patients with rheumatoid arthritis. Arthritis Rheum 1991; 34: 1125-1132.
37. Deleuran BW, Chu CQ, Field M et al. Localization of tumor necrosis factor receptors in the synovial tissue and cartilage-pannus junction in patients with rheumatoid arthritis. Implications for local actions of tumor necrosis factor α. Arthritis Rheum 1992a; 35: 1170-1178.
38. Williams RO, Feldmann M, Maini RN. Anti-tumor necrosis factor ameliorates joint disease in murine collagen-induced arthritis. Proc Nat Acad Sci U S A 1992; 89:9784-9788.
39. Thorbecke GJ, Shah R, Leu CH et al. Involvement of endogenous tumour necrosis factor α and transforming growth factor β during induction of collagen type II arthritis in mice. Proc Natl Acad Sci USA 1992; 89:7375-7379.
40. Piguet PF, Grau GE, Vesin C et al. Evolution of collagen arthritis in mice is arrested by treatment with anti-tumour necrosis factor (TNF) antibody or a recombinant soluble TNF receptor. Immunology 1992; 77:510-514.
41. Keffer J, Probert L, Cazlaris H et al. Transgenic mice expressing human tumour necrosis factor: a predictive genetic model of arthritis. EMBO J 1991; 10:4025-4031.
42. Fernandez-Botran R. Soluble cytokine receptors: their role in immunoregulation. FASEB J 1991; 5:2567-2574.
43. Arend W. Interleukin 1 receptor antagonist. A new member of the interleukin 1 family. J Clin Invest 1991; 5:1445-1451.
44. Cope AP, Aderka D, Doherty M et al. Increased levels of soluble tumor necrosis factor receptors in the sera and synovial fluid of patients with rheumatic diseases. Arthritis Rheum 1992; 35:1160-1169.

45. Brennan FM, Gibbons DL, Mitchell T et al. Enhanced expression of tumor necrosis factor receptor mRNA and protein in mononuclear cells isolated from rheumatoid arthritis synovial joints. Eur J Immunol 1992; 22:1907-1912.
46. Brennan FM, Gibbons D, Cope A et al. TNF inhibitors are produced spontaneously by rheumatoid and osteoarthritic synovial joint cell cultures: evidence of feedback control of TNF action (In press). Scand J Immunol 1995;
47. Balavoine J-F, de Rochemonteix B, Williamson K et al. Prostaglandin E2 and collagenase production by fibroblasts and synovial cells is regulated by urine derived human interleukin 1 and inhibitor(s). J Clin Invest 1986; 78:1120.
48. Roux-Lombard P, Modoux C, Vischer T et al. Inhibitors of interleukin 1 activity in synovial fluids and in cultured synovial fluid mononuclear cells. J Rheumatol 1992; 19:517-523.
49. Deleuran BW, Chu CQ, Field M et al. Localization of interleukin-1α, type 1 interleukin-1 receptor and interleukin-1 receptor antagonist in the synovial membrane and cartilage/pannus junction in rheumatoid arthritis. Br J Rheumatol 1992b; 31:801-809.
50. Firestein GS, Berger AE, Tracey DE et al. IL-1 receptor antagonist protein production and gene expression in rheumatoid arthritis and osteoarthritis synovium. J Immunol 1992; 149:1054-1062.
51. Symons JA, Eastgate JA, Duff GW. Purification and characterization of a novel soluble receptor for interleukin-1. J Exp Med 1991; 174:1251-1254.
52. Joyce DA, Gibbons D, Green P et al. Two inhibitors of pro-inflammatory cytokine release, IL-10 and IL-4, have contrasting effects on release of soluble p75 TNF receptor by cultured monocytes. Eur J Immunol 1994; 24:2699-2705.
53. Chantry D, Turner M, Abney E et al. Modulation of cytokine production by transforming growth factor-β. J Immunol 1989; 142:4295-4300.
54. Essner R, Rhoades K, McBride WH et al. IL-4 down-regulates IL-1 and TNF gene expression in human monocytes. J Immunol 1989; 142:3857-3861.
55. de Waal-Malefyt R, Yssel H, Roncarolo M-G et al. Interleukin-10. Curr Opin Immunol 1992; 4:314.
56. Turner M, Chantry D, Katsikis P et al. Induction of the interleukin 1 receptor antagonist protein by transforming growth factor β. Eur J Immunol 1991; 21:1635-1639.
57. Wong HL, Costa GL, Lotze MT et al. Interleukin (IL) 4 differentially regulates monocyte IL-1 family gene expression and synthesis in vitro and in vivo. J Exp Med 1993; 177:775-781.
58. Massague J. The TGFβ1 family of growth and differentiation factors. Cell 1987; 49:437-438.
59. Ranges GE, Figari IS, Espevik T et al. Inhibition of cytotoxic T cell development by transforming growth factor β, reversal by recombinant tumour necrosis factor. J Exp Med 1987; 166:991-998.

60. Kehrl JH, Roberts AB, Wakefield LM et al. Transforming growth factor β is an important immunomodulatory protein for human B lymphocytes. J Immunol 1986; 137:3855-60.
61. Coffman RL, Lebman DA, Shrader B. Transforming growth factor β specifically enhances IgA production by lipopolysaccharide-stimulated murine B lymphocytes. J Exp Med 1989; 170:1039-1044.
62. Allen JB, Manthey CL, Hand A et al. Transforming growth factor-β induces human T lymphocyte migration in vitro. J Exp Med 1990; 171:231.
63. Fava RA, Olsen NJ, Postlethwaite AE et al. Transforming growth factor β1 (TGF(β1) induced neutrophil recruitment to synovial tissues: implications for TGFβ-driven synovial inflammation and hyperplasia. J Exp Med 1991; 173:1121-1132.
64. Brandes ME, Allen JB, Ogawa Y et al. Transforming growth factor β1 suppresses acute and chronic arthritis in experimental animals. J Clin Invest 1991; 87:1108-1113.
65. Kuruvilla AP, Shah R, Hochwald GM et al. Protective effect of transforming growth factor β1. Proc Natl Acad Sci USA 1991; 88:2918-2921.
66. Wahl SM, Allen JB, Costa GL et al. Reversal of acute and chronic synovial inflammation by anti-transforming growth factor β. J Exp Med 1993; 177:225-230.
67. Lafyatis R, Thomson NL, Remmers ER et al. Transforming growth factor-β production by synovial tissues from rheumatoid patients and streptococcal cell wall arthritis rats. Studies on secretion by synovial fibroblast-like cells and immunohistological localisation. J Immunol 1989; 143:1142-1148.
68. Khalil N, Bereznay O, Sporn M et al. Macrophage production of transforming growth factor β and fibroblast collagen synthesis in chronic pulmonary inflammation. J Exp Med 1989; 170:727-737.
69. Lacraz S, Nicod I, Galve-de Rochemonteux B et al. Suppression of metalloproteinase biosynthesis in human alveolar macrophages by interleukin-4. J Clin Invest 1992; 90:382-386.
70. Miossec P, Briolay J, Dechanet J et al. The inhibition of the production of proinflammatory cytokines and immunoglobulins by interleukin-4 in an ex vivo model of rheumatoid synovitis. Arth & Rheum 1992; 35:874-883.
71. Cope AP, Gibbons DL, Aderka D et al. Differential regulation of tumour necrosis factor receptors (TNF-R) by IL-4; upregulation of P55 and P75 TNF-R on synovial joint mononuclear cells. Cytokine 1993; 5:205-12.
72. Spits H, Yssel H, Takebe Y et al. Recombinant interleukin-4 promotes growth of human T cells. J Immunol 1987; 139:1142-1147.
73. Defrance T, Vanbervliet B, Aubry JP et al. B cell growth-promoting activity of recombinant human interleukin 4. J Immunol 1987; 139:1135-41.
74. Noelle R, Krammer PH, Ohara J et al. Increased expression of Ia antigens on resting B cells: an additional role for B cell growth factor. Proc Natl Acad Sci USA 1984; 81:6149-6153.

75. Gerrard TL, Dyer DR, Mostowski HS. IL-4 and granulocyte-macrophage colony stimulating factor selectively increase HLA-DR and HLA-DP antigens but not HLA-DQ antigens on human monocytes. J Immunol 1990; 144:4670-4674.
76. Lewis-Faning E. Report on an enquiry into the aetiological factors associated with rheumatoid arthritis. Ann Rheum Dis 1950; 91:1-94.
77. Moore KW, Vieira P, Fiorentino DF et al. Homology of cytokine synthesis inhibitory factor (IL-10) to the Epstein-Barr virus gene BCRFI. Science 1990; 248:1230-1234.
78. Cush JJ, Splawski JB, Thomas R et al. Elevated interleukin-10 levels in patients with rheumatoid arthritis. Arth & Rheum 1995; 1:96-104.
79. Jinquan T, Gronhoj Larsen C, Gesser B et al. Human IL-10 is a chemoattractant for for CD8+ T lymphocytes and an inhibitor of IL-8-induced CD4+ T lymphocyte migration. J Immunol 1993; 151:4545-4551.
80. Te Velde AA, de Waal Malefyt R, Huijbens RJF et al. IL-10 stimulates monocyte Fcγ surface expression and cytotoxic activity. Distinct regulation of antibody-dependent cellular cytotoxicity by IFNγ, IL-4 and IL-10. J Immunol 1992; 149:4048.
81. Walmsley M, Katsikis PD, Abney ER et al. IL-10 inhibits progression of established collagen-induced arthritis. Arth & Rheum 1995; (Submitted).
82. Cope AP, Londei M, Chu NR et al. Chronic exposure to tumor necrosis factor (TNF) in vitro impairs the activation of T cells through the T cell receptor/CD3 complex; reversal in vivo by anti-TNF antibodies in patients with rheumatoid arthritis. J. Clin. Invest 1994; 94:749-760.
83. Feldmann M, Brennan FM, Maini RN. Role of cytokines in rheumatoid arthritis. Ann Rev Immunol 1996; (In press).
84. Elliott MJ, Maini RN, Feldmann M et al. Treatment of rheumatoid arthritis with chimeric monoclonal antibodies to TNFα. Arthritis Rheum 1993; 36:1681-1690.
85. Elliott MJ, Maini RN, Feldmann M et al. Randomised double blind comparison of a chimaeric monoclonal antibody to tumour necrosis factor α (cA2) versus placebo in rheumatoid arthritis. Lancet 1994; 344:1105-1110.
86. Seckinger P, Isaaz S, Dayer JM. A human inhibitor of tumor necrosis factor α. J Exp Med 1988; 167:1511-6.
87. Engelmann H, Aderka D, Rubinstein M, Rotman D, Wallach D. A tumor necrosis factor-binding protein purified to homogeneity from human urine protects cells from tumor necrosis factor toxicity. J Biol Chem 1989; 264:11974-80.
88. Olsson I, Lantz S, Nilsson E, Peetre C, Thysell H, Grubb A, Adolf G. Isolation and characterization of a tumor necrosis factor binding protein from urine. Eur J Haematol 1989; 42:270-5.

CHAPTER 3

CYTOKINES IN DIABETES

Janette Allison, Jacques Miller and Nora Sarvetnick

INTRODUCTION

Insulin dependent diabetes mellitus (IDDM) is an autoimmune disease, under polygenic control, manifested when more than 90% of islet β cells are destroyed.[1] In humans, rats and mice, T cells are of primary importance in disease initiation and studies with rodent models show that both CD4+ and CD8+ T cells are involved. Two models of spontaneous diabetes, the NOD mouse and BB rat, have provided much useful information on disease initiation and progression, which are almost impossible to follow in humans. Using these models it has become apparent that diabetes is a complex disease involving both the antigen-specific and nonspecific compartments of the immune system. Although antigen-specific T cells are essential, it is still not clear if β cell death occurs by direct MHC-restricted killing or by other less specific mechanisms resulting from the inflammatory response.

In regards to antigen specificity, it is accepted that autoreactive T cells can reside in the periphery and yet remain unresponsive or indifferent to self antigens.[2-4] For example, islet-reactive clones have been isolated from normal mouse strains[5] and diabetes could be induced in adult thymectomized, irradiated, normal rats.[6] Diabetes was prevented in these rats by injection of CD4+ T cells that displayed a Th$_2$ phenotype, the implication being that cytokine regulatory networks were involved in keeping potentially autoreactive T cells quiescent. In spontaneous diabetes rodent models, the disease process required both CD4+ and CD8+ T cell subsets. It has been proposed, however, that once initiated, diabetes progression or recurrence can be mediated entirely by CD4+ T cells through their production of cytokines and induction of free oxygen and nitric oxide radicals, which are very damaging to β cells.[7-11] Thus, an antigen-specific component, the islet-reactive CD4+ T cell, may lead to β cell destruction through nonspecific mechanisms involving induction of cytokines.

Cytokines in Autoimmunity, edited by Fionula M. Brennan and Marc Feldmann.
© 1996 R.G. Landes Company.

In support of a major role for CD4+ T cells, islet-reactive CD4+ T cell clones from NOD mice could themselves rapidly transfer diabetes to young, nondiabetic recipients depleted of CD8+ T cells,[12-13] and T cells expressing an islet-specific receptor from one such clone, introduced by transgenic technology, were spontaneously pathogenic in NOD mice.[14] Similarly, transfer of diabetogenic, pure, CD4+ T cells into NOD SCID mice that have no T and B cells, resulted in diabetes.[15] Wang et al,[9] using islet allografts depleted of antigen-presenting cells (APC), showed that such grafts which lacked NOD MHC-restriction elements suffered disease recurrence in NOD recipients. Thyroid allografts used as controls were unaffected, indicating that the allo-MHC when present on nonprofessional APCs did not induce an immune response. Lo et al[16] used a transgenic approach and reached a similar conclusion. Chimeric mice that expressed a foreign antigen (hemagglutinin, HA) on the islet β cells were engineered so that the H-2^d MHC molecule, needed to present the HA peptides to CD4+ T cells, was present on bone marrow-derived APCs but not on the islet β cells. When these chimeric mice were injected with H-2^d restricted T cells, primed for reactivity to HA, islets were infiltrated and destroyed. It is thus apparent from these studies in the NOD mouse model that islet antigens could be processed and presented to CD4+ T cells in the vicinity of the islets through the class II pathway, resulting in β cell damage, even though the β cells did not themselves express the relevant MHC-restriction element. How the CD4+ T cells might mediate this damage will be discussed in more detail below.

In spite of the pathogenicity of CD4+ T cells, it seems that CD8+ T cells are important both in the initiation and acceleration of disease, at least in the NOD mouse model. It has recently been found that NOD mice not expressing β2-microglobulin as a result of gene targeting, and therefore deficient in CD8+ T cells, did not develop insulitis,[17-19] thus establishing a critical role for CD8+ T cells in disease initiation. CD8+ T cells may also be important as effectors in diabetes progression. For example, although CD8+ T cells from diabetic donors could not transfer diabetes to NOD SCID recipients in the absence of CD4+ T cells, in their presence they accelerated the diabetes process normally achieved by CD4+ T cells alone in this system.[15] Similarly, although transfer of CD4+ T cells into nude NOD mice resulted in insulitis only, the subsequent addition of CD8+ T cells and cyclophosphamide rapidly led to diabetes onset in most animals.[20] This result agrees with earlier experiments by Charlton et al[21] who showed that cyclophosphamide-induced diabetes could be prevented by anti-CD8 antibodies. In addition, it has been found that some CD8+ T cell clones can induce diabetes, provided CD4+ splenocytes (depleted of CD8+ cells) were also transferred.[22] CD8+ T cells were likewise required for diabetes induction in irradiated, adult thymectomized normal rats.[6] It appears, therefore, that CD8+ T cells have a role in accelerating diabetes in rodent models. What is not clear, however, is whether these T cells perform their role by MHC-restricted killing of the β cells or through nonspecific effects, for example, by producing cytokines such as IFNγ.

THE ROLE OF CYTOKINES IN AUTOIMMUNE DIABETES

The role of cytokines in diabetes has been viewed from a number of aspects. Measurements of serum cytokine levels in humans or animals with diabetes have been done, but it has been difficult to determine if abnormal levels are a result of the ongoing disease or due to some primary defect in cytokine regulation. The systemic injection of recombinant cytokines or antibodies to specific cytokines has also been tested in rodent models (reviewed by Bowman et al).[23] In situ detection of cytokines in the islet β cells or cells of the infiltrate may be informative, although the presence of nonspecific lymphocytes recruited to a site of inflammation complicates interpretation of the results. The effects of recombinant cytokines on cultured islets and β cell lines has been extensively examined and the transgenic expression of a number of cytokine molecules has been tried. As our interests lie mainly in the local effects of cytokines on autoimmunity, this review will concentrate on these aspects.

LOCALLY PRODUCED CYTOKINES CAN INDUCE β CELL DAMAGE AND AUTOIMMUNITY

A number of studies have emphasized the role of cytokines in diabetes. Both antigen-specific and nonspecific mechanisms have been implicated and a survey of the effects of some relevant cytokines follows.

Interleukin 1: The free-radical effect

Interleukin 1 is an important proinflammatory cytokine that has been implicated as a major player in the destruction of islet β cells. There are two forms of IL-1, IL-1α and IL-1β, that are encoded by separate genes to give proproteins. The pro-IL-1α has biological activity but the pro-IL-1β has to be processed by the IL-1β converting enzyme (ICE) to attain its full biological potential.[24] IL-1α and β can bind to the same receptor on many different tissues and are produced by a range of cell types, the activated macrophage being a major source. In the case of IL-1β, however, it is possible that only the monocytic lineage possesses the ICE activity needed to provide mature IL-1β and is, therefore, the only source of the functional protein.

Much work has indicated that at certain concentrations, IL-1β is toxic to islet β cells with different sensitivities being recorded for mouse, rat and human islets.[8,25] These studies have been somewhat complicated by the lack of purity of β cell preparations which may still contain passenger macrophages that themselves produce cytokines as well as by the use of species-different recombinant cytokine preparations. In vitro studies with rat and mouse islet cells showed that IL-1β alone had serious consequences for glucose-stimulated insulin secretion and islet-cell morphology.[8] TNFα or IFNγ at high concentrations also affected glucose-stimulated insulin release from mouse whole islet preparations and in combination had very detrimental effects on islet integrity.[26] Human islets were not directly affected by IL-1β, but in combination with TNFα and IFNγ, IL-1β had effects on glucose-induced insulin secretion.[27,28]

The detrimental effect of cytokines on β cells is concentration dependent and may involve the induction of free-oxygen radicals[7,8,11] or the cytokine-induced expression of nitric oxide synthase, resulting in nitric oxide (NO) production by macrophages or by the β cells themselves.[8,10,27] Furthermore, unrelated studies on mouse T cell lines implicated Th$_1$ cell-derived NO as a mediator in immune responses.[29] Exposure of human islets to combinations of IL-1β, TNFα and IFNγ was associated with NO production by the β cells with subsequent effects on insulin biosynthesis and secretion.[27,28] Inhibitors of NO prevented the effects of the cytokines on insulin secretion, implying that NO generation was the mechanism by which cytokines damaged β cells.[27] Another study, however, found that NO inhibitors appeared to have no influence on the damaging effects of combinations of cytokines.[28] In the case of rat islets, direct exposure to IL-1β alone resulted in NO production by the islet β cells but not by islet α cells.[30] Another difference was reported between the α and β cells in that transformed mouse β cells, but not α cells, could be induced to produce TNFα.[31] The apparent specific destruction of β cells, but not other islet cells, in autoimmune diabetes is often quoted as evidence for the actions of islet-specific killer T cells. An alternative explanation is that the damage is mediated by the induced production of NO or TNFα by β cells or by the particular sensitivity of β cells to free oxygen radicals.[7,9-11] Such radicals may ultimately kill β cells by causing DNA fragmentation.[32-34]

A direct test of the toxicity of IL-1β could be done by generating transgenic mice that overexpress or ectopically express the mature form of the protein. So far, attempts to overexpress the precursor and mature forms of IL-1β in transgenic mice have proved difficult, most probably because this cytokine is lethal to the developing embryos.[35]

Interleukin 2: Can it abrogate peripheral tolerance?

Interleukin 2 (IL-2) is the exclusive product of T cells, encoded by a single gene.[36] In mice it has been shown that different strains have slightly different IL-2 sequences with variations in the length of the CAG repeat as well as other amino acid changes in the 5' region of the protein.[37-39] It seems, however, that these different IL-2 proteins have the same biological activity when used to promote the growth of IL-2-dependent CTLL cells.[37] In picomolar amounts IL-2 is a growth factor for activated T and B cells. In vitro, IL-2 at nanomolar levels also affects macrophages and NK cells. Thus, IL-2 can directly activate human macrophages[40] but in mice, in vitro studies showed that IFNγ was needed to synergize with IL-2 to do so.[41] As regards the effects of IL-2 on NK cells, in vivo studies showed that a recombinant vaccinia virus transfected with a murine IL-2 cDNA could cure nude mice of vaccinia infections by activating NK cells.[42] Transgenic overexpression of human IL-2 in mice resulted in large numbers of NK cells, provided the human IL-2R tac (α) chain was also present.[43]

The fact that elevated serum levels of IL-2 have been observed in certain autoimmune diseases[44] begs the question of whether IL-2 released by T cells responding to infectious agents stimulates previously silent cross-reactive autoantigen-specific T cells to become autoaggressive. In fact, in a number of experimental situations in vitro and in vivo IL-2 has interfered with immunological unresponsiveness. For example, in rats in which tolerance had been induced by blood transfusion,[45] T cells infiltrating tolerated kidney allografts could not produce biologically active IL-2. The state of tolerance was abrogated by giving IL-2 at the time of transplantation. Another in vivo situation in which IL-2 appears to have reversed tolerance occurred following thymectomy of infant mice of certain strains. These mice developed a variety of autoimmune diseases.[46,47] Presumably, autoreactive T cells released from the neonatal thymus, which otherwise would have been deleted or diluted,[48] were involved in the pathogenesis. In some cases, however, these T cells were deemed to be anergic[49,50] and could be activated in vivo by high levels of IL-2.[50]

The observation that IL-2 appeared to break tolerance in some in vivo situations, suggested that the onset of an autoimmune response might result from the inappropriate delivery of IL-2 to T cells which had not undergone negative selection, because the antigen for which these cells had a specific TCR was either not represented intrathymically or present there in too low an amount. Against the idea that IL-2 produced by bystander T cells can activate normally quiescent T cells to become autoreactive is the work of Ishida et al.[43] Transgenic overexpression of IL-2 resulted in strong NK cell activation but not self reactive T cell activation. We have undertaken a number of our own transgenic studies in which IL-2 was overexpressed by the β cell to investigate the role of this cytokine in autoimmune diabetes. Depending on the experimental system used, it appeared that locally produced IL-2 could induce damage to islets as a consequence of nonspecific inflammation or influence antigen-specific T cells to become autoaggressive.

Ectopic overexpression of IL-2 by islet β cells

The ectopic overexpression of IL-2 by islet β cells was investigated to determine whether a local source of IL-2 could break T cell tolerance to islet antigens.[51] This resulted in a massive inflammatory response surrounding the islets. Notably, a dose effect of the RIP-IL-2 transgene was found so that higher levels of expression resulted in such severe inflammatory damage with masses of macrophages that the acinar tissue was destroyed and mice did not survive beyond 15 days of age. At lower levels of IL-2, inflammation was localized to islets and adjoining acinar tissue. A breeding line was established from a founder that had only one copy of the RIP-IL-2 transgene. In these mice, at less than two weeks of age, the inflammatory lesion comprised mainly macrophages but as the lymphocyte compartment became established these cells were replaced or diluted by T and B lymphocytes. In general, the proportions of the different lymphocyte populations were similar to those found in normal spleen with the exception of some Thy1$^+$ CD3$^-$ IL-2R p55$^+$ cells which were unique to the pancreatic infiltrate. In fact, the infiltrates even demonstrated some organization with B cell and T cell areas as shown by immunohistology. Islets were broken up by the inflammation but β cells retained good staining for insulin. It was also demonstrated that lymphocytes were recruited from the circulation and did not proliferate at the local source of IL-2.

As a consequence of all this inflammation there was upregulation of MHC class I molecules on the β cells and infiltrate and of VCAM-1 and Meca 79 antigen on endothelium. In spite of the islet damage resulting from the chronic inflammation, mice of normal background (B6^{bm1}, CBA) did not progress to diabetes. Nor did they reject syngeneic islet grafts not expressing IL-2, implying that islet-specific T cells were not circulating in these animals. It seemed that the deleterious effects of local IL-2 involved nonspecific mechanisms that damaged the islets, for example through the activation of macrophages to produce free radicals and other cytokines such as TNFα, or because NK cells were activated to produce IFNγ. Indeed, when the RIP-IL-2 transgene was introduced into T cell-deficient CBA nude mice, the disease pathology was identical.[52] Diabetes did, however, occur in euthymic B6^{bm1} or CBA animals that carried two copies of the RIP-IL-2 transgene. It might be said that the higher amounts of IL-2 activated islet-specific T cells which killed all the β cells, but it seems more likely that diabetes resulted from the increased inflammation. Recently we have found that CB17 and CB17 SCID mice (which lack T or B cells) could progress to diabetes even with one copy of the RIP-IL-2 transgene. The CB17 background genes may in some way have contributed to the disease process since Scott et al[53] found that background genes from normal mouse strains were important in another transgenic mouse model of diabetes. At any rate, it seems likely from these results that T cells were not essential in the disease process initiated by β cell IL-2. Rather, IL-2 most probably acted on macrophages to induce production of IL-1, TNFα and possibly on NK cells to produce IFNγ. All this could ultimately lead to the production of free-oxygen or NO radicals that damaged β cells. Thus, artificial IL-2 production by β cells may simulate the activities of CD4+ T cells responding to islet antigens presented on dendritic cells in the vicinity of the islets.

Ectopic IL-2 production by NOD β cells

Since we had no clear demonstration that locally produced IL-2 could cause T cell activation to islet antigens in normal mouse strains, we wondered what would happen in the diabetes prone NOD mouse. In this case a single copy of the RIP-IL-2 transgene led to a dramatic acceleration of the diabetes process even in the very low incidence NOD WEHI strain and males were more susceptible than females.[54] In spite of this, circulating T cells reactive to syngeneic islet grafts not expressing IL-2 were absent. In mice backcrossed to the C57BL/6 genetic background, it was found that homozygosity of NOD Idd-1 and Idd-3/10 diabetes susceptibility genes was required for the progression to diabetes. This effect of locally expressed IL-2 in the NOD background was very similar to that of the Ins-IL-10 transgene described below.[55] In this case, however, only homozygosity at Idd-1 was required possibly because the genetic backcross was different, involving Balb/c genes. It is of relevance that the CB17 genetic background, which is similar to Balb/c, also potentiated the damaging effects of artificially expressed IL-2 (see above). If the NOD mice expressing local IL-2 lacked CD8+ T cells, by mating them to β2-microglobulin deficient NOD mice,[56] then the time of onset and incidence of diabetes was greatly reduced. So it seemed that the chronic inflammatory response induced by local IL-2 eventually led to diabetes in the NOD genetic background, but the presence of CD8+ T cells was needed for the acute onset. This result is rather contrary to the data that showed absence of islet-specific T cells circulating in the diabetic mice. Perhaps, islet-specific CD8+ T cells did exist, but they could not damage the β cells unless a local source of IL-2 was available to "help" them. IL-2 help could come in the form of a growth factor for T cells or indirectly as a consequence of the inflammatory response which could upregulate antigen-presenting machinery on the β cells. Syngeneic islet grafts not expressing IL-2 may therefore have levels of antigen too low to activate any islet-specific CD8+ T cells. Of course, we cannot yet discount that the influence of the CD8+ T cells may still have involved nonspecific mechanisms, for example their production of IFNγ. Backcrosses are in progress to make NOD SCID mice that express local IL-2 and a nonspecific TCR (anti-H-Y) on all CD8+ T cells. Such T cells should not accelerate diabetes onset if islet-specific CD8+ T cells are required. In conclusion, it appeared from these studies that much of the damage to the islets was mediated by the nonspecific inflammatory consequences of local IL-2 production that was potentiated in the NOD genetic background. CD8+ T cells had a role in accelerating the disease process.

Ectopic production of IL-2 by β cells of the C3H lpr/lpr mouse

The RIP-IL-2 transgene was backcrossed into the C3H *lpr/lpr* strain to see the influence of this genetic background on diabetes incidence (J. Allison, unpublished data). The *lpr* mutation results from insertion of the Etn retrotransposon into the second intron of the *Fas* gene,[57] and in the C3H genetic background homozygosity at this locus causes mice to develop severe lymphadenopathy starting at about 8-12 weeks of age. Of 12 RIP-IL-2 mice that displayed the lpr phenotype, only one developed diabetes but not until 250 days of age. The infiltrates in the islets of all 12 mutants showed massive accumulations of small resting lymphocytes that were similar to the types of cells found in the spleen or lymph nodes of the same animals. Apart from the huge accumulation of cells, the islet morphology was similar to that in nonmutant, RIP-IL-2 littermates, i.e., islets were broken apart and suffered damage but still contained some insulin. Apparently, the Fas death pathway was not involved in the process of β cell damage by in situ IL-2.

Ectopic IL-2 production with a known target antigen

So far, we were quite unsuccessful in proving that IL-2 could activate islet-specific T cells to kill islets directly. Most of the results pointed to nonspecific mechanisms of β cell killing by local IL-2. So we designed a transgenic mouse model in which a known target antigen (the class I H-2 K^b protein) was present on the islets and where most of the T cells expressed a receptor specific for this K^b autoantigen (Des-TCR) to give RIP-K^b x Des TCR double transgenic mice.[58] This was done by: (a) linking the K^b gene to the rat insulin promoter so it would be expressed on β cells;[59] and (b) by introducing the rearranged α and β chains of the Des TCR as a transgene.[60] This apparently simple approach resulted in two unexpected anomalies. Firstly, the Des TCR transgene proved interesting in that its α chain did not prevent the rearrangement and expression of endogenous α chains in all thymocytes. So some thymocytes actually expressed two TCRs, one being the Des TCR and the other being made up of the transgenic β chain with a rearranged endogenous α chain.[61] Because the density of TCR expression on the cell surface is controlled by the CD3 molecule, the density of the Des TCR was lower if the endogenous TCR was expressed at high levels. Secondly, it was expected that the K^b gene under the influence of the rat insulin promoter would be expressed only on the β cells but in fact a very low level was also expressed in the thymus. This amount was, however, sufficient, to induce the deletion of Des TCR cells that had the highest density of Des-TCR on their surface. Cells with a lower level of Des TCRs were not affected and migrated to the periphery. Although this low level, ectopic expression of the K^b transgene in the thymus created problems in studying our model, its effects may actually reflect what happens in a normal mouse. For example, Jolicoeur et al[62] have shown by PCR analysis that insulin, GAD67 and other pancreatic proteins are ectopically expressed in the young mouse thymus. Whether this occurs on thymus cells that could delete autoreactive thymocytes is not known, but it is possible that low level expression of self proteins by any thymus cells could negatively select T cells with receptors of high affinity for their target antigens. This would allow low affinity autoreactive T cells to escape thymus censorship and thus provide a source of potentially autoaggressive T cells.

In our RIP-K^b x Des TCR model, the lower density Des TCR cells that migrated to the periphery were quite capable of rejecting K^b-bearing skin grafts but did not infiltrate islets that expressed the K^b autoantigen. This was the case even when the transgenic mice were manipulated so that they had high density Des TCR cells circulating in the periphery (Heath et al, submitted). An explanation for this comes from the important work of Ohashi et al[2] and Oldstone et al[3] who transgenically expressed LCMV proteins on the β cells. Nothing happened to the β cells unless the animals were primed with wild type virus which would be presented on professional APCs. After this, the mice mounted a typical response to LCMV and islets expressing LCMV proteins were rapidly destroyed. Thus antigens expressed on nonprofessional APCs, like β cells, are not noticed by circulating T cells that have the ability to recognize the same antigens when presented on professional APCs. This might be for two reasons: firstly, because parenchymal cells lack costimulatory properties and secondly because tissues are protected from the immune system by an endothelial barrier. It has been shown that naive T cells do not normally circulate through tissues but preferentially migrate back to the lymph nodes.[63] Antigen-experienced cells, however, having upregulated levels of adhesion molecules, can interact with the endothelium and extravasate into tissues. Such experienced cells may not need to be supplied with help or costimulation provided they are of sufficiently high avidity. Priming of the RIP-K^b x Des TCR mice with professional APCs carrying K^b also resulted in β cell death, but only if high density Des TCR cells were present (Heath et al, submitted). So although low density, primed Des TCR cells could respond to K^b on professional APCs, they still could not respond to islet β cells presenting K^b.

Could local production of IL-2 allow the low density Des TCR cells to respond to islet K^b, for example, by attracting the cells into the islets or once there, by acting as a helper growth factor for them? It did so,[58] but so could locally produced TNFα which also induced a local inflammatory response around the islets (see below).[64] This result implies that IL-2 did not necessarily help the low density Des TCR cells by acting as a T cell growth factor, but more likely by inducing inflammation and leading to the upregulation of class I molecules and other antigen-presenting machinery on the β cells. These islets might then be recognized by the low density Des TCR cells.

So far, we have only discussed experiments involving mice in which nearly all T cells expressed a receptor specific for K^b. What happens in the case of a normal T cell repertoire? Such a repertoire might have been modified by the low level expression of K^b in the thymus of RIP-K^b mice but it is likely that low avidity K^b-specific CD8+ T cells escaped thymic deletion, since peripheral T cells from RIP-K^b mice could respond to K^b in vitro but only if IL-2 was present.[65] When RIP-K^b mice were crossed to RIP-IL-2 mice, however, autoimmunity to β cells expressing K^b did not occur. Ohashi et al reported similar results when LCMV proteins were expressed on the β cells in the presence of local TNFα:[66] no autoimmunity occurred unless the animals were primed. But the priming threshold was reduced because of the presence of local TNFα such that LCMV proteins expressed by vaccinia virus vectors were able to prime, whereas in the absence of local TNFα, whole virus was required. They concluded that the MHC haplotype, level of MHC expression, nature of the priming antigen and CTL precursor frequency could all influence diabetes induction. Likewise, von Herrath et al[67] found that when low avidity CD8+ T cells against LCMV proteins were present in the normal repertoire, CD4+ T cells were needed to help the primed response. When high avidity cells were present, they could respond on their own after priming.

To summarize, the presence of autoreactive T cells to islet antigens need not have any serious consequences for the mouse. They could circulate for life without ever gaining access to the islets. Even if access occurred, with local inflammation, they might still not respond unless optimally primed by a strong antigenic stimulus on professional APCs so that a high precursor frequency was obtained. It seems, therefore, that a number of factors must act in concert before autoimmune diabetes can occur.

Interleukin-6

IL-6 is a multifunctional cytokine made by a range of cell types such as T and B lymphocytes, macrophages, epidermal keratinocytes, endothelial cells, fibroblasts, and mesangial cells. Its many effects include promoting the maturation of activated B cells into antibody-forming plasma cells, induction of acute phase proteins from hepatocytes, regulation of myeloid cell growth and the stimulation of mesangial cell growth.[68,69] In certain autoimmune diseases some of the clinical symptoms could be explained by the abnormal production of IL-6. Hirano et al showed that patients with a cardiac myxoma tumor that was producing IL-6 had a number of autoimmune symptoms, including autoantibodies, hypergammaglobulinemia and an increase in acute phase proteins and these symptoms disappeared after the tumor was removed.[68] IL-6 is also thought to play a role in the pathogenesis of IDDM. Isolated mouse islet β cells can produce IL-6 in response to cytokines such as IFNγ and TNFα[70] and anti-IL-6 antibodies given to NOD mice could suppress the cyclophosphamide-induced diabetes in these animals.[71] Incubation of rat islets with human IL-6 resulted in stimulation of insulin secretion at lower IL-6 concentrations but degenerative changes in the β cells at higher concentrations.[72] These results are reminiscent of the effects of IL-1β on isolated islet cells and it is possible that since IL-1 is a potent stimulator of IL-6, some of its effects on the β cell may be mediated by IL-6.

Dysregulated expression of IL-6 in transgenic mouse β cells resulted in a progressive insulitis without diabetes.[73] The infiltrating cells were predominantly B cells with some T cells and macrophages. Islet architecture was altered and young animals showed evidence of islet hyperplasia with increased mitotic figures and neoductular formation. In spite of the presence of islet infiltrating cells, other cytokine mRNAs were not detected at significant levels in an RNAse protection assay implying that islet-specific autoimmune reactivity was not underway in this location. Consistent with one of the functions of IL-6, there were many IgG positive plasma cells around the islets. The presence of plasma cells seems unique to the local expression of IL-6, since they were not seen when IFNγ,[74] IL-2,[51] IL-10,[75] TNFα,[64,76] TNFβ,[77] or IFNα[78] were artificially made by β cells. In spite of the accumulation of plasma cells, it seemed that islet-reactive antibodies were not being made since the islets did not appear to have bound Ig molecules.

Effects of localized expression of IL-10

IL-10 inhibits macrophage dependent antigen-specific T cell proliferation and macrophage dependent production of cytokines by T cells.[79,80] In particular, IL-10 inhibits the development of Th_1 cells and their ability to secrete cytokines. To study these facets and to determine the role of this factor in IDDM in vivo, we expressed IL-10 in the islets of transgenic mice (Ins-IL-10 transgenic mice). Surprisingly, this cytokine induced pancreatic inflammation in most of the transgenic lines studied.[75] The histopathological phenotype was actually quite unique, comprising a purely peri-islet accumulation of inflammatory cells, and no detectable islet infiltration, islet-cell destruction or diabetes. This study included mice as old as 14 months of age and, in these, the large inflammatory infiltrates remained only in the peri-islet region. Analysis of the cells comprising these infiltrates revealed mainly CD4+ T lymphocytes, with some CD8+ cells, B lymphocytes, and macrophages accumulating in the peri-islet region. Studies with BrdU incorporation indicated the mitotic index of the infiltrating cells to be quite low as compared to the infiltrating cells in Ins-IFNγ transgenic mice or NOD Ins-IL-10 transgenic mice (see below). The low level of localized cell division, accompanied by very notable morphological changes in the vascular endothelium indicating activation, implied to us that the lymphocytes accumulated in the pancreas due to increased extravasation capacity of the pancreatic vascular endothelium. We further surmised that such regulatory cytokines might need to recruit lymphocytes and induce recirculation in order to amplify their regulatory effects. The lack of islet inflammation or destruction indicated that these cells had not been sensitized to islet antigens or if so, were not activated to a pathogenic capacity.

Effect of pancreatic IL-10 on IDDM models

Since IL-10 has immunoregulatory effects including the inhibition of Th_1 functions, we assessed the effects of localized production of IL-10 in several models of immune mediated islet destruction. The first example was the islet allograft model. In this study islets were engrafted across MHC barriers[81] and the status of the graft was assessed histologically. These studies revealed no delay in the rejection process in spite of the presence of in situ IL-10. In the second model we wished to determine if locally expressed IL-10 would prevent the destruction of islets expressing LCMV antigens that occurred after LCMV infection. In the Ins-LCMV transgenic lines utilized in our study, $CD4^+$ T cells were required to elicit islet destruction following virus infection[67] and the possibility exists that the IL-10 could have deviated their function to be less pathogenic. The results of this study indicated that the cytokine did not block the islet cell destruction.[82]

Effect of pancreatic IL-10 on diabetes in the NOD mouse

Whereas in the experiments described above the effect of IL-10 was judged to be neutral, a fascinating and quite unpredicted finding occurred when the transgene was introduced onto the NOD/Shi genetic background:[55] a dramatic acceleration of the disease was observed. In these experiments the blood glucose levels in Ins-IL-10 NOD x Balb/c F1 mice were normal in both transgenic and nontransgenic mice. Pancreata from the nontransgenic F1 mice showed no evidence of leukocyte infiltration as evaluated by hematoxylin and eosin staining, whereas pancreata from Ins-IL-10 F1 transgenic mice demonstrated morphological changes similar to those seen in the parental Ins-IL-10 lines.[75] However, on the first backcross to NOD/Shi (N2), a dramatic acceleration of diabetes was seen in the transgenic animals provided they were homozygous at the NOD MHC locus. We found that 84% of transgenic, homozygous NOD MHC, N2 mice were diabetic by 4-10 weeks of age, whereas all of the MHC-identical, nontransgenic littermates were normoglycemic. We did not observe diabetes in transgenic, heterozygous NOD MHC, N2 mice. In addition, none of the N2 nontransgenic littermates were diabetic at 10-13 weeks of age. Diabetes in homozygous NOD MHC transgenic N2 mice was accompanied by pronounced insulitis. This is in sharp contrast to the selective periinsulitis seen in the parental Ins-IL-10 transgenic strain.[75] Severe insulitis was found in homozygous NOD MHC transgenic N2 mice. When NOD diabetes susceptibility genes are present, localized IL-10 production did not protect the islets from inflammation. IL-10 induced infiltration of the islets since no islets with insulitis were demonstrated in MHC identical, but IL-10 negative mice.

Accelerated diabetes was also seen in the second backcross to NOD/Shi (N3). In this generation, 87% of homozygous NOD MHC, Ins-IL-10 transgenic mice of both genders were diabetic by 10 weeks of age, whereas none of the homozygous NOD MHC, nontransgenic littermates were diabetic at this time. As in the N2 generation increased insulitis was associated with the early onset of diabetes in homozygous NOD MHC, Ins-IL-10 mice. The localized IL-10 induced diabetes at 5 and 6 weeks of age in one third of mice heterozygous for the NOD MHC in the N3 generation, whereas none of the MHC identical, nontransgenic littermates were diabetic at 10 weeks of age. Along with the development of clinical diabetes in heterozygous NOD MHC, Ins-IL-10 mice insulitis increased from the N2 (13%) to N3 (37%) generation. Introduction of more diabetes susceptibility genes from N2 to N3 was demonstrated by the increased presence of peri-islet inflammation in nontransgenic littermates mice that were either heterozygous or homozygous at the NOD MHC. Recently our results were confirmed in a similar IL-10 transgenic model (in this case the glucagon promoter was used) by another group of investigators and led to nearly identical findings.[83]

Autoimmunity induced by expression of IFNγ in the islets

IFNγ is produced by antigen stimulated T lymphocytes. It is immune stimulatory and the prototypic Th_1 "proinflammatory" molecule. It induces the expression of MHC class I and class II antigens as well as costimulatory molecules such as B7. It can also activate macrophages and influence B cell responses. IFNγ was the first cytokine to be expressed transgenically in islet β cells[74] and this model has proved quite illuminating.[84-89] Islet expression of IFNγ induced both peri-islet and intra-islet inflammation, later developing into islet associated pancreatitis. Islet cell loss and diabetes were eventually observed. Treatment of these transgenic mice with anti-IFNγ prevented the development of inflammation. In addition to the immune cell infiltration, other signs of immune activation were present in the pancreas, including increased expression of MHC class I and II antigens, expression of costimulatory molecules and endothelial cell activation.

Proof of autoimmunity was attained through the engraftment of histocompatible islet or pituitary tissue into these transgenic mice. Only engrafted islets were rejected, indicating sensitization to (as yet unidentified) islet antigens in this transgenic model.[85] This finding was confirmed in subsequent experiments utilizing double transgenic mice expressing both LCMV antigens and IFNγ in the β cells.[82] In these experiments, lymphocytes from the periphery were studied in vitro to determine whether cells recognizing the LCMV antigens could be identified. These studies directly demonstrated the spontaneous development of cytotoxic T lymphocytes (CTL) that recognized this individual "islet" antigen. Thus, as opposed to the other models of ectopic cytokine expression, such as those using IL-2 (see above) and TNFα (see below), IFNγ is unique in its ability to abrogate tolerance.

While autoimmune diabetes and loss of islet tolerance were demonstrated in this model, the relationship between the induced disease and IDDM in humans is not entirely clear. In these mice a single genetic perturbation, inducing IFNγ overexpression in the islets, is sufficient to induce autoimmunity. In contrast, in the NOD model, it is clear that numerous interacting genes are needed to result in disease. Still, much can be learned from the naturally occurring and induced models of diabetes to help us learn the basic etiopathogenic mechanisms potentially involved in the development of human IDDM.

Islet regeneration occurs in mice expressing IFNγ in β cells
Cells within the adult pancreas show limited mitotic activity and the organ overall exhibits developmental stability. The turnover of cells in each cellular compartment, pancreatic ducts, islets, or exocrine of the adult pancreas is quite low. Thus, any attempt at cure for this disease has involved replacement of lost islet tissue by grafting. However, the lack of adequate sources of such tissue has limited its utility. Additionally, the risk of antirejection therapy could be more dangerous than the diabetes itself. While a great deal is known about how these cells might be destroyed in diseased individuals, there is relatively little known about the mechanism by which adult and neonatal islet cells proliferate. A greater understanding of these growth mechanisms would certainly contribute to therapeutic potential for IDDM, since the knowledge gained could potentially be exploited to induce the proliferation of new islet cells. If β cells could be induced to grow in situ one of the main limitations of this methodology could be overcome. A knowledge of the growth factors affecting islet proliferation could additionally be utilized to grow fetal cells in vitro.

Transgenic mice that expressed IFNγ in the pancreatic β cells also underwent a remarkable regenerative process where duct proliferation and islet cell neogenesis was apparent in the adult mice. The continued differentiation of endocrine cells from duct epithelial cells has been demonstrated. These new endocrine cells were incorporated into islet-like structures which were found adjacent to ducts or protruding into the duct lumen.[88] This continuous proliferation occurred in the absence of mature T and B lymphocytes indicating that it did not result directly from T cell mediated islet destruction. The ontogeny of the new β cells appeared to recapitulate embryonic development since cells containing multiple islet hormones have been identified as well as cells coexpressing both amylase and insulin.[89] However, the identity of the islet stem cell from which these new islet cells are derived has not been defined. The study of the factors regulating this process will further our understanding how the duct and β cells grow and differentiate.

Expression of IFNα in islet β cells

IFNα shows antiviral properties and can be found in the pancreas of recent onset diabetes patients. To determine the effect of this cytokine on islet integrity the IFNα gene was targeted to the pancreatic β cells.[78] The resulting transgenic mice demonstrated leukocyte infiltration into the islets and diabetes occurred. Treatment with anti-IFNα prevented the disease indicating that the expressed protein mediated the diabetic effects. The role of direct toxicity of IFNα versus that of the immune system remains to be investigated in this model. Additionally, the pathway to activation of autoreactivity is not yet defined. A role for IFNα in diabetes induction was recently proposed from using two nontransgenic rodent models of IDDM in which islet expression of this cytokine preceded any infiltration.[90] The idea of a β cell virus precipitating IFNα production is always appealing as a mechanism for starting off the diabetic process but it remains to be seen if this is fact what happens.

Expression of TNF in islet β cells

TNFα is elicited from activated macrophages and is an important inflammatory mediator. TNFα and TNFβ are known to induce the expression of MHC class I and II antigens as well as leukocyte-associated adhesion molecules. TNFα shares multiple activities ascribed to interleukin-1 and can also act synergistically with other cytokines. Since it is a potent inflammatory mediator, it is important to understand the in vivo function and regulation of this molecule. Islet expression of TNFα led to extravasation of lymphocytes into the islet region.[64,76] The inflammatory infiltrates consisted largely of T lymphocytes which accumulated in the periphery of the islets and within the islet itself. In fact, the pathology was very like that described for β cell expression of IL-2 (see above). Similar infiltrates can be observed with islet expression of TNFβ,[77] however, the inflammatory cells accumulated largely within the peri-islet space, with lower numbers of accumulating cells. In both cases, no hyperglycemia was observed although the TNFα mice showed some degree of islet cell destruction as evidenced by the partial obliteration of islet cell structures from the pancreas.

Transgenic expression of TNFα or LT in islets did not result in autoimmunity. Insufficient numbers of islet cells were destroyed to elicit diabetes, implying that no islet-specific effector cells were generated in this model. Lafferty has proposed that the β cell, being a parenchymal cell, lacks costimulatory activity. For example, islets depleted of professional APCs were not recognized by naive T cells when grafted into allogeneic recipients.[91] Similarly, Markmann et al[92] using a transgenic model showed that β cells expressing transgenic I-E molecules were not recognized by I-E⁻ hosts, but if such hosts were primed with spleen cells expressing I-E then the I-E⁺ β cells were rejected. These data along with other transgenic experiments,[2,3] support the idea that professional priming is required before a T cell can see antigens on parenchymal cells like the β cell. To determine whether the failure to induce autoimmunity by TNFα was due to the lack of induction of appropriate costimulatory molecules, the experimental system was manipulated so that human B7.1 was artificially expressed by pancreatic β cells. Less than 2% of the animals developed spontaneous diabetes.[93] If TNFα was coexpressed by the β cells then diabetes onset was very rapid, within 3-5 weeks indicating the presence of islet-reactive effector cells.[94] These studies suggest that TNFα could induce the recruitment of lymphocytes into the pancreas but this signal was insufficient to induce autoimmunity. When B7.1 was added, the islet cell antigens could be perceived by inflammatory cells and autoimmunity resulted.

In related experiments the potential role of TNFα in accelerating autoimmunity induced by LCMV infection of mice harboring an islet-targeted LCMV protein was investigated. In the presence of the TNFα transgene, the frequency of diabetes following infection was much higher.[66] TNFα may have played a dual role in this pathogenesis: firstly, by recruiting naive T cells into the islets from which they are normally excluded by the endothelial barrier[95] and secondly, by indirectly upregulating antigen-presenting machinery on the islets as a consequence of the inflammatory response. Thus one important role of cytokines in the periphery is their ability to attract appropriate effector cells both through activation of the endothelium and chemotaxis.

Expression of TGFβ in islet β cells

TGFβ, like most other cytokines, has a quite complex series of traits defined mainly in vitro. Some of these are clearly proinflammatory: it fosters adhesion, recruitment and activation of immature cells. However, it suppresses functions mediated by lymphocytes.[96] Additionally, it inhibits IL-1 dependent lymphocyte proliferation[97] and IL-2 mediated induction of IL-2 receptors on T cells.[98] It is a chemotaxin for monocyte/macrophages, potent at subpicomolar levels and induces the expression of the growth factors PDGF, TNFα and FGF.[97]

To determine whether TGFβ could have therapeutic potential, it was targeted to the pancreatic β cells of transgenic mice.[99] Histological analysis of these mice revealed phenotypic changes, but in no case was any significant accumulation of inflammatory cells detected. This finding was somewhat unexpected since TGFβ had originally been associated with specific lymphocyte recruitment activities, which apparently may be tissue specific in vivo or subject to the ability of the molecule to induce appropriate activation of the endothelium, enabling leukocyte adhesion and extravasation.

Several transgenic lines showed severe fibrosis of the exocrine pancreas and eventual loss of large regions of the exocrine pancreas. Fibrosis was apparent by 2 weeks of age. The overall organization of the pancreas, both exocrine and endocrine, appeared disrupted in these pancreata with islet cells being present in clusters rather than in distinct circumscribed structures. In the severely fibrosed lines the islet structure appeared disrupted, although the overall islet mass was quite substantial. The number of insulin-producing cells, while not quantitated, appeared quite high. Clusters of cells expressing the other islet hormones could also be found among these disrupted islet fragments. It is not currently known whether the islet structure was disrupted as a result of fibrosis or whether this represented a developmental defect in these animals.

Several additional lines exhibited a much milder disruption with a relatively normal organization of the pancreas.[99] Fibrosis would certainly have been predicted from the expression of this transgene, since TGFβ has been demonstrated to elicit growth factor release from cells of the monocyte/macrophage lineage. Further studies on the potential of this molecule to elicit local immunosuppression are underway.

REGULATION OF AUTOIMMUNITY BY CYTOKINES

After activation it has been shown that different subsets of CD4+ T cells produce distinct cytokine repertoires.[99] The Th_1 subset, responsible for delayed type hypersensitivity (DTH) and for IgG2a production, produces IFNγ, TNFα and IL-2. The murine Th_2 subset, which stimulates IgG1, 2b, and IgE antibody production, makes IL-4, -5, -6, -10 and -13. Most individual cells of a subset may only make one of the cytokines, but on a population basis the complete range of cytokines can form part of the repertoire.[100] The drive to either phenotype does not appear to depend on antigen specificity[101] but may relate to the type of stimulating APC in the primary response[102] and to the ligand density.[103-105] Once primed, the availability of specific cytokines drives the cells towards either the Th_1 (with IFNγ) or Th_2 (with IL-4) subset. The Th_1 cytokines are proinflammatory and responsible for inducing much of the tissue damage during their production; the Th_2 cytokines, IL-4, IL-10 and IL-13 inhibit the proliferation of Th_1 cells. This division in helper subsets has led to the idea that various autoimmune diseases may mirror the skewing towards either the Th_2 or Th_2 profile. Systemic diseases such as SLE in which autoantibody production predominates might indicate the involvement of Th_2 cells (see chapter 7), whereas organ-specific inflammatory diseases such as IDDM may result from the activity of Th_1 cells (reviewed in Liblau et al, 1995).[106]

Evidence for a role of Th_1 cells in IDDM comes from a number of studies. In NOD mice, a high frequency of IFNγ producing cells are found in recently infiltrated islet grafts suffering disease recurrence[107] and injection of mice with antibody to IFNγ reduced the incidence of

It is recently canvassed that protection from organ-specific autoimmunity may result from regulatory T cell networks. Diversion of pathogenic T cells from Th_1 repertoire to Th_2 cytokines seems to protect against diabetes onset. By preventing the local production of pro-inflammatory (Th_1) cytokines by islet-specific T cells the damage to β cells may be reduced. Whether the rescue from diabetes allows other pathologies to develop in animals or humans prone to autoimmunity must be a consideration.

Finally, it will be of interest to determine the mechanisms of β cell death by cytokines and T cells. Is it primarily through cytokines produced by $CD4^+$ T cells responding to islet antigens? Is perforin mediated killing by $CD8^+$ T cells an important mechanism or could even the Fas-Fas ligand pathway be involved? It is possible that all mechanisms are important or that one scenario may predominate in a particular patient giving rise to different kinetics or disease outcome or recovery.

Acknowledgments

The work performed in the author's laboratories was supported by grants from the National Health and Medical Research Council of Australia, the US National Institute of Health, Diabetes Australia, The Ian Potter Foundation and the Rebecca Cooper Foundation, The Juvenile Diabetes Foundation International and the Danish Medical Research Council.

References

1. Cooke A. An overview on possible mechanisms of destruction of the insulin-producing beta cell. Curr Top Microbiol Immunol 1990; 164:125-42.
2. Ohashi PS, Oehen S, Buerki K et al. Ablation of "tolerance" and induction of diabetes by virus infection in viral antigen transgenic mice. Cell 1991; 65:305-17.
3. Oldstone MB, Nerenberg M, Southern P et al. Virus infection triggers insulin-dependent diabetes mellitus in a transgenic model: role of anti-self (virus) immune response. Cell 1991; 65:319-31.
4. Miller JFAP, and Heath WR. Self ignorance in the peripheral T cell pool. Immunol Rev 1993; 133:131-50.
5. Burtles SS, Trembleau S, Drexler K et al. Absence of T cell tolerance to pancreatic islet cells. J Immunol 1992; 149:2185-93.
6. Fowell D, Mason D. Evidence that the T cell repertoire of normal rats contains cells with the potential to cause diabetes. Characterization of the $CD4^+$ T cell subset that inhibits this autoimmune potential. J Exp Med 1993; 177:627-36.
7. Nomikos IN, Wang Y and Lafferty KJ. Involvement of O_2 radicals in 'autoimmune' diabetes. Immunol Cell Biol 1989; 67:85-7.
8. Mandrup-Poulsen T, Helqvist S, Wogensen LD et al. Cytokines and free radicals as effector molecules in the destruction of pancreatic beta cells. Curr Top Microbiol Immunol 1990; 165:169-93.

9. Wang Y, Pontesilli O, Gill RG et al. The role of CD4+ and CD8+ T cells in the destruction of islet grafts by spontaneously diabetic mice. Proc Natl Acad Sci USA 1991; 88:527-31.
10. Kolb H, Kolb BV. Nitric oxide: a pathogenetic factor in autoimmunity. Immunology Today. 1992; 13:157-60.
11. Horio F, Fukuda M, Katoh H et al. Reactive oxygen intermediates in autoimmune islet cell destruction of the NOD mouse induced by peritoneal exudate cells (rich in macrophages) but not T cells. Diabetologia 1994; 37:22-31.
12. Haskins K, McDuffie M. Acceleration of diabetes in young NOD mice with a CD4+ islet-specific T cell clone. Science 1990; 24:1433-6.
13. Bradley BJ, Haskins K, La RF et al. CD8+ T cells are not required for islet destruction induced by a CD4+ islet-specific T-cell clone. Diabetes 1992; 41:1603-8.
14. Katz JD, Wang B, Haskins K et al. Following a diabetogenic T cell from genesis through pathogenesis. Cell 1993; 74:1089-100.
15. Christianson SW, Shultz LD and Leiter EH. Adoptive transfer of diabetes into immunodeficient NOD-scid/scid mice. Relative contributions of CD4+ and CD8+ T cells from diabetic versus prediabetic NOD.NON-Thy-1a donors. Diabetes 1993; 42:44-55.
16. Lo D, Reilly CR, Scott B et al. Antigen presenting cells in adoptively transferred and spontaneous autoimmune diabetes. Eur J Immunol 1993; 23:1693-8.
17. Katz J, Benoist C and Mathis D. Major histocompatibility complex class I molecules are required for the development of insulitis in nonobese diabetic mice. Eur J Immunol 1993; 23: 3358-60.
18. Serreze DV, Leiter EH, Christianson GJ et al. Major histocompatibility complex class I deficient NOD β2m(null) mice are diabetes and insulitis resistant. Diabetes 1994; 43:505-9.
19. Wicker LS, Leiter EH, Todd JA et al. Beta-2-microglobulin deficient NOD mice do not develop insulitis or diabetes. Diabetes 1994; 43:500-4.
20. Yagi H, Matsumoto M, Kunimoto K et al. Analysis of the roles of CD4+ and CD8+ T cells in autoimmune diabetes of NOD mice using transfer to NOD athymic nude mice. Eur J Immunol 1992; 22:2387-93.
21. Charlton B, Bacelj A and Mandel TE. Administration of silica particles or anti-Lyt2 antibody prevents beta-cell destruction in NOD mice given cyclophosphamide. Diabetes 1988; 37: 930-5.
22. Nagata M, Santamaria P, Kawamura T et al. Evidence for the role of CD8+ cytotoxic T cells in the destruction of pancreatic beta-cells in nonobese diabetic mice. J Immunol 1994; 152:2042-50.
23. Bowman MA, Leiter EH and Atkinson MA. Prevention of diabetes in the NOD mouse: implications for therapeutic intervention in human disease. Immunology Today 1994; 15:115-20.
24. Howard AD, Kostura, MJ, Thornberry, N et al. IL-1-converting enzyme requires aspartic acid residues for processing of the IL-1 beta precursor at two distinct sites and does not cleave 31-kDa IL-1 alpha. J Immunol 1991; 47: 2964-9.

25. Mandrup-Poulsen T, Zumsteg U, Reimers J et al. Involvement of interleukin 1 and interleukin 1 antagonist in pancreatic beta cell destruction in insulin dependent diabetes mellitus. Cytokine 1993; 5:185-91.
26. Campbell IL, Iscaro A and Harrison LC. IFN-gamma and tumor necrosis factor-alpha. Cytotoxicity to murine islets of Langerhans. J Immunol 1988; 141:2325-9.
27. Corbett JA, Sweetland MA, Wang JL et al. Nitric oxide mediates cytokine-induced inhibition of insulin secretion by human islets of Langerhans. Proc Natl Acad Sci USA 1993; 90:1731-5.
28. Eizirik DL, Sandler S, Welsh N et al. Cytokines suppress human islet function irrespective of their effects on nitric oxide generation. J Clin Invest 1994; 93:1968-74.
29. Taylor-Robinson AW, Liew FY, Severn A et al. Regulation of the immune response by nitric oxide differentially produced by T helper type 1 and T helper type 2 cells. Eur J Immunol 1994; 24:980-4.
30. Corbett JA, Kwon G, Misko TP et al. Tyrosine kinase involvement in IL 1 beta induced expression of INOS by beta cells purified from islets of Langerhans. Am J Physiol 1994; 267:C48-54.
31. Yamada K, Takane N, Otabe S et al. Pancreatic beta-cell-selective production of tumor necrosis factor-alpha induced by interleukin-1. Diabetes 1993; 42:1026-31.
32. Uchigata Y, Yamamoto H, Kawamura A et al. Protection by superoxide dismutase, catalase, and poly(ADP-ribose) synthetase inhibitors against alloxan- and streptozotocin-induced islet DNA strand breaks and against the inhibition of proinsulin synthesis. J Biol Chem 1982; 257:6084-8.
33. Fehsel K, Jalowy A, Qi S et al. Islet cell DNA is a target of inflammatory attack by nitric oxide. Diabetes 1993; 42:496-500.
34. Ankarcrona M, Dypbukt JM, Brune B et al. Interleukin-1 beta-induced nitric oxide production activates apoptosis in pancreatic RINm5F cells. Exp Cell Res 1994; 213:172-7.
35. Csaikl FF, Csaikl UM and Durum SK. Strategies for modulation of interleukin-1 in vivo: knockout and transgenics. In: Overexpression and knockout of cytokines in transgenic mice. Academic Press: CO Jacob, 1994:1-13.
36. Smith KA. Interleukin-2. Curr Op Immunol 1992; 4:271-6.
37. Chesnut K, She JX, Cheng I et al. Characterizations of candidate genes for IDD susceptibility from the diabetes-prone NOD mouse strain. Mammalian Genome 1993; 4:549-54.
38. Ghosh S, Palmer SM, Rodrigues NR et al. Polygenic control of autoimmune diabetes in nonobese diabetic mice. Nature Genetics 1993; 4:404-9.
39. Matesanz F, Alcina A and Pellicer A. Existence of at least five interleukin-2 molecules n different mouse strains. Immunogenetics 1993; 38:300-3.
40. Malkovsky M, Loveland B, North M et al. Recombinant interleukin-2 directly augments the cytotoxicity of human monocytes. Nature 1987; 325:262-5.

41. Cox GW, Mathieson BJ, Giardina SL et al. Characterization of IL-2 receptor expression and function on murine macrophages. J Immunol 1990; 145:1719-26.
42. Karupiah G, Blanden RV and Ramshaw IA. Interferon gamma is involved in the recovery of athymic nude mice from recombinant vaccinia virus/interleukin 2 infection. J Exp Med 1990; 172:1495-503.
43. Ishida Y, Nishi M, Taguchi O et al. Expansion of natural killer cells but not T cells in human interleukin 2/interleukin 2 receptor (Tac) transgenic mice. J Exp Med 1989; 170:1103-15.
44. Kroemer G, Andreu JL, Gonzalo JA et al. Interleukin-2, autotolerance, and autoimmunity. Adv Immunol 1991; 50:147-235.
45. Dallman MJ, Shiho O, Page TH et al. Peripheral tolerance to alloantigen results from altered regulation of the interleukin 2 pathway. J Exp Med 1991; 173:79-87.
46. Kojima A and Prehn RT. Genetic susceptibility to post-thymectomy autoimmune diseases in mice. Immunogenetics 1981; 14:15-27.
47. Taguchi O and Nishizuka Y. Autoimmune oophoritis in thymectomized mice: T cell requirement in adoptive cell transfer. Clin Exp Immunol 1980; 42:324-31.
48. Smith H, Chen IM, Kubo R et al. Neonatal thymectomy results in a repertoire enriched in T cells deleted in adult thymus. Science 1989; 245:749-52.
49. Jones LA, Chin LT, Merriam GR et al. Failure of clonal deletion in neonatally thymectomized mice: tolerance is preserved through clonal anergy. J Exp Med 1990; 172:1277-85.
50. Andreu-Sánchez JL, Moreno-de-Alborán IM, Marcos MA et al. Interleukin 2 abrogates the nonresponsive state of T cells expressing a forbidden T cell receptor repertoire and induces autoimmune disease in neonatally thymectomized mice. J Exp Med 1991; 173:1323-9.
51. Allison J, Malcolm L, Chosich N et al. Inflammation but not autoimmunity occurs in transgenic mice expressing constitutive levels of interleukin-2 in islet beta cells. Eur J Immunol 1992; 22:1115-21.
52. Allison J, Oxbrow L, Miller JFAP. Consequences of in situ production of IL-2 for islet cell death. Int Immunol 1994; 6:541-9.
53. Scott B, Liblau R, Degermann S et al. A role for non-MHC genetic polymorphism in susceptibility to spontaneous autoimmunity. Immunity 1994; 1:73-82.
54. Allison J, McClive P, Oxbrow L et al. Genetic requirements for acceleration of diabetes in non-obese diabetic mice expressing interleukin-2 in islet β cells. Eur J Immunol 1994; 24:2535-41.
55. Wogensen L, Lee MS, Sarvetnick N. Production of interleukin 10 by islet cells accelerates immune mediated destruction of beta cells in nonobese diabetic mice. J Exp Med 1994; 179:1379-84.
56. Zijlstra M, Bix M, Simister NE et al. Beta 2-microglobulin deficient mice lack CD4-8+ cytolytic T cells. Nature 1990; 344: 742-6.
57. Wu J, Zhou T, He J et al. Autoimmune disease in mice due to integration of an endogenous retrovirus in an apoptosis gene. J Exp Med 1993; 178:461-8.

58. Heath WR, Allison J, Hoffmann MW et al. Autoimmune diabetes as a consequence of locally produced interleukin-2. Nature 1992; 359:547-9.
59. Allison J, Campbell IL, Morahan G et al. Diabetes in transgenic mice resulting from over-expression of class I histocompatibility molecules in pancreatic beta cells. Nature 1988; 333:529-33.
60. Schönrich G, Kalinke U, Momburg F et al. Down-regulation of T cell receptors on self-reactive T cells as a novel mechanism for extrathymic tolerance induction. Cell 1991; 65:293-304.
61. Heath WR, Miller JF. Expression of two alpha chains on the surface of T cells in T cell receptor transgenic mice. J Exp Med 1993; 178:1807-11.
62. Jolicoeur C, Hanahan D, Smith KM. T-cell tolerance toward a transgenic beta-cell antigen and transcription of endogenous pancreatic genes in thymus. Proc Natl Acad Sci USA 1994; 91:6707-11.
63. Mackay CR, Marston WL, Dudler L. Naive and memory T cells show distinct pathways of lymphocyte recirculation. J Exp Med 1990; 171:801-17.
64. Higuchi Y, Herrera P, Muniesa P et al. Expression of a tumor necrosis factor alpha transgene in murine pancreatic beta cells results in severe and permanent insulitis without evolution towards diabetes. J Exp Med 1992; 176:1719-31.
65. Morahan G, Allison J, Miller JFAP. Tolerance of class I histocompatibility antigens expressed extrathymically. Nature 1989; 339:622-4.
66. Ohashi PS, Oehen S, Aichele P et al. Induction of diabetes is influenced by the infectious virus and local expression of MHC class I and tumor necrosis factor alpha. J Immunol 1993; 150:5185-94.
67. von Herrath MG, Dockter J, Oldstone MBA. How virus induces a rapid or slow onset insulin-dependent diabetes mellitus in a transgenic model. Immunity 1994; 1:231-42.
68. Hirano T. Interleukin-6 and its relation to inflammation and disease. Clin Immunol Immunopathol 1992; 62:S60-5.
69. Yoshizaki K, Kuritani T, Kishimoto T. Interleukin-6 in autoimmune disorders. Seminars in Immunol 1992; 4:155-66.
70. Campbell IL, Cutri A, Wilson A et al. Evidence for IL-6 production by and effects on the pancreatic beta-cell. J Immunol 1989; 143:1188-91.
71. Campbell IL, Kay TW, Oxbrow L et al. Essential role for interferon-gamma and interleukin-6 in autoimmune insulin-dependent diabetes in NOD/Wehi mice. J Clin Invest 1991; 87:739-42.
72. Buschard K, Aaen K, Horn T et al. Interleukin 6: a functional and structural in vitro modulator of beta-cells from islets of Langerhans. Autoimmunity 1990; 5:185-94.
73. Campbell IL, Hobbs MV, Dockter J et al. Islet inflammation and hyperplasia induced by the pancreatic islet-specific overexpression of interleukin-6 in transgenic mice. Am J Path 1994; 145:157-66.
74. Sarvetnick N, Liggitt D, Pitts SL et al. Insulin-dependent diabetes mellitus induced in transgenic mice by ectopic expression of class II MHC and interferon-gamma. Cell 1988; 52:773-82.

75. Wogensen L, Huang X, Sarvetnick N. Leukocyte extravasation into the pancreatic tissue in transgenic mice expressing interleukin 10 in the islets of Langerhans. J Exp Med 1993; 178:175-85.
76. Picarella DE, Kratz A, Li CB et al. Transgenic tumor necrosis factor (TNF)-alpha production in pancreatic islets leads to insulitis, not diabetes. Distinct patterns of inflammation in TNF-alpha and TNF-beta transgenic mice. J Immunol 1993; 150:4136-50.
77. Picarella DE, Kratz A, Li CB et al. Insulitis in transgenic mice expressing tumor necrosis factor beta (lymphotoxin) in the pancreas. Proc Natl Acad Sci U S A 1992; 89:10036-40.
78. Stewart TA, Hultgren B, Huang X et al. Induction of type I diabetes by interferon-alpha in transgenic mice. Science 1993; 260:1942-6.
79. Malefyt RDW, Haanen J, Spits H et al. Interleukin 10 and viral IL-10 strongly reduce antigen-specific human T cell proliferation by diminishing the antigen-presenting capacity of monocytes via downregulation of class II major histocompatibility complex expression. J Exp Med 1991; 174:915-24.
80. Fiorentino DF, Zlotnik A, Vieira P et al. IL-10 acts on the antigen-presenting cell to inhibit cytokine production by Th_1 cells. J Immunol 1991; 146:3444-51.
81. Lee MS, Wogensen L, Shizuru J et al. Pancreatic islet production of murine interleukin 10 does not inhibit immune mediated destruction. J Clin Invest 1994; 93:1332-8.
82. Lee MS, von Herrath M, Reiser H et al. Sensitization to self (virus) antigen by in situ expression of murine interferon gamma. J Clin Invest 1995; 95:486-92.
83. Moritani M, Yoshimoto K, Tashiro F et al. Transgenic expression of IL10 in pancreatic islet α cells accelerates autoimmune insulitis and diabetes in non-obese diabetic mice. Int Immunol 1994; 6:1927-36.
84. Sarvetnick N. Transgenic models of diabetes. Curr Op Immunol 1989; 2:604-6.
85. Sarvetnick N, Shizuru J, Liggitt D et al. Loss of pancreatic islet tolerance induced by beta-cell expression of interferon-gamma. Nature 1990; 346:844-7.
86. Lee MS and Sarvetnick N. Induction of vascular addressins and adhesion molecules in the pancreas of IFN gamma transgenic mice. J Immunol 1994; 152:4597-603.
87. Wogensen L, Molony L, Gu D et al. 1994; Postnatal anti-interferon-gamma treatment prevents pancreatic inflammation in transgenic mice with beta-cell expression of interferon-gamma. J Interferon Res 14:111-6.
88. Gu DL, Sarvetnick N. Epithelial cell proliferation and islet neogenesis in IFNγ transgenic mice. Development 1993; 118:33-46.
89. Gu D, Lee MS, Krahl T et al. Transitional cells in the regenerating pancreas. Development 1994; 120:1873-81.
90. Huang XJ, Hultgren B, Dybdal N et al. Islet expression of interferon alpha precedes diabetes in both the BB rat and streptozotocin treated mice. Immunity 1994; 1:469-78.

91. Lafferty KJ, Prowse SJ, Simeonovic CJ et al. Immunobiology of tissue transplantation: a return to the passenger leukocyte concept. Ann Rev Immunol 1983; 1:143-73.
92. Markmann J, Lo D, Naji A et al. Antigen presenting function of class II MHC expressing pancreatic beta cells. Nature 1988; 336:476-9.
93. Guerder S, Meyerhoff J, Flavell R. The role of the T cell costimulator B7-1 in autoimmunity and the induction and maintenance of tolerance to peripheral antigen. Immunity 1994; 1:155-66.
94. Guerder S, Picarella DE, Linsley PS et al. Costimulator B7-1 confers antigen-presenting-cell function to parenchymal tissue and in conjunction with tumor necrosis factor alpha leads to autoimmunity in transgenic mice. Proc Natl Acad Sci USA 1994; 91:5138-42.
95. Mackay CR. Immunological memory. Adv Immunol 1993; 53:217-65.
96. Roberts AB, Flanders KC, Heine UI et al. Transforming growth factor-beta: multifunctional regulator of differentiation and development. Phil Trans Roy Soc London Series B 1990; 327:145-54.
97. Wahl SM, McCartney FN, Mergenhagen SE. Inflammatory and immunomodulatory roles of TGF-beta. Immunology Today 1989; 10:58-61.
98. Kehrl JH, Wakefield LM, Roberts AB et al. Production of transforming growth factor beta by human T lymphocytes and its potential role in the regulation of T cell growth. J Exp Med 1986; 163:1037-50.
99. Lee MS, Gu DL, Feng L et al. Accumulation of extracellular matrix and development dysregulation in the pancreas by transgenic production of TGF-β1. Am J Pathol 1995; 147: 42-52.
100. Bucy RP, Panoskaltsismortari A, Huang GQ et al. Heterogeneity of single cell cytokine gene expression in clonal T cell populations. J Exp Med 1994; 180:1251-62.
101. Hsieh CS, Heimberger AB, Gold JS et al. Differential regulation of T helper phenotype development by interleukins 4 and 10 in an alpha beta T-cell-receptor transgenic system. Proc Natl Acad Sci USA 1992; 89:6065-9.
102. Duncan DD, Swain SL. Role of antigen-presenting cells in the polarized development of helper T cell subsets: evidence for differential cytokine production by Th0 cells in response to antigen presentation by B cells and macrophages. Eur J Immunol 1994; 24:2506-14.
103. Rocken M, Muller KM, Saurat JH et al. Central role for TCR/CD3 ligation in the differentiation of CD4⁺ T cells toward A Th$_1$ or Th$_2$ functional phenotype. J Immunol 1992; 148:47-54.
104. Bottomly K. A functional dichotomy in CD4⁺ T lymphocytes. Immunology Today 1988; 9:268-74.
105. Murray JS, Ferrandis-Edwards D, Wolfe CJ et al. Major histocompatibility complex regulation of T helper functions mapped to a peptide C terminus that controls ligand density. Eur J Immunol 1994; 24:2337-44.
106. Liblau RS, Singer SM, McDevitt HO. Th$_1$ and Th$_2$ CD4⁺ T cells in the pathogenesis of organ specific autoimmune disease. Mol Cell Biol 1995; 9:3151-4.

107. Shehadeh NN, LaRosa F, Lafferty KJ. Altered cytokine activity in adjuvant inhibition of autoimmune diabetes. J Autoimmunity 1993; 6:291-300.
108. Campbell IL, Kay TW, Oxbrow L et al. Essential role for interferon-gamma and interleukin-6 in autoimmune insulin-dependent diabetes in NOD/Wehi mice. J Clin Invest 1991; 87:739-42.
109. Harada M, Kishimoto Y, Makino S. Prevention of overt diabetes and insulitis in OD mice by a single BCG vaccination. Diabetes Res Clin Prac 1990; 8:85-9.
110. Sadelain MW, Qin HY, Lauzon J et al. Prevention of type I diabetes in NOD mice by adjuvant immunotherapy. Diabetes 1990; 39:583-9.
111. Baxter AG, Horsfall AC, Healey D et al. Mycobacteria precipitate an SLE-like syndrome in diabetes-prone NOD mice. Immunology 1994; 83:227-31.
112. Baxter AG, Healey D, Cooke A. Mycobacteria precipitate autoimmune rheumatic disease in NOD mice via an adjuvant-like activity. Scand J immunol 1994; 39:602-6.
113. Diaz-Gallo C, Moscovitch-Lopatin M, Strom TB et al. An anergic, islet-infiltrating T-cell clone that suppresses murine diabetes secretes a factor that blocks interleukin2/interleukin 4-dependent proliferation. Proc Natl Acad Sci USA 1992; 89:8656-60.
114. Miller JFAP, Flavell RA. T cell tolerance and autoimmunity in transgenic models of central and peripheral tolerance. Curr Op Immunol 1994; 6:892-9.
115. Singer SM, Tisch R, Yang XD et al. An $A_\beta(d)$ transgene prevents diabetes in nonobese diabetc mice by inducing regulatory T cells. Proc Natl Acad Sci USA 1993; 90:9566-70.
116. Slattery RM, Miller JFAP, Heath WR et al. Failure of a protective major histocompatibility complex class II molecule to delete autoreactive T cells in autoimmune diabetes. Proc Natl Acad Sci USA 1993; 90:10808-10.
117. Locksley RM. Immunology of Leishmaniasis. Curr Op Immunol 1992; 4:413-8.
118. Trembleau S, Penna G, Bosi E et al. Interleukin 12 administration induces T helper type 1 cells and accelerates autoimmune diabetes in NOD mice. J Exp Med 1995; 181:817-21.

CHAPTER 4

CYTOKINES IN MULTIPLE SCLEROSIS

David Baker, Lawrence Steinman, and Koenraad Gijbels

DISEASE COURSE OF MULTIPLE SCLEROSIS

Multiple sclerosis (MS) is a disease of unknown etiology which is characterized by chronic inflammation and demyelination of the central nervous system (CNS). Once triggered there is increasing evidence that disease results from autoimmune attack on the CNS myelin and on the oligodendrocyte which produces the myelin sheath.[1] Whilst the clinical course of this disease is unpredictable, it is typically associated with acute attacks of neurological dysfunction separated by periods of disease stabilization or slow remission. In a high proportion of relapsing-remitting (RRMS) patients, disease may then enter a chronic-progressive (CPMS) course where the patient's condition increasingly deteriorates without remission. Histologically MS is associated with the presence of mononuclear cell perivascular-cuffs within the CNS white-matter. These expand into the surrounding parenchyma and produce a wave of inflammation-mediated myelin destruction. Repeated inflammatory insults generate the formation of large demyelinated plaques containing astrocytic scars (sclerosis). Both acute inflammation as well as demyelinated astrocytic scar tissue can be associated with neurological dysfunction, depending on the anatomical location of the lesion. Similar histopathological lesions are also observable in experimental autoimmune encephalomyelitis (EAE) which serves as an experimental model of MS. EAE has a known autoimmune etiology and is induced in animals by active sensitization to CNS autoantigens or by the transfer of neuroantigen-specific CD4$^+$ T lymphocytes.[2] EAE is one of the most extensively studied experimental autoimmune models and provides an opportunity to identify and dissect the immunopathological events occurring in vivo during chronic

Cytokines in Autoimmunity, edited by Fionula M. Brennan and Marc Feldmann.
© 1996 R.G. Landes Company.

inflammatory reactions, especially in relation to those of the CNS (Fig. 4.1). Although autoimmune diseases are induced by leukocytes, it is becoming increasingly evident that some of their biological effects are mediated by the para- or endocrine actions of the cytokines they secrete (Table 4.1).

Table 4.1. Detection of cytokines in the CNS during demyelinating disease

Cytokine	Possible Source	Detection in Disease
IL-1	M, Mi, A, E, T, B	MS, EAE
IL-2	T	MS, EAE
IL-3	T, MI	EAE
IL-4	T	MS, EAE
IL-5	T	EAE
IL-6	M, Mi, A, E, T	MS, EAE
IL-8	T	EAE
IL-10	T, M, B, A	MS, EAE
IL-12	M	EAE
M-CSF	T, A	MS, EAE
G-CSF	T, A	MS, EAE
GM-CSF	T, A	MS, EAE
IFNγ	T	MS, EAE
TNFα	M, Mi, A, T	MS, EAE
LT	T, Mi	MS, EAE
MCP-1	M, Mi, A	EAE
MCP-3	M	EAE
TCA3	T	EAE
MIP1α	T, M	MS, EAE
MIP1β	T, M	EAE
RANTES	T	MS, EAE
IP-10	M, A	EAE
TGFβ1	T, F, M, Mi, A, E	MS, EAE
TGFβ2	T, F, M, Mi, A, E	MS, EAE

Cytokine secretion potential has been detected either in vitro or in vivo[3-17] in T = T cells, B = B cells, M = monocytes/macrophages, Mi = microglia, A = astrocytes, E = CNS endothelia, F = fibroblasts

Fig. 4.1 (opposite). Cytokine involvement in the immunopathological processes occurring during the development of demyelination in multiple sclerosis. Following the generation of autoreactive T cells within peripheral lymphoid tissue, circulating 'activated' memory cells enter the CNS. Upon recognition of myelin antigens presented by resident perivascular microglia/macrophages these cells are activated to release a variety of cytokines. These activate the vascular endothelium to upregulate adhesion molecules and induce a secondary recruitment of additional mononuclear cells. Recruited B lymphocytes may secrete myelin reactive antibodies which could induce demyelination by either complement-mediated lysis or antibody-dependent cell cytotoxicity. Macrophages strip myelin off the axons and engulf myelin debris. Oligodendrocytes may be a target for killing by T cells or cytotoxic cytokines. Astrocytes proliferate to form a scar surrounding the demyelinated axons.

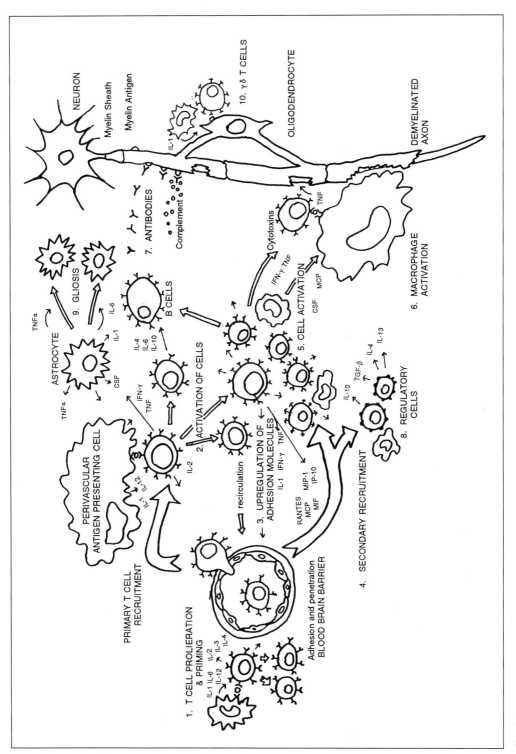

Fig. 4.1.

ANALYSIS OF CYTOKINES IN MS

Analysis of cytokine action in MS has been limited to some clinical experiments and is confined mainly to the analysis of blood and cerebrospinal fluid (CSF), and the histological analysis of postmortem CNS tissue. Although dependent on the detection protocol, it has been invariably possible to detect cytokines (Table 4.1) within the CNS, CSF or serum of MS patients.[3-17] However conflicting observations have been consistently noted between different studies and patient groups,[17] and this serves to underscore the difficulties in analyzing limited samples of human tissue within the context of an unpredictable natural history. The short half-lives in plasma and rapid uptake of cytokines by their receptors on cells, or in soluble form inhibits assessment of the cytokine profile. Cytokine analysis following ex vivo mitogenic stimulation may show the propensity of the cells to produce cytokines in vivo, and has been informative.[17-20] However cytokine analysis of such cultures may merely reflect the relative levels of the cell phenotypes present. These fluctuate during remission and active disease. Furthermore it is clear that at the population level, the phenotypes of cells within the peripheral blood bear little resemblance to those present within CNS lesions.[20] In experimental models of MS, clinical disease is associated with distinct inflammatory events within the CNS which allows the kinetics to be studied systematically. Cytokine production during EAE is actively regulated during lesion formation and resolution.[12,13] Similar systematic analysis of cytokine function in MS is extremely complicated, not only by the inability to sequentially sample target tissue, but also by patient, disease and lesion heterogeneity. Magnetic resonance imaging (MRI) can be used noninvasively to assess lesion load, development and activity. Clinically active attacks are associated with gadolinium-enhancing lesions. MRI studies also suggest that MS is associated with the production of substantial numbers of clinically silent lesions.[21,22] Therefore this suggests that disease is rarely silent at the lesion level. Using gadolinium enhancement these individual lesions take from days to months to resolve and may be developing and resolving simultaneously.[21,22] Analysis of mRNA production within different plaques have indicated that whilst some lesions may preferentially express IL-2 mRNA others produced IL-4 mRNA mainly or both IL-2 and IL-4 mRNA.[23] Lesion heterogeneity is further indicated by immunocytochemical analysis of the lesions themselves, including their cellular components and cytokine components. The average effects of this heterogeneity and degree of activity and regulation may then be reflected in serum and CSF samples and may account for some of the heterogeneity reported.[17] Nevertheless it is consistently indicated that increased cytokine activity is associated with clinically active disease and that cytokine activity is concentrated within the CNS compared with the peripheral blood. Animal models of autoimmune demyelinating disease provide a means to model the relative roles of these cytokines during neuroimmunological diseases (Fig. 4.1).

CYTOKINES IN DISEASE INITIATION

Genetic analysis of MS patients has as yet to unequivocally implicate the role of any nonmajor histocompatibility complex (MHC) locus in MS susceptibility.[24] However comparisons between individuals show a marked heterogeneity in the levels of cytokine production in response to stimulation. Phenotypic differences in IL-2 and TNFα secretion between EAE responder and nonresponder rat strains have been identified. In addition EAE susceptibility loci have been mapped to regions which encode cytokines.[25,26] Cytokines are clearly involved in the effector process, in cell recruitment to lesions and in leukocyte hematopoesis (Fig. 4.1). Therefore genetically-controlled differences in cytokine production could contribute to the intensity of the neuro-immunological disease process. Normal human individuals harbor autoreactive myelin-specific T cells. However the initial essential component of disease development is the clonal expansion and priming of these cells outside homeostatic control mechanisms. Cytokines are intimately involved in this immune process. In EAE this occurs following sensitization to myelin antigens but may also be the result of responses to environmental stimuli inducing a cross-reactive myelin-specific immune response, which could also occur in MS.[1,27] In contrast to other autoimmune diseases, MS is different in that the target tissue (CNS) is normally shielded from the events in the systemic environment by the presence of the blood-brain barrier (BBB). This is formed by endothelial cells which possess tight junctions, and by adjacent CNS-derived glial cells. These CNS endothelia express low levels of adhesion molecules and serve to limit migration of leukocytes and serum products into the CNS.[5] Disease-inducing cells must be activated prior to neurological disease development.[28] Cytokine induced activation (Fig. 4.1) serves to upregulate the expression of adhesion molecules such as the integrins LFA-1 (CD11b:CD18) and VLA-4 (CD49d:CD29) which are involved in leukocyte extravasation into the CNS. Although IL-2 is an integral component of encephalitogenic T cell activation, and inhibition of T cell IL-2 receptor expression can prevent the development of clinical EAE,[29] other cytokine components common to the generation of other immune responses undoubtedly play a role in this aspect (see other chapters). In relation to the development of EAE in vivo these can be shown to include IL-1, IL-3 and IL-12 which increase encephalitogenicity of myelin-reactive T cells.[30,31] After activation IL-2 receptor (IL-2R) appears on the surface of T cells and soluble IL-2R (sIL-2R) is released from activated T cells. Some authors report that occasionally CSF levels of both IL-2 or sIL-2R are increased in patients with MS particularly during clinically active disease.[17,32-35] Furthermore an increased frequency of activated (IL-2R+) myelin-reactive T cells can be detected in the blood and more so in the CSF compared to normal individuals.[36] This serves to indicate that progression of MS is associated with T cell activity and may further add to evidence supporting an autoimmune component in disease. Once activated, T cells irrespective of their specificity, can cross the BBB[28] and, upon recognition of myelin or other CNS derived antigens presented by MHC class II+ perivascular microglia/pericytes, are stimulated to elaborate a cascade of events resulting in the activation of resident CNS-cells, and the recruitment of additional mononuclear leukocytes within the perivascular space and surrounding parenchyma (Fig. 4.1).

CELLULAR RECRUITMENT DURING NEUROIMMUNOLOGICAL DISEASE

Once T cells become activated by specific antigen within the CNS, they induce BBB dysfunction, extravasation of serum proteins and small molecules and the secondary recruitment of mononuclear leukocytes (Fig. 4.1). In rodent systems in vitro, T cell clones can be functionally divided into those of the T helper 1 (Th_1) phenotype, which preferentially secrete IL-2, IFNγ and TNFα and stimulate cell mediated immune reactions, and the Th_2 phenotype which preferentially secrete IL-4, IL-6, IL-10, IL-13 and facilitate antibody synthesis.[37] In humans such a functional distinction is less clear cut and T cells often exhibit a Th_0 cytokine response, releasing both Th_1 and Th_2 cytokines. However the observations that T cells which induce EAE belong to the Th_1 phenotype suggests that IL-2, IFNγ and TNFα may be of particular relevance to proinflammatory events. This is further supported by the observation that the capacity of T cell clones to induce EAE has been correlated with the ability to produce TNFα following antigen or superantigen activation.[27,38] Intrathecal IL-2 and sIL-2R levels have been correlated with BBB impairment during MS,[33] which is probably reflective of leukocyte activation and the cytokine cascade (see other chapters).

IFNγ producing cells, particularly in response to myelin antigens, are concentrated in the CSF of MS patients[20] and the increased capacity to produce IFNγ following mitogenic stimulation in vitro may precede exacerbations.[39] This, coupled with the observation that treatment of MS patients with IFNγ induces clinical relapse, indicates that this is an important proinflammatory cytokine in MS.[40] IFNγ activates monocytes, macrophages and resident CNS-glial cells to produce additional cytokines including TNFα, IL-1 and IL-6 which may in turn upregulate the production of additional cytokine products including M-CSF, GM-CSF and chemokines to form a cytokine milieu which may exhibit additional proinflammatory capabilities (Fig. 4.1). IFNγ is also a potent regulator of immunologically relevant surface antigens. IFNγ induces the upregulation of MHC class I and class II molecules on astrocytes, endothelia and microglia in vitro. Likewise TNFα can mediate the expression of MHC class I products on astrocytes, endothelial cells and oligodendrocytes and synergizes with IFNγ induced class II antigen expression on astrocytes.[17,41] This in turn could amplify the immune response by local antigen presentation and provide potential targets for CD4+ cytolytic and CD8+ cytotoxic cells. However, an important feature in the development of clinical disease is the recruitment of additional mononuclear cells into the CNS. This is facilitated by the upregulation of vascular adhesion molecules. IL-1, IFNγ and TNFα induce the upregulation of intracellular adhesion molecule (ICAM-1) on CNS endothelium, and also in some instances on astrocytes. IFNγ and TNFα are also known to induce the upregulation of vascular cell adhesion molecule 1 (VCAM-1) on CNS endothelia which is an important ligand for T cell extravasation into the CNS.[5,42] Whilst injection of IL-1 into the CNS parenchyma may have some minimal effect on CNS leukocyte recruitment, injection of TNFα or IFNγ can induce BBB dysfunction and leukocyte recruitment in experimental animals.[43,44] Neutralization of IL-1 activity has inhibited the development of EAE.[45] Likewise neutralization of IFNγ after the adoptive transfer of myelin-reactive cells has also been reported to inhibit EAE. This was attributed to the inhibition of upregulation of VCAM-1, but not ICAM-1 preventing the secondary recruitment of cells and further supports the particular importance of VCAM-1 in CNS autoimmune inflammation.[46] However a number of reports in EAE have clearly indicated that IFNγ may have regulatory effects.[29,47-49] Lesions in MS are almost exclusively mononuclear in composition and early lesions in MS and EAE contain many macrophages and CD4+ memory/primed (CD45RO+), whereas the cells within the circulation contain a higher frequency of naive CD45RA+ cells.[50] While this may to some extent be reflective of increased adhesion molecules on these cells, chemotactic cytokines including MCP, MIP-1, IP-10 and RANTES (see other chapters) are now being identified in EAE and MS (Table 4.1) which will serve to recruit and retain certain inflammatory phenotypes within the CNS enviroment.[7,13,15] Although the functional significance of the expression of these molecules within the CNS requires further elucidation a preliminary report suggests that neutralization of macrophage inflammatory protein-1 alpha (MIP-1α) can inhibit the development of clinical EAE.[51]

ROLE OF TNFα AS AN IMPORTANT PATHOGENIC MEDIATOR OF CELLULAR RECRUITMENT

TNFα is an important mediator in the pathogenesis of autoimmune disease both by direct receptor-ligand interactions and by the triggering of secondary mediators, including IL-1, CSF and IL-6 (see other chapters). In addition to definitive evidence in EAE, there is increasing circumstantial evidence to suggest that TNFα also plays an important role in the pathogenesis of MS. Elevated levels of TNFα have been detected both in the sera and CSF of some RRMS and CPMS patients compared with normal and noninflammatory neurological disease controls.[17,52-54] The CSF levels of TNFα have most notably been correlated with clinical disease activity and were associated with BBB dysfunction.[54,55] During TNFα activation extracellular domains of the TNF-receptors (TNF-R) are proteolytically cleaved to produce soluble receptor. Increased sTNFR-1 and sTNFR-2 have been detected in MS patients. sTNFR-1 have been reported to correlate with TNF production within the CSF and may also correlate with disease activity.[56] T cell clones derived from MS patients produce large amounts of TNFα, and the observation that these were significantly more prevalent in the CSF than the blood[54] further indicates that a major source of TNFα activity occurs in the CNS. In addition to leukocyte TNFα production, TNFα can be synthesized in the CNS by neurons, astrocytes and microglia. In all areas of acute and chronic active MS lesions TNFα is associated with astrocytes and macrophages. Lymphotoxin (LT) is additionally produced by infiltrating T cells and microglia within MS lesions. Similar expression of TNFα is observed within EAE lesions,[58] where further in vivo evidence of the pathogenic nature of TNFα has been established. Injection of TNFα directly into the CNS parenchyma can induce inflammatory lesions, edema and cerebrospinal fluid leukocytosis typical of MS and EAE.[44] In animals containing primed myelin-specific T lymphocytes such TNFα injection serves to exacerbate EAE.[59] The importance of TNFα in the pathogenesis of disease has been implicated by direct inhibition of TNFα activity using specific monoclonal antibodies (Fig. 4.2) and sTNFR-1 and sTNFR-2.[46,58,60] Neutralization of TNFα activity has been associated with the inhibition of effector cell function and a major activity appears to be the prevention of recruitment of inflammatory cells along the neuroaxis due to inhibition of ICAM-1, and VCAM-1 upregulation.[46] Furthermore neutralization of TNFα activity within the CNS exhibits significantly improved effect compared to systemic neutralization and underscores the importance of locally produced cytokines (Fig. 4.2) which are not only involved in cellular recruitment but also myelin pathology.

CYTOKINES IN MYELIN PATHOLOGY

Although the initiation of the inflammatory response is related to T cell function, myelin pathology is a result of synergy between different mononuclear cell subsets. The macrophage plays a major role in effector function by receptor mediated phagocytosis (Fig. 4.1). Demyelination in EAE may be mediated by myelin-specific antibodies either by direct complement-mediated lysis or antibody dependent cellular cytotoxicity (Fig. 4.1). The Th$_2$ cytokines including IL-4, IL-6, IL-10 and IL-13 are involved in B cell proliferation, differentiation and immunoglobulin class switching (see other chapters). Later stages of relapsing demyelinating EAE are associated with increased B cell activity. IL-4 can induce class switching from IgM to IgG, and can be detected in the CSF of MS patients, particularly following stimulation of CSF T cells with myelin antigens.[20] Likewise secretion of IL-6 has

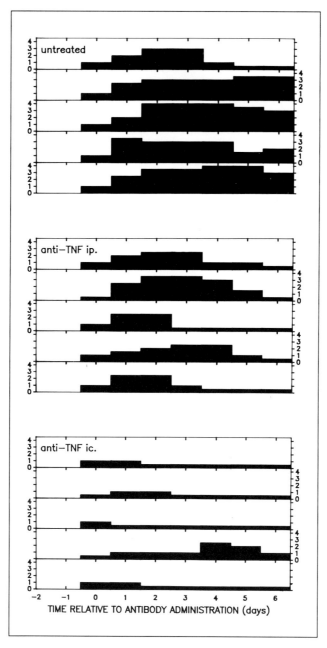

Fig. 4.2. Neutralization of TNF activity within the CNS inhibits the progression of EAE. The figure represents the clinical course of five individual animals per group which were either untreated or injected with 150 µg of TNF-neutralising antibody either directly into the CNS (intracerebrally; i.c.) or systemically (intraperitoneally; i.p.) at the onset (grade 1) of clinical disease. Animals also received saline either i.p. or i.c. respectively.[58] Y axis = clinical grade: 1 = limp tail, 2 = impaired righting reflex, 3 = partial paralysis, 4 = complete paralysis.

been reported to be more frequent in cultures of unstimulated monocytes from CPMS patients than in controls,[19] although other studies have shown no differences.[52,55] The CSF of MS patients contains elevated levels of immunoglobulin (Ig) and a well known feature of MS is the detection of oligoclonal immunoglobulin bands within the CSF. In some instances the CSF has been shown to contain myelin-specific antibodies. However the in vivo function of cytokines in antibody development in MS must be speculated from their in vitro biology (see other chapters).

In addition to increased levels of IL-4 producing cells, IFNγ producing T cells are elevated within the CNS of MS patients, particularly when stimulated with myelin antigens.[20] IFNγ is a potent activator of macrophages and microglia which induces the production of additional cytokines into the local microenvironment. M-CSF and GM-CSF can be produced by cytokine-activated astrocytes and may be involved in myeloid cell differentiation and activation (see other chapters). GM-CSF has been reported to be elevated in the CSF during clinical relapse.[62] Activation of macrophages induces upregulation of Fc and complement receptors, phagocytic capacity, the production of TNFα, nitric oxide, reactive oxygen species and proteases[63] which may lead to myelin damage (Fig. 4.1). For example, matrix metalloprotease (MMP) production is induced in macrophages and other cell types by IL-1 and TNFα, whereas LT and IL-6 induce the production of their natural inhibitors α2-macroglobulin and the TIMPs (tissue inhibitors of matrix metalloproteases).[64] The MMPs play an important role in the pathogenesis of inflammatory demyelinating CNS disease as is demonstrated by their presence in CSF and lesions in both MS and EAE,[65-67] their ability to degrade type IV collagen in the basement membrane surrounding the capillaries as well as myelin basic protein, and the fact that EAE can be reversed by administration of a specific MMP inhibitor.[68] Soluble TNFα and particularly LT are cytotoxic for oligodendrocytes and myelin sheaths in vitro.[69-71] Microglia also produce a membrane-bound form of TNFα which could be involved in myelin attack. Furthermore in vivo injection of TNFα into the CNS can induce demyelination.[72] Clinical experiments in MS patients using bothdepleting CD4 and CD52-specific monoclonal antibodies have induced a transient deterioration in MS patients, particularly in relation to reactivating previous neurological dysfunction.[73,74] These have been associated with an increase in serum TNFα levels suggesting that TNFα may induce conduction block in previously demyelinated axons, possibly by vasogenic edema. This indirect evidence suggests that TNFα may exhibit a pathogenic in vivo role in MS.[73,74] Although acute lesions are associated with the recruitment of T cell receptor α, β+ T cells, chronic lesions contain numerous T cell receptor γ, δ+ T cells. IL-1 may induce the expression of heat shock proteins on oligodendrocytes. These may act as recognition elements for T cell receptor γ, δ+ T cells, which have been shown to be lytic to oligodendroglia and thus may contribute to the demyelinating process.[75]

Furthermore TNFα, IL-1 and IL-6 can also induce astrocyte proliferation in vitro and may contribute to the gliotic process.[72,76] IL-6 has been detected in the CSF of MS patients in a few studies and is present in the CNS of animals with EAE.[10,49] This may serve to inhibit local IL-1 and TNFα production and in some instances ameliorates EAE.[49a,49b] Although IL-6 can be detected in both MS and EAE lesions in infiltrating mononuclear cells and microglia, the major source at least in EAE, may be from reactive astrocytes (D.B. unpublished. Fig. 4.3). IL-6 may thus function in an autocrine growth pathway for the development of the gliotic lesion.

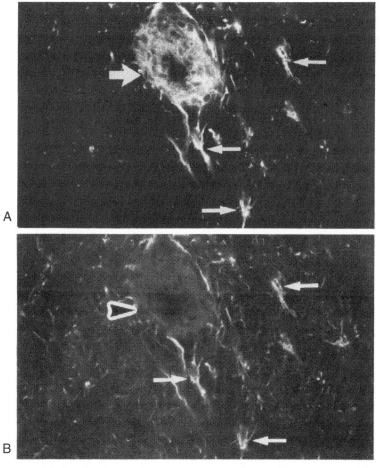

Fig. 4.3. Interleukin-6 activity in reactive astrocytes during EAE. Double immunofluorescence staining of IL-6 (A) and glial acid fibrillary protein positive astrocytes (B) during relapse phase EAE in the mouse. While mononuclear cells within the perivascular cuff (➜) may express IL-6, within the CNS parenchyma astrocytes (→) are the major source of IL-6.

CYTOKINE INDUCED REGULATION OF DISEASE

Although current data indicate an important pathogenic role for TNFα, the production of this and other cytokines activates the production of soluble receptors, which have the capacity to regulate cytokine action, and trigger natural feed-back loops. Intravenous administration of TNFα or IL-1 results in increased plasma levels of corticotrophin.[77] Systemic administration of steroids which can suppress TNFα and other leukocyte activities is well known to induce clinical improvement in MS and EAE. Glucocorticoid responses may serve to induce the development of Th$_2$ immunoregulatory responses[78] which are suggested from mRNA cytokine profiles extracted from the CNS during disease development. Cytokine expression is developmentally regulated during lesion formation whilst LT, IL-12, IL-1, IL-6, IFNγ, IL-2, and IL-4 mRNA detection can be correlated with the onset, influx of mononuclear cells and development of clinical EAE. Remission has been associated with the production of TGFβ and IL-10 mRNA.[12,13,79] Likewise periods of stabilization of MS have been reported to correlate with an increased capacity to produce TGFβ and IL-10.[55] This suggests the possible down regulation of disease-inducing Th$_1$ responses by Th$_2$ cytokines. A clinical trial administering IFNγ subcutaneously was ceased as it seemed to cause relapses in MS patients, indicating that it was disease promoting at least in these pharmacological doses.[40] Although subcutaneous administration of IFNγ may also exhibit adjuvant activity in rodents, in marked contrast to that suggested in MS, both systemic and intraventricular administration of IFNγ can inhibit EAE.[47,48] Furthermore systemic IFNγ neutralization increases susceptibility to EAE and exacerbates disease.[29,47,48] This effect may have been mediated by inhibiting the generation and function of effector cells within the periphery. Alternatively this could point to a fundamental difference between the animal model and the human disease. However, the effects of cytokines are complex and dose-dependent and the critical determinant for IFNγ induced enhancement or suppression could be due to timing of cytokine/antibody administration relative to disease induction and expression.[80]

Whilst IL-4 mRNA expression from cells within the CNS during EAE does not appear to correlate with clinical recovery during the normal course of EAE,[12,13,79] other recent studies have suggested that it is possible for IL-4 administered in vivo to inhibit myelin-specific Th$_1$ T cells from inducing EAE.[81] Likewise it has been suggested that when IL-4 neutralizing antibodies were administered during sensitization the clinical signs expressed were elevated compared to controls.[82] These data suggest that IL-4 may exhibit some regulatory capabilities, at least during early T cell development and activation within the periphery. IL-4 producing cells have readily been detected within the CSF of MS patients, particularly when stimulated with antigen.[20] Recently IL-13, which shares many functions with IL-4, has also been shown to inhibit EAE.[83] In addition to IL-4 and IL-13, IL-10 can exhibit marked inhibitory action on the production of Th$_1$-like cytokines, particularly by inhibiting macrophage function (see other chapters). Interleukin-10 producing cells have been detected in the CSF and blood of MS patients and have been associated with astrocytes and perivascular cells in MS lesions.[5,84] Assessment of the in vivo function of IL-10 in neuroimmunological disease is in its early stages but reports suggest that it may either inhibit,[85] have minimal effect[49] or enhance[86] the development of EAE. This suggests that while there may possibly be a balance between Th$_1$ and Th$_2$ cytokines, at least in EAE, as demonstrated with IFNγ, there is a complex relationship between the different cytokines which can either exert proinflammatory or anti-inflammatory roles dependent on the relevant microenvironment within which they are acting.

Experimental data to date has more consistently suggested that TNFα exhibits a major proinflammatory function within neuroimmunological disease, whereas transforming growth factor β has most consistently downregulated disease. Immunocytochemically TGFβ1 and TGFβ2 have been detected in leukocytes and within the perivascular matrix in EAE and MS and can be produced in vitro by glial cells.[3,5,16] TGFβ is reported to be upregulated in animals showing clinical resolution,[78] and disease regression during MS has been associated with the production of TGFβ.[18,55] Both TGFβ1 and TGFβ2 have been shown to inhibit the development of EAE, exacerbate disease and also induce relapse following TGFβ neutralization.[16,87,88] This serves to suggest that TGFβ forms an integral part of the normal regulatory process. TGFβ serves to inhibit proinflammatory mononuclear cell responses, endothelial cell function and cytokine-induced astrocyte proliferation and in many respects serves to antagonize the proinflammatory effects of TNFα. Upon culture of MS peripheral blood lymphocytes it has been suggested that the production of active forms of TGFβ decreased below normal levels during exacerbation of clinical disease. However, this may be secondary due to a lower frequency of TGFβ producing CD8+, CD45RA+ cells within the blood of MS patients.[18] Significantly elevated numbers of IFNγ, IL-4 and TGFβ mRNA expressing cells have been detected in the blood and CSF of MS patients compared with controls.[20] The potential therapeutic role of TGFβ in MS is currently being evaluated in pilot clinical trials.

INHIBITION OF THE PROGRESSION OF MULTIPLE SCLEROSIS WITH INTERFERONS

Clinical relapses in MS patients can often be associated with antecedent viral infections, e.g., upper respiratory tract infections.[27] This observation and the idea that MS could be initiated by some as yet unidentified virus prompted the establishment of clinical trials using interferons in MS. As has already been mentioned, the trial with IFNγ was terminated due to the rapid, unexpected deterioration of some patients. In contrast a number of clinical trials involving type I (α/β) interferons have been undertaken. The systemic administration of IFNα in MS patients has been studied in three major trials[89-91] which have suggested neither significant benefit or activation of disease. Intrathecal IFNβ showed beneficial effects in patients with RRMS in an initial placebo-controlled trial.[92] However, the relapse rate was increased compared with placebo in a more recent study administering intrathecal IFNβ, which also included patients with CPMS.[93] Nevertheless these trials suggested a potential role for IFNβ in the treatment of MS. Recently major clinical trials involving over 600 patients have been completed.[94-96] These have indicated that either the systemic administration of IFNβ1a or IFNβ1b can result in a modest, dose-dependent reduction in the exacerbation rate in RRMS patients (Fig. 4.4). Although the rate of relapse frequency was reduced by only 30-40%, this difference was highly significant compared to the placebo group, and is the first treatment to have shown a beneficial effect of this magnitude in MS. However, it was the significant reduction in the number of gadolinium-enhanced, MRI-detected CNS lesions by an impressive 50-70%[95] that prompted approval and widespread use of these interferons as a specific MS therapy. The significance of these MRI findings for the long-term evolution of the clinical disease remains to be proven. Experimentally type I interferon (IFNα/β) has been reported to exhibit a inhibitory effect on the development of EAE.[47] However it is not clear if IFNβ is involved in the natural regulatory processes occurring during neuroimmunological disease and its mechanisms of action are unknown. It seems that the positive effect of IFNβ on the course of MS is not attributable to a direct effect on viral infections,[97] but may influence immune responsiveness to such stimuli by inhibiting monocyte and T cell activation including IFNγ, TNFα and lymphotoxin production, or by upregulation of TGF-β or IL-10.[98,99] Nevertheless these data show that cytokine therapy can make a significant impact on disease development.

CONCLUSIONS

In the absence of definitive clinical trials, the implication of cytokines within any inflammatory or regulatory role in MS must be hypothesized from circumstantial evidence. Cytokine analysis of body fluids from MS patients clearly indicates that there are abnormalities in immune function during the course of MS and points to the CNS as the major site and target of the immune response. However even if the results obtained by many authors infer the diagnostic and prognostic capabilities of some cytokine, none as yet appear to have diagnostic or prognostic value with our current detection systems and understanding of the disease process.

The effects of cytokine interactions may be subtle and are highly complex. Although the in vitro analysis of cytokine function with cells

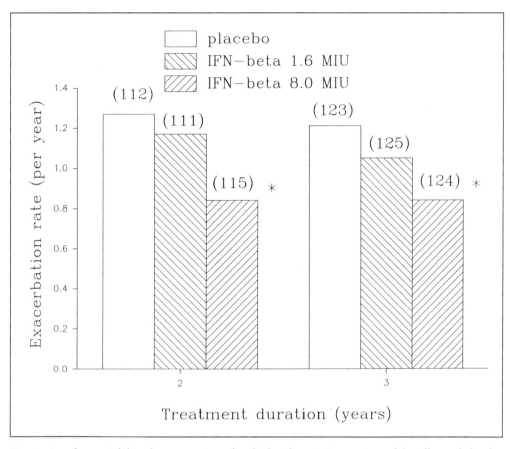

Fig. 4.4. Interferon-β inhibits the progression of multiple sclerosis. Comparison of the effects of placebo and interferon β-1b, 1.6 or 8 million international units (MIU), given intramuscularly every second day on exacerbations of multiple sclerosis. The number of patients being assessed at each time point is indicated in parentheses. A significant (*p<0.0001) dose-dependent inhibition was observed compared with placebo.[94]

of the CNS may provide indications of potential in vivo activity this may not necessarily reflect what is actually occurring during the disease process in vivo. IFNγ can induce the upregulation of MHC class II on endothelia, astrocytes and microglia in vitro. While IFNγ and TNFα may synergize to upregulate class II antigen expression on astrocytes, TNFα inhibits IFNγ induced class II expression by cerebral endothelia.[41] However, during both MS and EAE, both endothelial cells and astrocytes fail typically to express MHC class II antigens which are present mainly on activated microglia and infiltrating macrophages.[100,101] This serves to indicate further the complex relationship of the cytokine cascade. The balance of pro- or anti-inflammatory cytokine effects is therefore likely to determine the net outcome. It is also likely that the actual function induced will be dependent on the stage of development of the immune response and the location of interacting cells, either in the circulation or tissue. Furthermore, function will depend on the current local microenvironment produced by cytokine secretion, adjacent leukocytes expressing appropriate receptors and the nature of cell-cell contact which provides the interface for local cytokine action.

Nevertheless, as has been demonstrated in rheumatoid arthritis (see other chapters), there may be a hierarchy of cytokines involved in pro- and anti-inflammatory events. Tumor necrosis factor appears to play a pivotal role in the immunopathological events and may provide a target for immunotherapy. Novel anticytokine strategies, such as synthetic low molecular weight TNF-convertase inhibitors, may offer new therapeutic approaches for MS.[102,103] The recent studies with interferon β have shown that it is possible to manipulate the cytokine cascade with beneficial effect in multiple sclerosis. Once the immune system can be effectively regulated, the use of transplantation of oligodendrocyte precursors and cytokine modulating therapy to induce remyelination may then be of value in repairing the tissue damage induced by the disease process.

References

1. Steinman L. Autoimmune disease. Sci Am 1993; 269:74-82.
2. Brocke S, Gibjels K, Steinman S. Experimental autoimmune encephalomyelitis in the mouse. In: IR Cohen, A Miller, eds. Autoimmune disease models: a guidebook. Orlando, FL: Academic Press Inc, 1994:1-14.
3. Woodroofe MN, Cuzner ML. Cytokine mRNA expression in inflammatory multiple sclerosis lesions:Detection by non-radioactive in situ hybridization. Cytokine 1993; 5:583-588.
4. Correale J, Gilmore W, McMillan M et al. Patterns of cytokine secretion by autoreactive proteolipid protein specific T cell clones during the course of multiple sclerosis. J Immunol 1995; 154:2959-2968.
5. Cannella B, Raine CS. The adhesion molecule and cytokine profile of multiple sclerosis lesions. Ann Neurol 1995; 37:424-435.
6. Rieckmann P, Albrecht M, Ehrenreich H et al. Semi-quantitative analysis of cytokine gene expression in blood and cerebrospinal fluid cells by reverse transcriptase polymerase chain reaction. Res Exp Med 1995: 195:17-29.
7. Hvas J, Sindling JR, Oksenberg JR et al. Expression of the cytokine RANTES in multiple sclerosis lesions. J Neuroimmunol 1994; 54:169.
8. Baker D, O'Neill JK, Turk JL. Cytokines in the central nervous system of mice during chronic relapsing experimental allergic encephalomyelitis. Cell Immunol 1991; 134:505-510.
9. Merrill JE, Kono DH, Clayton J et al. Inflammatory leukocytes and cytokines in the peptide-induced disease of experimental allergic encephalomyelitis in SJL and B10.PL mice. Proc Natl Acad Sci USA 1992; 89:574-578.

10. Gijbels K, Van Damme J, Proost P et al. Interleukin 6 production in the central nervous system during experimental autoimmune encephalomyelitis. Eur J Immunol 1990; 20:233-235.
11. Khoury SJ, Hancock WW, Weiner HL. Oral tolerance to myelin basic protein and natural recovery from experimental autoimmune encephalomyelitis are associated with downregulation of inflammatory cytokines and differential upregulation of transforming growth factor beta, interleukin 4, and prostaglandin E expression in the brain. J Exp Med 1992; 176:1355-1364.
12. Kennedy MK, Torrance DS, Picha KS et al. Analysis of cytokine mRNA expression in the central nervous system of mice with experimental autoimmune encephalomyelitis reveals that IL-10 mRNA expression correlates with recovery. J Immunol 1992; 149:2496-2505.
13. Issazadeh S, Ljungdahl A, Hojeberg B et al. Dynamics of cellular cytokine mRNA expression in the central nervous syetm during experimental autoimmune encephalomyelitis in Lewis rats. J Neuroimmunol 1994; 54:187.
14. Hulkower K, Brosnan CF, Aquino DA et al. Expression of CSF-1, c-fms and MCP-1 in the central nervous system of rats with experimental allergic encephalomyelitis. J Immunol 1993; 150:2525-2533.
15. Godiska R, Chantry D, Dietsch GN et al. Chemokine expression in murine experimental allergic encephalomyelitis. J Neuroimmunol 1995; 58:167-176.
16. Racke MK, Sriram S, Carlino J et al. Long term treatment of chronic relapsing experimental allergic encephalomyelitis by transforming growth factor β2. J Neuroimmunol 1993; 46:175-184.
17. Carrieri PB. The role of cytokines in the pathogeneis of multiple sclerosis. Int MSJ 1994; 1:53-59.
18. Mokhtarian F, Shi Y, Shirazian D et al. Defective production of anti-inflammatory cytokine, TGF-β by T cell lines of patients with active multiple sclerosis. J. Immunol 1994; 152:6003-6010.
19. Maimone D, Reder AT, Gregory S. T cell lymphokine-induced secretion of cytokines by monocytes from patients with multiple sclerosis. Cell Immunol 1993; 146:96-106.
20. Link J, Soderstrom M, Olsson T et al. Increased transforming growth factor-beta, interleukin-4, and interferon-γ in multiple sclerosis. Annals Neurol 1994; 36:379-386.
21. Kermode AG, Thompson AJ, Tofts P et al. Breakdown of the blood brain barrier precedes symptoms and other MRI signs of new lesions in multiple sclerosis. Pathogenic and clinical implications. Brain 1990; 113:1477-1489.
22. Harris JO, Frank JA, Patronas N et al. Serial gadolinium-enhanced magnetic resonance imaging scans in patients with early, relapsing-remitting multiple sclerosis: Implications for clinical trials and natural history. Ann Neurol 1991; 29:548-555.
23. Wucherpfennig KW, Newcombe J, Li H et al. T cell receptor Vα-Vβ repertoire and cytokine gene expression in active multiple sclerosis lesions. J Exp Med 1992; 175:993-1002.

24. Ebers G, Sadovnick AD. The role of genetic factors in multiple sclerosis susceptibility. J Neuroimmunol 1994; 54;1-17.
25. Chung IY, Norris JG, Benveniste EN. Differential tumor necrosis factor alpha expression by astrocytes from experimental allergic encephalomyelitis-susceptible and -resistant rat strains. J Exp Med 1991; 173:801-811.
26. Baker D, Rosenwasser OA, Simpson E et al. Genetic analysis of experimental autoimmune encephalomyelitis in mice. J. Neuroimmunol 1994; 54:150.
27. Brocke S, Veromaa T, Weissman IL et al. Infection and multiple sclerosis: A possible role of superantigens? Trends Microbio 1994; 2:250-254.
28. Wekerle H, Linnington C, Lassman H et al. Cellular immune reactivity within the CNS. Trens Neurosci 1986; 9:271-277.
29. Duong TT, St. Louis J, Gilbert J et al. Effect of anti-interferon γ and anti-interleukin-2 monoclonal antibody treatment on the development of actively and passively induced experimental allergic encephalomyeltis in the SJL/J mouse. J Neuroimmunol 1992; 35:105.
30. Zhoa ML, Xia JQ, Fritz RB. Interleukin 3 and encephalitogenic activity of SJL/J myelin basic protein-specific T cell lines. J Neuroimmunol 1993; 43:69-78.
31. Leonard JP, Waldburger KE, Goldman SJ. Prevention of experimental autoimmune encephalomyelitis by antibodies against interleukin 12. J Exp Med 1995; 181:381-386.
32. Adachi K, Kumamoto T, Araki S. Elevated sIL-2R in patients with active multiple sclerosis. Ann Neurol 1990; 28:687-691.
33. Sharief MK, Hentges R, Ciardi M et al. In vivo relationship of interleukin-2 and soluble IL-2 receptor to blood-brain barrier impairment in patients with active multiple sclerosis. J Neurol 1993; 240:46-50.
34. Trotter JL, Collins KG, Van der Veen RC. Serum cytokine levels in chronic progressive multiple sclerosis: Interleukin-2 levels parallel tumor necrosis factor-α levels. J Neuroimmunol 1991; 33:29-36.
35. Gallo P, Piccinno MG, Tavolato B et al. A longitudinal study on IL-2, sIL-2R, IL-4 and gamma IFNγ in multiple sclerosis CSF and serum. J Neurol Sci 1991; 101:227-232.
36. Zhang J, Markovic-Plese S, Lacet et al. Increased frequency of interleukin 2 responsive T cells specific for myelin basic protein and proteolipid protein in the peripheral blood and cerebrospinal fluid of patients with multiple sclerosis. J Exp Med 1994; 179:973-984.
37. Mosmann TR, Coffman RL. Th_1 and Th_2 cells: different patterns of lymphocyte secretion lead to different functional proterties. Ann Rev Immunol 1988; 7:145-173.
38. Powell MB, Mitchell D, Lederman J et al. Lymphotoxin and tumor necrosis factor-α production by myelin basic protein specific T cell clones correlates with encephalitogenicity. Int Immunol 1990; 2:539-544.
39. Beck J, Rondot P, Catinot L et al. Increased production of interferon γ and tumor necrosis factor precedes clinical manifestation in multiple sclerosis: D cytokines trigger off exacerbations? Acta Neurol Scand 1988; 78:318-323.

40. Panitch HS, Hirrsch RL, Haley AS et al. Exacerbations of multiple sclerosis in patients treated with interferon γ. Lancet 1987; 1:893-895.
41. Tanaka M, McCarron RM. The inhibitory effect of tumor necrosis factor and interleukin-1 on Ia induction by interferon γ on endothelial cells from murine central nervous system microvessels. J Neuroimmunol 1990; 27:209-215.
42. Yednock TA, Cannon C, Fritz LC et al. Prevention of experimental autoimmune encephalomyelitis by antibodies against α4β1 integrin. Nature 1992; 356:63-66.
43. Andersson PB, Perry VH, Gordon S. Intracerebral injection of pro-inflammator cytokines or leukocyte chemotaxins induces minimal myelomonocytic cell recruitment to the parenchyma of the central nervous system. J Exp Med 1992; 176:255-259.
44. Simmons RD, Willenborg DO. Direct injection of cytokines into the spinal cord causes autoimmune encephalomyelitis-like inflammation. J Neurol Sci 1990; 100:37-42.
45. Jacobs CA, Baker PE, Roux ER et al. Experimental autoimmune encephalomyelitis is exacerbated by IL-1α and suppressed by soluble IL-1 receptor J. Immunol 1991; 146:2983-2989.
46. Barten DM, Nuddle NH. Vascular cell adhesion molecule-1 modulation by tumor necrosis factor in experimental allergic encephalomyelitis. J Neuroimmunl 1994; 51:123-133.
47. Billiau AH, Heremans H, Vandekerckhove et al. Enhancement of experimental allergic encephalomyelitis in mice by antibodies against IFNγ. J Immunol 1988; 140:1506-15010.
48. Voorrthuis JAC, Uitdehaag BMJ, De Groot CJA et al. Suppression of experimental allergic encephalomyelitis by intraventricular administration of interferon γ in Lewis rats. Clin Exp Immunol 1990; 81:183-188.
49a. Willenborg DO, Fordham SA, Cowden WB et al. Cytokines and murine autoimmune encephalomyelitis: Inhibition or enhancement of disease with antibodies to select cytokines, or by delivery of exogenous cytokines using a recombinant vaccinia virus system. Scand J Immunol 1995; 41:31-41.
49b. Gijbels K, Brocke S, Abrams JS, Steinman L. Administration of neutralizing antibodies to interleukin-6 (IL-6) reduces experimental autoimmune encephalomyelitis and is associated with elevated levels of IL-6 bioactivity in central nervous system and circulation. Mol Med 1995; in press.
50. Hafler DA, Weiner HL. Multiple Sclerosis: a CNS and systemic disease. Immunol Today 1989; 9:195-199.
51. Karpus WJ, Lukacs NW, McRae BL. Prevention and treatment of PLP-peptide induced EAE by anti-MIP-1α administration. J Neuroimmunol 1994; 54:171.
52. Hauser SL, Doolittle TH, Lincoln R et al. Cytokine accumulations in CSF of multiple sclerosis patients:Frequent detection of interleukin-1 and tumor necrosi factor but not interleukin-6. Neurology 1990; 40:1735-1739.
53. Benvenuto R, Paroli M, Buttinelli C et al. Tumour necrosis factor α synthesis by cerebrospinal fluid-derived T cell clones from patients with multiple sclerosis. Clin Exp Immunol. 1991; 84:97-102.

54. Sharief MK, Thompson EJ. In vivo relationship of tumor necrosis factor-to blood-brain barrier damage in patients with active multiple sclerosis. J Neuroimmunol 1992; 38:27-34.
55. Rieckmann P, Albrecht M, Kitze B et al. Tumor necrosis factor α messenger RNA expression in patients with relapsing remitting multiple sclerosis is associated with disease activity. Ann Neurol 1995; 37:82-88.
56. Matsuda M, Tsukada N, Miyagi K et al. Increased levels of soluble tumor necrosis factor receptor in patients with multiple sclerosis and HTLV-1-associated myelopathy. J Neuroimmunol 1994; 52:33-40.
57. Selmaj K, Raine CS, Cannella B et al. Identification of lymphotoxin and tumor necrosis factor in multiple sclerosis lesions. J Clin Invest 1991; 87:949-954.
58. Baker D, Butler D, Scallon BJ et al. Control of established allergic encephalomyelitis by inhibition of tumor necrosis factor (TNF) activity within the central nervous system using monoclonal antibodies and TNF receptor-immunoglobulin fusion proteins. Eur J Immunol 1994; 24:2040-2048.
59. Kuroda Y, Shimamoto Y. Human tumor necrosis factor-α augments experimental allergic encephalomyeltis in rats. J Neuroimmunol 1991; 34:159-164.
60. Ruddle NH, Bergman CM, McGrath KM et al. An antibody to lymphotoxin and tumor necrosis factor prevents transfer of experimental allergic encephalomyelitis. J Exp Med 1990; 172:1193-2000.
61. Nitta T, Sato K, Allogretta M et al. Expression of granulocyte colony stimulating factor and granulocyte macrophage colony stimulating factor in human astrocytoma cell lines and glioma specimens. Brain Res 1992; 571:19-29.
62. Perrella O, Carrieri PB, De Mercato R et al. Markers of activated T-lymphocytes and T cell receptor gamma delta+ in patients with MS. Eur Neurol 1993; 33:152-155.
63. MacMicking JD, Willenborg DO, Weidemann MJ et al. Elevated secretion of reactive nitrogen and oxygen intermediates by inflammatory leukocytes in hyperacute experimental autoimmune encephalomyelitis: Enhancement by the soluble products of encephalitogenic T cells. J Exp Med 1992; 176:303-307.
64. Krane SM. Clinical importance of metalloproteinases and their inhibitors. Ann NY Acad Sci 1994; 732:1-10.
65. Gijbels K, Masure S, Carton H et al. Gelatinase in the cerebrospinal fluid of patients with multiple sclerosis and other inflammatory neurological disorders. J Neuroimmunol 1992; 41:29-34.
66. Gijbels K, Proost P, Masure S et al. Gelatinase B is present in the cerebrospinal fluid during experimental autoimmune encephalomyelitis and cleaves myelin basic protein. J Neurosci Res 1993; 36:432-440.
67. Gijbels K, Steinman L. Gelatinase B producing cells in multiple sclerosis lesions. J Cell Biochem 1994; Suppl 18D:143.

68. Gijbels K, Galardy RE, Steinman L. Reversal of experimental autoimmune encephalomyelitis with a hydroxamate inhibitor of matrix metalloproteases. J Clin Invest 1994; 94:2177-2182.
69. Robbins DS, Shirazi Y, Drysdale BE et al. Production of cytotoxic factor for oligodendrocytes by stimulated astrocytes. J Immunol 1987; 139:2593-2597.
70. Selmaj K, Raine CS. Tumor necrosis factor mediates myelin and oligodendrocyte damage in vitro. Ann Neurol 1988; 23:339-346.
71. Selmaj K, Raine CS, Cannella B et al. Cytokine cytotoxicity against oligodendrocytes. Apoptosis induced by lymphotoxin. J Immunol 1991; 147:1522-1529.
72. Butt AM, Jenkins HG. Morphological changes in oligodendrocytes in the intact mouse optic nerve following intravitreal injection of tumour necrosis factor. J Neuroimmunol 1994; 51:27-33.
73. Racadott E, Herve P, Wijdenes J. Treatment of multiple sclerosis with anti-CD4 monoclonal antibody. A preliminary report on B-F5 in 21 patients. J Autoimmun 1993:6:771-786.
74. Compston A. Future prospects for the management of multiple sclerosis. Annal Neurol Suppl 1 1994; 36:S146-S150.
75. D'Souza SD, Antel JP, Freedman MS. Cytokine induction of heat shock protein expression in human oligodendrocytes: An interleukin-1-mediated mechanism. J Neuroimmunol 1994; 50:17-24.
76. Selmaj KW, Farooq M, Norton WT et al. Proliferation of astrocytes in vitro in response to cytokines. A primary role for tumor necrosis factor. J Immunol 1990; 144:129-135.
77. Butler LD, Layman NK, Riedl PE et al. Neuroendocrine regulation of in vivo cytokine production and effects: I. In vivo regulatory networks involving the neuroendocrine system, interleukin-1 and tumor necrosis factor-α. J Neuroimmunol 1989; 24:143-153.
78. Mason DW. Genetic variation in the stress response: susceptibility to experimental allergic encephalomyelitis and implications for human inflammatory disease. Immunol Today 1992; 12:57-61.
79. Issazadeh S, Mustafa M, Ljungdahl A et al. Interferon γ, interleukin 4 and transforming growth factor β in experimental autoimmune encephalomyelitis in Lewis rats: Dynamics of cellular cytokine mRNA expression in the central nervous system and lymphoid cells. J Neurosci Res 1995; 40:579-590.
80. Jacob CO, Holoshitz J, van der Meide P et al. Heterogeneous effects of IFNγ in adjuvant arthritis. J Immunol 1989; 142:1500-1505.
81. Racke MK, Bonomo A, Scott DE et al. Cytokine-induced immune deviation as a therapy for inflammatory autoimmune disease. J Exp Med 1994; 180:1961-1966.
82. Van Der Veeen RC. Myelin specific Th$_2$ cells in EAE. J Neuroimmunol 1994; 54:202.
83. Cash E, Minty A, Ferrara P et al. Macrophage-inactivating IL-13 suppresses experimental autoimmune encephalomyelitis in rats. J Immunol 1994; 153:4258-4267.

84. Navikas V, Link J, Palasik W et al. Increased mRNA expression of IL-10 in mononuclear cells in multiple sclerosis and optic neuritis. Scand J Immunol 1995; 41:171-178.
85. Rott O, Fleischer B, Cash E. Interleukin-10 prevents experimental allergic encephalomyelitis in rats. Eur J Immunol 1994; 24:1434-1440.
86. Cannella B, Gao Y-L, Brosnan CF et al. IL-10 enhances experimental allergic encephalomyelitis. J Neuroimmunol 1994; 54:154.
87. Racke MK, Dhib-Jalbut S, Cannella B et al. Prevention and treatment of chronic relapsing experimental allergic encephalomyelitis by transforming growth factor-β1. J Immunol 1991; 146:3012-3017.
88. Santambrogio L, Hochwald GM, Saena B et al. Studies on the mechanisms by which transforming growth factor-beta (TGF-β) protects against allergic encephalomyelitis: Antagonism between TGF-β and tumor necrosis factor. J Immunol 1993; 151:1116-1127.
89. Knobler RL, Panitch HS, Braheeny SL. Controlled clinical trial of systemic interferon α in multiple sclerosis. Neurology 1984; 34:1273-1279.
90. Camenga DL, Johnson KP, Alter M et al. Systemic recombinant α-2 interferon therapy in relapsing multiple sclerosis. Arch Neurol 1986; 43:1239-1246.
91. AUSTIMS Research Group. Interferon-α and transfer factor in the treatment of multiple sclerosis: a double-blind, placebo controlled-trial. J Neurol Neurosurg Psychiatry 1989; 52:566-574.
92. Jacobs L, Salazar AM, Herndon R et al. Multicentre double blind-study of the effect of intrathecally administered natural human fibroblast interferon on exacerbations of multiple sclerosis Lancet 1986; 2:1411-1413.
93. Milanese C, Salmaggi A, La Mantia L et al. Double-blind study of intrathecal beta-interferon in multiple sclerosis: clinical and laboratory results. J Neurol Neurosurg Psychiatry 1990; 54:554-557.
94. IFNβ MS Study Group. Interferon beta-1b is effective in relapsing-remitting multiple sclerosis: I Clinical results of a multicentre, randomized, double blind, placebo-controlled trial. Neurology 1993; 43:655-661.
95. Paty DW, Li DKB, UBC MS/MRI Study Group et al. Interferon beta-1b is effective in relapsing-remitting multiple sclerosis: II MRI analysis results of a multicentre randomized, double-blind, placebo-controlled trial. Neurology 1993; 43:662-667.
96. Jacobs L, Cookfair D, Rudick R et al. Results of a phase III trial of IM recombinant interferon β as treatment for MS. J Neuroimmunol 1994; 54:170.
97. Panitch HS. Influence of infection on exacerbations of multiple sclerosis. Annal Neurol Suppl 1994; 36:S25-S28.
98. Arnason BGW, Reder AT. Interferons and multiple sclerosis. Clin Neuropharm 1994; 17:495-547.
99. Porrini AM, Gambi D and Reder AT. Stimulation of IL-10 secretion may be one mechanism of the therapeutic effect of recombinant human interferon β (rIFN β^{ser}) J Neuroimmunol 1994; 54:190.

100. Raine CS, Lee SC, Scheinberg LL et al. Adhesion molecules on endothelial cells in the central nervous system: an emerging area in the neuroimmunology of multiple sclerosis. Clin Immunol Immunopathol 1990; 57:173-187.
101. Butter C, O'Neill JK, Baker D et al. Immunoelectron microscopical study of the expression of class II major histocompatibility complex during experimental allergic encephalomyelitis in Biozzi AB/H mice. J Neuroimmunol 1991; 33:37-42.
102. Gearing AJH, Beckett P, Christodoulon M et al. Processing of tumour necrosis factor α precursor by metalloproteinases. Nature 1994; 370:555-557.
103. Sommer N, Loschmann PA, Northoff GH et al. The antidepressant rolipram suppresses cytokine production and prevents autoimmune encephalomyelitis. Nature Med 1995; 1:244-248.

CHAPTER 5

THE ROLE OF CYTOKINES IN THYROID HEALTH AND DISEASE

Beatrix Grubeck-Loebenstein

Cytokines are produced in the normal as well as in the diseased thyroid gland. In both conditions they have important regulatory functions. They mediate growth processes and are involved in the control of thyroid hormone production. A whole variety of different cytokines are produced by the inflammatory infiltrate typically present in thyroid autoimmune disorders. These cytokines are of major importance for the initiation and perpetuation of the immune response directed against thyroid tissue. It is the aim of this review to summarize what is known about the production and regulatory role of cytokines in the thyroid gland under different conditions. Special emphasis is given to studies performed in the human system. Data from animal systems are referred to for comparison. The review also includes a section on the special importance of cytokines in the development of Graves' ophthalmopathy, a condition frequently associated with thyroid autoimmune disease.

INTRODUCTION

Cytokines are involved in many biological functions and are major mediators of the immune response. They have been implicated also to play a role in autoimmune disease.[1] As the thyroid gland is frequently a target organ of autoimmune processes, the understanding of the production and effects of cytokines in thyroid health and disease is of interest. Although important information has been derived from animal models of thyroid autoimmune disease and from studies on animal cells, the vast majority of studies on the production and effects of cytokines in the thyroid gland published over the last couple of years has been performed in the human system. It is, therefore, the

---

Cytokines in Autoimmunity, edited by Fionula M. Brennan and Marc Feldmann.
© 1996 R.G. Landes Company.

increased in both disorders[4,5,17] and cytokines not detectable in normal thyroid tissue such as IL-1α and TNFα may be produced.[2,4,11] However, TEC from patients with GD do not differ from nonautoimmune cells when kept in tissue culture.[2] This suggests that cytokine production is not constitutively impaired in TEC in thyroid autoimmune disease, but may rather be the result of increased stimulation exerted by inflammatory factors produced by adjacent immune cells. This assumption is supported by the fact that IL-1α and TNFα are also produced by other types of epithelial cells such as keratinocytes or hepatocytes under inflammatory conditions such as psoriasis or hepatitis.[18,19] Cytokines may also stimulate the production of one another. IL-1 has for instance been shown to stimulate IL-6 and IL-8 production in TEC.[3,15]

TEC transformation may also lead to alterations in the spectrum and concentrations of cytokines produced. Thus, a whole variety of different cytokines such as IL-6, IL-1α, IL-8 and granulocyte colony stimulating factor (G-CSF) have been reported to be produced by thyroid carcinoma cells.[20-22] Cytokine production by transformed TEC may have functional consequences as suggested by the observation of a marked neutrophilia in a patient with anaplastic thyroid carcinoma positive for G-CSF production.[21]

TEC from nontoxic goiter, a benign thyroid enlargement, which endemically occurs in iodine deficient areas, also have an impaired cytokine production pattern. Although they contain normal concentrations of IL-6[2-5] and IL-8,[5,15] they characteristically have a deficient production of TGFβ1.[7] This defect may be related to a lack of iodine exposure in vivo, as iodide has been shown to increase TGFβ1 production in TEC in vitro.[7,8]

The importance of the presence of an inflammatory infiltrate for cytokine production by TEC has been pointed out above. It seems thus of interest to define which kind of cytokines are produced by inflammatory cells in different thyroid disorders. A great number of different studies performed over the last 10 years has indicated that a whole variety of different cytokines may be produced by mononuclear cells infiltrating the thyroid gland under inflammatory conditions (Table 5.2).[2,4,5,7,11,17,23-26] The quantities of cytokines produced seem to correlate well with the size of the respective inflammatory infiltrate, but do not seem to depend on its pathogenetic origin.[2,5,17,25,26] Thus, a similar spectrum of cytokines, although at different concentrations, has been observed in the thyroid tissues from patients with autoimmune disorders—GD and HT—and nontoxic goiter thyroids, for which small nonspecific inflammatory infiltrates are characteristic.[27] Whereas there is general agreement on the production of most cytokines listed in Table 5.2, TNFα, which is important in the pathogenesis of rheumatoid arthritis,[28] has been detected by some,[2,11] but not by other investigators.[12] The reason for this discrepancy is not yet understood.

Another finding deserves particular attention. Apart from a recent study in which relatively low concentrations of IL-4 message were detected in the thyroids of a few patients with HT and GD,[17] IL-4 has so far not been detected in the thyroid gland.[5] This seems particularly surprising, as GD is characteristically accompanied by autoantibody production, whereas hardly any tissue destruction is detectable.[29] Accordingly, an increased occurrence of Th$_2$ T cells would be expected in this condition. Studies were, therefore, performed to analyze cytokine production in T cell clones derived from the thyroids of patients with GD and HT. Not surprisingly, CD4+ and CD8+ clones from HT, a disorder which is characterized by tissue destruction, were Th$_1$ with a preferential secretion of IFNγ and TNFα [30-33] (Table 5.3). Clones from

Table 5.2. Cytokines produced by intrathyroidal lymphocytic infiltrates in thyroid diseases[1]

	CYTOKINES												
	IL-1α	IL-1β	IL-2	IL-4	IL-5	IL-6	IL-8	IL-10	IFNγ	TNFα°	LT	TGFβ	PDGF
Graves' disease	+	+	+	±	–	+	+	+	+	+	+	+	+
Hashimoto's thyroiditis	++	++	++	+	+	++	N.D.	++	++	+	++	N.D.	+
Nontoxic goiter	±	±	±	–	N.D.	+	±	+	±	±	±	±	±

±, positive in some cases; +, positive; ++, high production; N.D., not determined
[1]Cytokines never detected or not yet studied in the thyroid are not listed. Quantifications refer to values given in the majority of studies performed.
Data on Graves' disease and on nontoxic goiter from refs. 2,4,5,7,11,17,23-25; on Hashimoto's thyroiditis from refs. 2,4,11,17.
° TNFα production was found by some,[2,11] but not by others.[12]

Table 5.3. Cytokines produced by T cell lines and clones expanded from surgically removed thyroid tissue[1]

	CYTOKINES						
	IL-2	IFNγ	TNFα	LT	IL-4	IL-6	TGFβ
Graves' disease	+	+	+	+	±	+	+
Hashimoto's thyroiditis	+	++	++	+	±	±	+
Nontoxic goiter	+	+	+	+	N.D.	+	+

±, detected in a small minority of lines/clones; +, number of positive lines/clones comparable to control tissues; ++, high production in the majority of lines/clones; N.D., not determined
[1] Cytokines never detected or not yet studied in thyroid derived T cell clones are not listed. Quantifications refer to values given in the majority of studies performed. Data on Graves' disease from refs. 32,34; on Hashimoto's thyroiditis from refs. 30-34; and on nontoxic goiter from ref. 34.

GD thyroids were mainly CD4+ and produced a spectrum of different cytokines including IL-2, IFNγ as well as IL-6, but mimimally IL-4.[32,34] True Th$_2$ T cell clones were thus not present in the autoimmune thyroid gland. One could speculate that this might be the result of autoantigen presentation by TEC, which may as "nonprofessional" antigen-presenting cells favor the stimulation of a certain spectrum of cytokines in T cells, as suggested for keratinocytes.[35] Th$_2$ clones might still reside in the draining lymph nodes, where they could provide the help needed for autoantibody production by B cells.

EFFECTS OF CYTOKINES IN THE THYROID GLAND

EFFECTS OF CYTOKINES IN THYROID PHYSIOLOGY

As mentioned above, a certain spectrum of cytokines is also produced in the normal thyroid gland. Cytokines seem to be primarily involved in the maintenance of normal growth and hormone production. IL-6 has been shown to have a weak, but statistically significant suppressive effect on cyclic AMP generation in human TEC.[3] It may thus play a role as a local regulator of thyroid function responsible for protecting the thyroid gland from increased stimulation by thyroid stimulating hormone (TSH) or related substances. TGFβ1 may play a similar role, as it inhibits TSH induced iodine metabolism[36] and has been shown to be a potent inhibitor of thyroid cell growth.[6,7,36] By downregulating the expression of potential thyroid autoantigens such as thyroid peroxidase (TPO) and MHC class II molecules, it may also protect the thyroid gland from the attack of autoreactive cells.[37] In this context it is also of interest that the transformation of TGFβ1 into its biologically active form is dependent on the presence of plasminogen activator in TEC.[38] Nothing is yet known about the role of IL-8 in TEC physiology. As it has, in addition to its chemotactic properties for neutrophils and lymphocytes, been shown to stimulate growth in keratinocytes,[39] it may also be involved in growth regulatory processes in the thyroid gland.

EFFECTS OF CYTOKINES IN THYROID DISEASE

Three main features characterize thyroid pathology, i.e.: (a) inflammation, immunity; (b) impaired thyroid hormone production; (c) impaired growth. The importance of these entities for the different thyroid disorders is outlined in Table 5.4. The role of cytokines for the generation and maintenance of the different conditions are summarized in Table 5.5 and dissscussed below.

a. Inflammation, immunity

Lymphocytic infiltration of the thyroid gland is the hallmark of thyroid autoimmune conditions such as HT and GD, but is also present in subacute thyroiditis (de Quervain's) and may occur in thyroid carcinoma and nontoxic goiter. In the latter condition it represents nonspecific inflammation,[40] in the former ones it is the correlate of a specific immune response directed against thyroid tissue.[40-44] Cytokines are involved in every part of an immune response, for the processing and the presentation of the specific antigens, for the activation and the clonal expansion of immune cells as well as for effector functions such as cytotoxicity or helper activity by cells of the immune system.

Table 5.4. Main pathological features characterizing thyroid disorders

	Graves' disease	Hashimoto's thyroiditis	Nontoxic goiter	Malignoma	Thyroiditis de Quervain
Inflammation, immunity	++	+++	+	+	++
Impaired hormone production → hyperthyroidism	+++	−	−	−	+[s]
→ hypothyroidism	−	++	±	−	+[s]
Impaired growth	±	±	+	+++	−

+, impairment may occur; ++, medium to severe impairment; +++, severe impairment; [s], transient

Table 5.5. Role of cytokines for the generation and maintenance of intrathyroidal inflammation/immunity and impairments of thyroid hormone production and TEC growth^

Cytokines	Inflammation/Immunity			Hormone production	TEC growth
	antigen presentation and T cell activation	cytotoxicity	helper function		
IL-1 (α and β)	s	s	−	si[a]	si[a]
IL-2	s	s	s	−	−
IL-4	s	−	s	−	−
IL-6	s	−	s	i	s?
IL-10	i	i	s	N.D.	N.D.
IFNγ	s	s	is[ϙ]	si[a]	i
TNF (α and LT)	s	s	−	si[a]	si[a]
TGFβ	i	i	i	i	i
G-CSF	N.D.	N.D.	N.D.	N.D.	s?

s, stimulation; i, inhibition; −, no effect; N.D., not determined
^Cytokines not yet studied in the context of the thyroid are not listed
[a] stimulatory as well as inhibitory properties have been described in different systems
[ϙ] inhibitory on IgG^1 and IgE, stimulatory on complement fixing IgG^2
Data from refs. 3,6,7,10,36,37,40,47-59,66 and 74-86.

Antigen processing and presentation

Antigens need to be processed and presented to T lymphocytes. This can be done by conventional antigen presenting cells such as dendritic cells or macrophages, which may reside in the thyroid itself or in the draining lymph nodes. Alternatively, antigenic peptides may also be presented by TEC themselves, which have been shown to be able to present foreign peptides as well as autoantigen to T cells.[41,45] As antigenic peptides are presented in the context of MHC molecules, sufficient expression of the latter molecules is a prerequisite for satisfactory antigen presentation. IFNγ has been shown to be a potent inducer of MHC class I and class II expression in "professional" and "nonprofessional" antigen presenting cells.[46] TEC, which constitutively do not express class II molecules, are among the latter ones.[40,47-51] IFNγ may additionally affect the intracellular sorting of antigenic peptides by the induction of heat shock proteins[52] and also augments the expression of adhesion molecules such as CD54[53] which strengthen the intercellular contact between antigen presenting cells and T cells. IFNγ effects may be amplified by the presence of TNFα which has been shown to synergize with IFNα.[54-57] The induction of immunoregulatory molecules by IFNγ can also be augmented by TSH.[58,59] The result of antigen/autoantigen presentation is the activation and clonal expansion of antigen specific T cells.

Activation and clonal expansion of antigen specific T cells

In this process IL-1 and IL-6 have been shown to act as important costimulators.[60] As both factors are produced by TEC, the microenvironment for T cell activation by "nonprofessional" antigen presenting cells seems to be extremely good in the thyroid. Activated T cells produce IL-2, which is found in abundance in intrathyroidal lymphocytic infiltrates.[2,5,17] IL-2 effects seem of special interest in the context of the development of autoimmunity, as IL-2 has been shown to be constitutively overproduced in animals with genetic susceptibility for the development of thyroid autoimmune disease.[61,62] IL-2 induces T cell proliferation and is thus responsible for the clonal expansion of antigen specific T cells.[63] It also enhances the secretion of other lymphokines by activated T cells and heightens the expression of membrane receptors for other growth factors such as the transferrin or the insulin receptor.[63] IL-2 effects can be enhanced by other cytokines such as IL-7,[64] IL-11[65] and IL-15 which have not yet been described, but are presumably also present in the inflamed thyroid gland.

Effector functions

Tissue destruction is the main feature of HT. It is brought about by the target cell directed cytotoxicity of autoaggressive immune cells. Cytokines are of major importance in this process. IL-2 plays an important role in supporting the development of antigen stimulated cytotoxic T lymphocyte precursors into functional cytotoxic effector T cells. It also enhances NK cell activity.[63] TNFα and lymphotoxin (LT) exert cytotoxic effects on a wide range of cells and have been shown to be cytotoxic on cultured TEC.[66] IL-12 may also be of relevance in this context, as it induces cytotoxic lymphocyte differentiation and enhances NK function.[67]

As pointed out above, the clinical picture of GD is dominated by the production of "thyroid stimulating immunoglobulins" (TSI), a subclass of autoantibodies with the capacity to stimulate the TSH receptor.[29] T cell help is thus required. In most immunological reactions it is provided by CD4+ cells of the Th$_2$ type, which produce IL-4, IL-5, IL-6 and IL-10, cytokines which promote B cell growth and/or maturation.[68] IL-4 has so far only rarely been detected in the inflamed thyroid gland (Table 5.2) and is hardly produced by thyroid derived T cell clones (Table 5.3). The possibility that it is produced in the draining lymph node has been mentioned. Alternatively, other cytokines such as IL-6 and IL-2, which are present in the autoimmune thyroid gland, might in a certain microenvironment exert sufficient helper function in the absence of IL-4. IL-13, which has not yet been detected in the thyroid gland, may also be of relevance in this context.[69]

An interesting phenomenon is the fact that suppressors of the immune response such as TGFβ or IL-10 have been found in high concentrations in the inflamed thyroid gland.[5,7,17,26] The inhibitory effects of TGFβ on autoantigen expression and the antigen presenting capacity of thyroid cells have been pointed out.[37] TGFβ additionally counteracts IL-2, TNFα and IL-1.[70] IL-10 has also been described to be a general suppressor of the immune response.[71] It has, for instance, been shown to inhibit the production of TNFα and LT[72] and to diminish antigen presentation.[73] The presence of the two inhibitory cytokines at the site of heavy lymphocytic infiltration and active disease suggest the activation of counter-regulatory mechanisms which may be decisive for the determination of an immune response or the induction of remission in patients with autoimmune disease.

b. Impaired thyroid hormone production

As mentioned earlier in this article, a similar spectrum of cytokines is present in extreme hypo- as well as hyperthyroidism. Cytokines seem thus not to be decisive for the development of a certain thyroid hormone status. They may still affect processes involved in thyroid hormone production and thus aggravate a certain pre-existent defect. Potential effects on hormone production exerted by TGFβ and IL-6 have been pointed out in the section entitled 'Effects of cytokines in thyroid physiology,' above. Cytokines typically present in the inflammatory infiltrate have also been reported to affect hormone production in TEC. Depending on the cell and assay system used, stimulatory as well as inhibitory influences have been described for IL-1,[3,74-76] TNFα[76-80] and IFNγ.[76,81-84]

c. Impaired growth

Physiological growth regulatory mechanisms exerted by cytokines have been discussed in the section entitled 'Effects of cytokines in thyroid physiology'. Cytokines only present in the inflamed thyroid gland have also been suggested to have effects on thyroid cell proliferation. Thus, IL-1 has, for instance, been demonstrated to stimulate thyroid cell growth and increase the concentration of the c-*myc* proto-oncogene in thyroid cells.[10,85] In a different system it has, however, been shown to be inhibitory.[74] TNFα has also been reported to affect thyroid cell proliferation. In different systems it has been attributed growth stimulatory as well as growth inhibitory properties.[56,77,80] IFNγ has been shown to suppress thyroid cell growth.[81,86] The possibility of aberrant cytokine production by transformed thyroid cells has been referred to earlier in this article. Cytokines such as G-CSF or IL-6 expressed at extremely high concentrations may be of importance in the autocrine growth regulation of tumor cells.[20-22]

IN VIVO EFFECTS OF CYTOKINES ON THE THYROID GLAND

Recently clinical trials have been performed in which patients with malignancies such as melanomas, renal carcinomas or neoplastic hematological diseases were treated with IFNγ, IL-2, lymphokine-activated killer (LAK) cells or combinations of IL-2 and IFNγ. Many of these patients consecutively developed thyroid dysfunction.[87-92] Whereas an initial hyperthyroid state was observed in some,[92] transient hypothyroidism associated with high TSH concentrations and high titers of thyroid autoantibodies was the dominant clinical feature. Patients with a predisposition for autoimmunity seemed to be particularly prone to develop hypothyroidism after cytokine treatment.[91] Thyroid dysfunction was accompanied by lymphocytic infiltration of the thyroid gland and MHC class II expression in thyroid cells.[88-90,92] Although the pathogenic mechanism of this impairment is not fully understood, it will have to be anticipated in future clinical trial.

ROLE OF CYTOKINES IN GRAVES' OPHTHALMOPATHY

GD is frequently associated with Graves' ophthalmopathy. The reason for this coincidence is not yet fully understood, but antigenic crossreactivity seems to be involved.[93] Histological examination of the retrobulbar tissue of patients with endocrine ophthalmopathy reveals severe lymphocytic infiltrations and the presence of a whole spectrum of different cytokines including IFNγ, TNFα and β and IL-1α and β.[94,95] These cytokines have been shown to be potent stimulators of glycosaminoglycan (GAG) production by orbital fibroblasts in vitro.[96,97] Orbital fibroblasts can also be stimulated to proliferate in vitro following treatment with IL-1α, IL-4 and TGFβ1.[98] This mechanism may in part be responsible for the fibrosis of orbital tissue in Graves' ophthalmopathy.

Cytokines seem thus to be of major importance for the development of the disease. Attempts have recently been made to characterize the profile of cytokines secreted by T cells infiltrating the retrobulbar tissue in Graves' ophthalmopathy. The results are still controversial. Whereas a Th_1-like cytokine production profile has been reported by one group based on the analysis of T cell clones of unknown specificity,[99] a Th_2-like T cell spectrum has been suggested by another group on the basis of the detection of IL-4, IL-5 and IL-10 by PCR mRNA amplification of unpurified tissue samples.[100] Our laboratory has recently succeeded in establishing $CD8^+$ T cell lines from the retrobulbar tissues of patients with Graves' ophthalmopathy.[101] These lines have specific reactivity towards autologous fibroblasts and produce an unusual combination of cytokines. They secrete IFNγ as well as IL-4 and IL-10. Substantial IL-4 production by $CD8^+$ cells is a rare finding,[68] but has been shown to be a feature of $CD8^+$ suppressor T cell clones.[102] Suppressor functions may thus have been operative in our T cell lines. The immunosuppressive function of IL-10 has been pointed out above. It seems possible that some of the typical functions of Th_1 cells may have been attenuated or lost in $CD8^+$ T cell populations capable of simultaneous IL-10, IL-4 and IFNγ production. This may provide an explanation for the fact that most of our $CD8^+$ class I restricted lines proliferated in response to stimulation with autologous fibroblasts, but failed to exert target cell cytotoxicity. This in vitro observation is in good agreement with in vivo findings which demonstrate fibroblast proliferation with no indication of target cell damage in spite of the presence of $CD8^+$ cells in the retrobulbar tissues from patients with Graves' ophthalmopathy.[93]

In summary, Graves' ophthalmopathy is a good example how a clinical picture can be brought about by a complex network of cytokine interactions. Our concept of the sequence of events leading to Graves' ophthalmopathy is depicted in Figure 5.1.

CONCLUSION

A complex network of cytokines seems to be operative in thyroid health and disease. Whereas in thyroid health cytokines are involved in the maintenance of normal thyroid cell growth and function, cytokines may exert a variety of different effects in thyroid disease. Their concentrations and interactions may determine whether an inflammatory process is terminated or perpetuated, whether autoantibodies with dominant metabolic functions such as TSI are produced or whether tissue injury is predominant. Various disturbances of thyroid hormone production and growth typically present in the different thyroid disorders may also be influenced by cytokines. Therapeutic approaches based on the inhibition of cytokines such as recently tried in rheumatoid arthritis[104] may be envisaged in the future, although at present the molecular target is unclear.

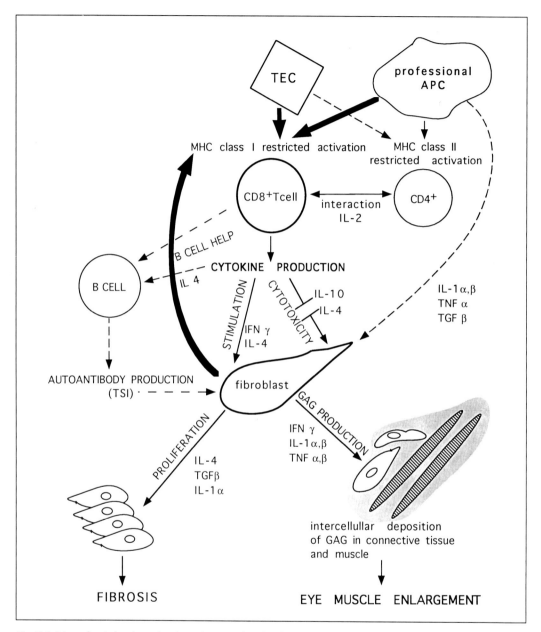

Fig. 5.1. Hypothesis for the role of cytokines in the development of endocrine ophthalmopathy: MHC class I restricted CD8⁺ T cells with reactivity to thyroid autoantigen(s) crossreact with retrobulbar fibroblasts. Upon activation they secret IL-4, IL-10 and IFNγ. IL-1α and β as well as TNFα and TGFβ1 may be produced by other infiltrating cells such as macrophages. IL-4 and IL-10 attenuate or suppress cytotoxic effector functions leading to undisturbed fibroblast survival. IFNγ may alone or in synergy with TNFα increase the antigen presenting capacity of fibroblasts. Fibroblast proliferation may be stimulated by cytokines such as IL-4, IL-1α and TGFβ1, leading to retrobulbar fibrosis. IFNγ, IL-1α and β and TNFα and LT increase the production of glycosaminoglycans (GAG) by fibroblasts. GAG is deposited in the intercellular space in the connective tissue and in the eye muscles, leading to secondary eye muscle enlargement. Autoantibodies with stimulatory activity for the TSH receptor which may be expressed in fibroblasts[103] could exert an additional stimulatory influence.

REFERENCES

1. Feldmann M, Brennan FM, Chantry D et al. Detection of cytokines. Immunol Rev 1991; 119:106-123.
2. Grubeck-Loebenstein B, Buchan G, Chantry D et al. Analysis of intrathyroidal cytokine production in thyroid autoimmune disease: Thyroid follicular cells produce interleukin-1α and interleukin-6. Clin Exp Immunol 1989; 77:324-330.
3. Bendtzen K, Buschard K, Diamant M et al. Possible role of IL-1, TNFα, and IL-6 in insulin-dependent Diabetes mellitus and autoimmune thyroid disease. Lymphokine Research 1989; 8:335-340.
4. Zheng RQH, Abney E, Chu CQ et al. Detection of interleukin-6 and interleukin-1 production in human thyroid epithelial cells by non-radioactive in situ hybridization and immunohistochemical methods. Clin Exp Immunol 1991; 83:314-319.
5. Weetman AP, Pickerill AP, Davies R et al. Cytokine gene expression in intrathyroidal lymphocytes from Graves' disease. J Endocrinol Invest 1994; 17:28.
6. Morris JC III, Ranganathan G, Hay ID et al. The effects of transforming growth factor-β on growth and differentiation of the continuous rat thyroid follicular cell line, FRTL-5. Endocrinology 1988; 123:1385-1394.
7. Grubeck-Loebenstein B, Buchan G, Sadeghi R et al. Transforming growth factor beta regulates thyroid growth. Role in the pathogenesis of nontoxic goitre. J Clin Invest 1989; 83:764-770.
8. Cowin AJ, Davis JRE, Bidey SP. Transforming growth factor-beta 1 production in porcine thyroid follicular cells: Regulation by intrathyroidal organic iodine. J Mol Endocrinol 1992; 9:197-205.
9. Hirose W, Kawagoe M, Hara M et al. Production of thymocyte-stimulating activity by cultured human thyroid epithelial cells. Clin Exp Immunol 1987; 70:102-109.
10. Kawabe Y, Eguchi K, Shimomura C et al. Interleukin-1 production and action in thyroid tissue. J Clin Endocrinol Metab 1989; 68:1174-1183.
11. Zheng RQ, Abney ER, Chu CQ et al. Detection of in vivo production of tumour necrosis factor-alpha by human thyroid epithelial cells. Immunology 1992; 75:456-462.
12. Paschke R, Kist A, Jännicke R et al. Lack of intrathyroidal tumor necrosis factor in Graves' disease. J Clin Endocrinol Metab 1993; 76:97-102.
13. Dinarello CA, Savage N. Interleukin-1 and interleukin-1 antagonism. Blood 1991; 77:1627-1652.
14. van Snick J. Interleukin 6: An overview. Annu Rev Immunol 1990;8:253-278.
15. Weetman AP, Bennett GL, Wong WLT. Thyroid follicular cells produce interleukin-8. J Clin Endocrinol Metab 1992; 75:328-330.
16. Moore K, O'Garra A, de Waal Malefyt R et al. Interleukin-10. Annu Rev Immunol 1993; 11:165-172.
17. Paschke R, Schuppert F, Taton M et al. Intrathyroidal cytokine gene expression profiles in autoimmune thyroiditis. J Endocrinol 1994; 141:309-315.

18. Krueger JG, Gottlieb AB. Growth factors, cytokines, and eicosanoids. In: Dubertret L, ed. Psoriasis. Bresca, Italy: ISED Publishing Co., 1994:18-28.
19. González-Amaro R, García-Monzón C, García-Buey L et al. Induction of tumor necrosis factor α production by human hepatocytes in chronic viral hepatitis. J Exp Med 1994; 179:841-848.
20. Yoshida A, Asaga T, Masuzawa C et al. Production of cytokines by thyroid carcinoma cell lines. J Surg Oncol 1994; 55:104-107.
21. Oka Y, Kobayashi T, Fujita S et al. Establishment of a human anaplastic thyroid cancer cell line secreting granulocyte colony-stimulating factor in response to cytokines. In vitro Cell Dev Biol 1993; 29A:537-542.
22. Yoshida M, Matsuzaki H, Sakata K et al. Neutrophil chemotactic factors produced by a cell line from thyroid carcinoma. Cancer Res 1992; 52:464-469.
23. Hamilton F, Black MA, Farquharson MA et al. Spatial correlation between thyroid epithelial cells expressing class II molecules and interferon-γ containing lymphocytes in human thyroid autoimmune disease. Clin Exp Immunol 1991; 83:64-68.
24. Margolick JB, Weetman AP, Burman KD. Immunohistochemical analysis of intrathyroidal lymphocytes in Graves' disease: Evidence of activated T cells and production of interferon-γ. Clin Immunol Immunop 1988; 47:208-218.
25. Rutenfranz I, Kruse A, Rink L. In situ hybridization of the mRNA for interferon-γ, interferon-αE, interferon-β, interleukin-1β and interleukin-6 and characterization of infiltrating cells in thyroid tissues. J Immunol Methods 1992; 148:233-242.
26. Runkle I, Chafer-Vilaplana J, Biro A et al. Interleukin-10 in human thyroid disease. J Endocrinol Invest 1994; 17:28.
27. Grubeck-Loebenstein B, Derfler K, Kassal H et al. Immunological features of nonimmunogenic hyperthyroidism. J Clin Endocrinol Metab 1985; 60:150-155.
28. Brennan FM, Chantry D, Jackson A et al. Inhibitory effect of TNFα antibodies on synovial cell interleukin-1 production in rheumatoid arthritis. Lancet 1989; ii:244-250.
29. Weetman AP. Thyroid autoimmune disease. In: Braverman LE, Utiger RD, eds. Werner and Ingbar's The Thyroid: A Fundamental and Clinical Text. 6th ed. Philadelphia, New York, London, Hagerstown: JB Lippincott Company, 1991:1295-1310.
30. del Prete GF, Tiri A, Mariotti S et al. Enhanced production of γ-interferon by thyroid-derived T cell clones in Hashimoto's thyroiditis. Clin Exp Immunol 1987a; 69:323-331.
31. del Prete GF, Tiri A, de Carli M et al. High potential to tumor necrosis factor-α (TNFα) production of thyroid infiltrating T lymphocytes in Hashimoto's thyroiditis: A peculiar feature of destructive thyroid autoimmunity. Autoimmunity 1989; 4:267-276.
32. Mariotti S, del Prete GF, Mastromauro C et al. The autoimmune infiltrate of Basedow's disease: Analysis at clonal level and comparison with Hashimoto's thyroiditis. Exp Clin Endocrinol 1991; 97:139-146.

33. Turner M, Londei M, Feldmann M. Human T cells from autoimmune and normal individuals can produce tumor necrosis factor. Eur J Immunol 1987; 17:1807-1816.
34. Grubeck-Loebenstein B, Turner M, Pirich K et al. CD4⁺ T-cell clones from autoimmune thyroid tissue cannot be classified according to their lymphokine production. Scand J Immunol 1990; 32:433-440.
35. Nickoloff BJ, Turka LA. Immunological functions of non-professional antigen-presenting cells: New insights from studies of T-cell interactions with keratinocytes. Immunol Today 1994; 15:464-469.
36. Tsushima T, Arai M, Saji M et al. Effects of transforming growth factor-β on deoxyribonucleic acid synthesis and iodine metabolism in porcine thyroid cells in culture. Endocrinology 1988; 123:1187-1194.
37. Widder J, Dorfinger K, Wilfing A et al. The immunoregulatory influence of transforming growth factor beta in thyroid autoimmuity: TGF β inhibits autorecativity in Graves' disease. J Autoimmun 1991; 4:689-701.
38. Cowin AJ, Bidey SP. The proteolytic processing of iodide-responsive latent transforming growth factor-β1 by goitrous human thyroid follicular cells in monolayer is dependent upon plasminogen activation. J Endocrinol Invest 1994; 17:33.
39. Durum K, Oppenheim JJ. Proinflammatory cytokines and immunity. In: Paul WE, ed. Fundamental Immunology. 3rd ed. New York: Raven Press, Ltd., 1989:801-835.
40. Grubeck-Loebenstein B, Londei M, Greenall C et al. Pathogenetic relevance of HLA class II expressing thyroid follicular cells in nontoxic goiter and in Graves' disease. J Clin Invest 1988; 81:1608-1614.
41. Londei M, Bottazzo GF, Feldmann M. Human T cell clones from autoimmune thyroid glands: Specific recognition of autologous thyroid cells. Science 1985; 228:85-89.
42. Dayan CM, Londei M, Corcoran AE et al. Autoantigen recognition by thyroid-infiltrating T cells in Graves' disease. Natl Acad Sci USA 1991; 88:7415-7419.
43. del Prete GF, Mariotti S, Tiri A et al. Characterization of thyroid infiltrating lymphocytes in Hashimoto's thyroiditis: Detection of B and T cells specific for thyroid antigens. Acta Endocrinol Cop 1987b; 281 Suppl:111-114.
44. Nikolai TF. Silent thyroiditis and subacute thyroiditis. In: Braverman LE, Utiger RD, eds. Werner and Ingbar's The Thyroid: A Fundamental and Clinical Text. 6th ed. Philadelphia, New York, London, Hagerstown: JB Lippincott Company, 1991:710-727.
45. Londei M, Lamb JR, Bottazzo GF et al. Epithelial cells expressing aberrant MHC class II determinants can present antigen to cloned human T cells. Nature 1984; 312:639-641.
46. Trinchieri G, Perussia B. Immune interferon: A pleiotropic lymphokine with multiple effects. Immunol Today 1985; 6:131-142.
47. Todd I, Pujol-Borrell R, Hammond LJ et al. Interferon-gamma induces HLA-DR expression by thyroid epithelium. Clin Exp Immunol 1985; 61:265-273.

48. Weetman AP, Volkman DJ, Burman KD et al. The in vitro regulation of human thyrocyte HLA-DR antigen expression. J Clin Endocrinol Metab 1985; 61:817-824.
49. Asakawa H, Hanafusa T, Katsura H et al. Interferon-γ inhibits thyroid-stimulating hormone-induced morphological changes and induces the expression of major histocompatibility complex class II antigen in thyroid follicles in suspension culture. Endocrinology 1991; 128: 1409-1413.
50. Saji M, Moriarty J, Ban T et al. Major histocompatibility complex class I gene expression in rat thyroid cells is regulated by hormones, methimazole, and iodide as well as interferon. J Clin Endocrinol Metab 1992; 75:871-878.
51. Iwatani Y, Gerstein HC, Iitaka M et al. Thyrocyte HLA-DR expression and interferon-γ production in autoimmune thyroid disease. J Clin Endocrinol Metab 1986; 63:695-708.
52. Sztankay A, Trieb K, Lucciarini P et al. Interferon gamma and iodide increase the inducibility of the 72kD heat shock protein in cultured human thyroid epithelial cells. J Autoimmun 1994; 7:219-230.
53. Zheng RQH, Abney ER, Grubeck-Loebenstein B et al. Expression of intercellular adhesion molecule-1 and lymphocyte function-associated antigen-3 on human thyroid epithelial cells in Graves' and Hashimoto's diseases. J Autoimmun 1990; 3:727-736.
54. Kissonerghis AM, Grubeck-Loebenstein B, Pirich K et al. Tumour necrosis factor synergises with gamma interferon on the induction of mRNA from DR alpha chain on thyrocytes from Graves' disease and non toxic goitre. Autoimmunity 1989; 4:255-266.
55. Buscema M, Todd I, Deuss U et al. Influence of tumor necrosis factor-α on the modulation by interferon-γ of HLA class II molecules in human thyroid cells and its effect on interferon-γ binding. J Clin Endocrinol Metab 1989; 69:433-439.
56. Weetman AP, Rees AJ. Synergistic effects of recombinant tumor necrosis factor and interferon-gamma on rat thyroid cell growth and Ia antigen exprssion. Immunology 1988; 63:285-289.
57. Zakarija M, Hornicek FJ, Levis S et al. Effects of gamma interferon and tumor necrosis factor alpha on thyroid cells: Induction of class II antigen and inhibition of growth stimulation. Mol Cell Endocrinol 1988; 58:329-336.
58. Todd I, Pujol-Borrell R, Hammond LJ et al. Enhancement of thyrocyte HLA class II expression by thyroid stimulating hormone. Clin Exp Immunol 1987; 69:524-531.
59. Platzer M, Neufeld DS, Piccinini LA et al. Induction of rat thyroid cell MHC class II antigen by thyrotropin and gamma interferon. Endocrinology 1987; 121:2087-2092.
60. Houssiau FA, Coulie PG, Olive D et al. Synergistic activation of human T cells by interleukin 1 and interleukin 6. Eur J Immunol 1988; 18:653-656.

61. Wick G, Möst J, Schauenstein K et al. Spontaneous autoimmune thyroiditis—a bird's eye view. Immunol Today 1985; 6:359-364.
62. Gonzalo JA, Cuende E, Alés-Martínez JE et al. Interleukin-2: A possible trigger for autoimmunity. Int Arch Allergy Immunol 1992; 97:251-257.
63. Smith KA. Interleukin-2: Inception, impact and implications. Science 1988; 240:1169-1176.
64. Lynch DH, Miller RE. Interleukin 7 promotes long-term in vitro growth of antitumor cytotoxic T lymphocytes with immunotherapeutic efficacy in vivo. J Exp Med 1994; 179:31-42.
65. Paul S, Bennett F, Calvetti J et al. Molecular cloning of a cDNA encoding interleukin 11, a stromal cell-derived lymphopoietic and hematopoietic cytokine. Natl Acad Sci USA 1990; 87:7512-7516.
66. Taverne J, Rayner DC, van der Meide PH et al. Cytotoxicity of tumor necrosis factor for thyroid epithelial cells and its regulation by interferon-γ. Eur J Immunol 1987; 17:1855-1858.
67. Gately M, Wolitzky A, Quinn P et al. Regulation of human cytolytic lymphocyte responses by interleukin-12. Cell Immunol 1992; 143:127-142.
68. Romagnani S. Human Th_1 and Th_2 subsets: Regulation of differentiation and role in protection and immunopathology. Int Arch Allergy Immunol 1992; 98:279-285.
69. Zurawski SM, de Vries JE. Interleukin 13, an interleukin-4 like cytokine that acts on monocytes and B cells, but not on T cells. Immunol Today 1994; 15:19-26.
70. Fontana A, Constam DB, Frei K et al. Modulation of the immune response by transforming growth factor beta. Int Arch Allergy Immunol 1992; 99:1-7.
71. Spits H, de Waal Malefyt R. Functional characterization of human IL-10. Int Arch Allergy Immunol 1992; 99:8-15.
72. Hsu DH, Moore KW, Spits H. Differential effects of interleukin-4 and γ 10 on IL-2 induced interferon-γ synthesis and lymphokine-activated killer activity. Int Immunol 1992; 4:563-569.
73. de Waal Malefyt R, Haanen J, Spits H et al. Interleukin 10 (IL-10) and viral IL-10 strongly reduce antigen-specific human T cell proliferation by diminishing the antigen-presenting capacity of moncytes via downregulation of class II major histocompatibility complex expression. J Exp Med 1991; 174:915-924.
74. Rasmussen A, Kayser L, Bech K et al. Differential effects of interleukin 1α and 1β on cultured human and rat thyroid epithelial cells. Acta Endocrinol Cop 1990; 122:520-526.
75. Westermark K, Nilsson M, Karlsson FA. Effects of interleukin 1 alpha on porcine thyroid follicles in suspension culture. Acta Endocrinol Cop 1990; 122:505-512.
76. Sato K, Satoh T, Shizume K et al. Inhibition of ^{125}I organification and thyroid hormone release by interleukin-1, tumor necrosis factor-α, and interferon-γ in human thyrocytes in suspension culture. J Clin Endocrinol Metab 1990; 70:1735-1743.

CHAPTER 6

CYTOKINES IN SJÖGREN'S SYNDROME

F. N. Skopouli and H. M. Moutsopoulos

INTRODUCTION

Sjögren's syndrome (SS) is a chronic, slowly progressive, autoimmune disease, characterized by lymphocytic invasion of exocrine glands which results in xerostomia and keratoconjunctivitis sicca. It usually affects middle-aged women and is the second commonest autoimmune rheumatic disease after rheumatoid arthritis (RA). It can occur alone (primary SS) or in association with other autoimmune disorders, such as rheumatoid arthritis, systemic lupus erythematosus (SLE) and systemic sclerosis (secondary SS).[1]

Primary SS presents with a wide clinical spectrum: from exocrinopathy to systemic disease and finally to B cell neoplasia. Thus, it is unique among autoimmune rheumatic diseases since it evolves from a benign autoimmune process to B lymphoid malignancy. In fact, the relative risk of lymphoma development in SS patients is 44 times higher than that observed in the normal population.[2] The syndrome is characterized as autoimmune because it manifests two autoimmune phenomena: lymphocytic infiltration of the exocrine glands and B lymphocyte autoreactivity. In this chapter the autoimmune phenomena of the disorder will be summarized and studies on the physiology of cytokines in the serum and tissues will be presented.

THE HISTOLOGIC LESION

The common lesion of all organs affected in patients with SS is a potentially progressive lymphocytic infiltration. The salivary glands are the best studied organs in SS since they are affected in almost all patients, and are easily accessible.

Cytokines in Autoimmunity, edited by Fionula M. Brennan and Marc Feldmann.
© 1996 R.G. Landes Company.

The typical histopathologic characteristics of minor salivary gland biopsy in SS include:
1. focal aggregates of at least 50 lymphocytes and plasma cells adjacent to normal appearing acini.
2. larger foci, often exhibiting formation of germinal centers.[3] The focal round cell infiltrate starts around the ductal epithelium (Fig. 6.1); in more advanced and chronic lesions it extends and occupies the acinar epithelium and leads through unknown mechanisms to glandular dysfunction. The infiltrates consist predominantly of CD4⁺ T cells bearing CD45RO markers of memory and adhesion molecules. B cells constitute approximately 20% of the total infiltrating cells and produce IgM and IgG immunoglobulins with rheumatoid factor activity. The number of macrophages is small and the presence of natural killer cells (NK cells) is negligible. The T lymphocytes are activated since they express on their surface HLA class II antigens and *c-fos* and *c-jun* proto-oncogenes in the cell nucleus. The ductal and acinar epithelial cells inappropriately express HLA class II molecules. Using in situ hybridization it was shown that mRNA of the *c-myc* proto-oncogene is selectively expressed in epithelial cells of the salivary glands.[4] These findings pose the question of whether the epithelial cell plays a role in this pathologic process, or simply is an innocent bystander whose activation can be attributed to the signals of the inflammatory milieu.

B LYMPHOCYTE HYPERACTIVITY

B cell activation is the most consistent immunoregulatory abnormality in SS patients. The commonest serologic finding is hypergammaglobulinemia. The immunoglobulins of SS patients often contain a number of autoantibodies directed against nonorgan specific antigens such as immunoglobulins (rheumatoid factor, RF) cellular antigens and organ specific antigens such as salivary ductal cells, thyroid gland cells and gastric mucosa. The commonest autoantibodies to cellular antigens in SS patients are directed against two ribonucleoprotein antigens known as Ro (or also known as SSA) and La (or SSB).

The spectrum of B cell hyperactivity in SS patients is very interesting and unique since it follows the same pattern as the clinical picture. In the localized form of the syndrome, polyclonal B cell autoreactivity is evident, while in the systemic form of this syndrome polyclonal with oligomonoclonal B cell process is present. In fact circulating monoclonal immunoglobulins or light chains are often found in the serum and urine of these patients together with histologically benign lymphoid infiltrates in salivary glands which exhibit B cell clonal expansion.[5] Approximately 10 per cent of the patients develop atypi-

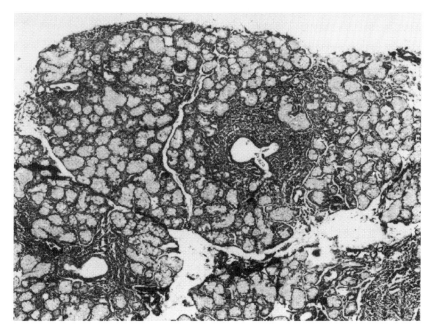

Fig. 6.1. Focal periductal lymphocytic infiltrates in the labial salivary gland biopsy of a patient with primary SS. (H&E, magnification x200).

cal lymphoid hyperplasia or malignant lymphoma of B cell origin. Longitudinal studies have shown that the oligomonoclonal B cell expansion proceeds to overt lymphoma in which associated karyotypic alterations (*bcl-2* translocation: t[14; 18]) have been detected. This suggests that SS lymphoma develops as a multistep process.[6]

ETIOPATHOGENESIS

Genetic and viral factors seem to be the main players in the pathogenesis of SS. Numerous investigators have shown an association of primary SS with molecules encoded by the major histocompatibility complex (MHC) such as HLA-B8 and -DR3.[7] Recent studies have shown that autoantibody production directed against La(SSB) and Ro(SSA) antigens strongly correlate with heterozygosity for HLA-DQw1/DQw2, suggesting that the presence of these autoantibodies is dependent on the specific linear structure of the antigen binding groove of the DQα and DQβ chains.[8] What activates the immune system is not known. Viral infection or activation of endogenous viruses have been suspected of being major contributing factors in SS. The cross-reactivity with retroviral antigens observed in the sera of pSS patients and the retroviral and herpesviral sequences detected in the salivary glands argue for some type of viral infection in pSS patients during the course of the disease.[9]

Other factors that play important role in the pathogenesis of SS are endocrine factor and stress. The ability of sex hormones to modulate immune and autoimmune responses is well known, while the ability of neuropeptides to modify the immune response is under vigorous investigation.

CYTOKINE STUDIES

Cytokine research in SS has followed three main directions:
1. Studies looking for cytokine production by peripheral blood mononuclear cells. These studies tried to evaluate indirectly the function of B and T lymphocytes and the effect of T cells on B cell hyperactivity as well as the monoclonal expansion.
2. Studies evaluating the expression of cytokines in the affected exocrine glands of SS patients. These studies attempt to delineate the activation status of the immunocytes and epithelial cells in the inflammatory lesion of SS patients, the cross-talk between the cells and the signals responsible for the initiation and perpetuation of the autoimmune lesion.
3. Studies on tissues of experimental animal models for SS. These studies attempted to correlate the time sequence of cytokine expression with the disease progression. In addition, these models have been used for therapeutic intervention using cytokines.

IMMUNOREGULATORY CYTOKINES

Several studies on the immunoregulatory cells have been carried out in the peripheral blood and in the salivary tissues. The absolute number of the peripheral blood total lymphocytes, T cells and B cells of SS patients do not differ substantially from that observed in normal individuals. Studies on T cell subsets in SS have ended up with inconclusive results.[10,11] Some patients, however, present with immunoregulatory aberrations such as decreased autologous mixed lymphocyte reaction and impaired NK cell activity.[12]

In 1986 Miyasaka et al[13] showed that IL-2 production of the peripheral blood mononuclear cells (PBMC) was significantly impaired in patients with SS. However, impaired IL-2 production could be partially restored by adding phorbol myristic acetate (PMA). Furthermore the response of PBMC to IL-2 was not disturbed in these patients.

In another study[14] exogenous recombinant IL-2 did not significantly enhance the depressed anti-CD2 induced response of SS patients PBMC, as it did in normal PBMC. At the same time Manoussakis et al[15] showed that soluble IL-2 receptor levels were highly increased in the sera of SS patients and correlated well with disease activity, and especially with disease progression to pseudolymphoma or lymphoma (Table 6.1). Soluble IL-2R release may be regarded as a marker of immune cell activation. However, it is not presently known whether this phenomenon has any pathophysiologic significance. Soluble IL-2R molecules retain the capacity to bind to IL-2; therefore, the possibility of interfering with physiologic IL-2 activity has been suggested. In patients with SS the presence of increased serum levels of soluble IL-2R molecules appeared to denote the progression of the disease to extraglandular involvement and finally to pseudolymphoma or lymphoma. Given that primary SS is a slowly evolving disorder with additive symptoms and signs that frequently results in frank lymphoid neoplasia, the early demonstration of a neoplastic lymphocytic expansion would be of paramount importance. More recently, diminished ability to mobilize intracellular calcium and activate protein kinase C in response to PHA and PMA were demonstrated in SS peripheral blood lymphocytes.[16] Complete activation of the IL-2 gene requires the synergistic interaction of five transcription factors reacting with known oligonucleotide promoter sequences. The ability of one of these factors (called Oct-1) to bind to its DNA oligonucleotide promoter is greatly diminished in the majority of SS patients, but not in SLE patients even when the latter patients produce antibodies to Ro(SSA) and La(SSB) autoantigens. Furthermore, the addition of phophatase to the transcription factor-containing nuclear extract reveals a cryptic DNA binding activity in SS that was not previously apparent.[16] Since phosphorylation is an important mechanism in kinase activation and in many protein-protein interactions including those involving suppressor proto-oncogenes, this observation may be of considerable importance and a clue to possible genetic/viral mechanisms operative in SS.

On the other hand, immunohistochemical studies to identify cytokine expression on the surface of the mononuclear cells infiltrating exocrine glands in SS have resulted in conflicting data.[17-19] Recently using reverse transcriptase-polymerase chain reaction (RT-PCR) analysis as well as in situ hybridization technique[22] for the detection of mRNA, it was demonstrated that many cells in the salivary gland tissue from almost all the SS patients tested produce IL-2 mRNA and express IL-2 receptor (IL-2R) (Fig. 6.2, Table 6.2).

Table 6.1. Incidence of elevated soluble IL-2R levels in the various clinical subgroups of patients with primary Sjögren's syndrome (pSS)

Sjögren's syndrome	Patients (number)	Elevated soluble IL-2R levels (percent)
Glandular	19	5
Systemic	28	29
Pseudolymphoma or lymphoma	5	80*

* $p < 0.005$

The results are more confusing on the production of interferon γ (IFNγ). Fox et al[20] found IFNγ message in all 10 patient's biopsies (submandibular and parotid glands) tested, compared to Ogawa et al[21] in four out of thirteen tested (minor salivary glands) and Boumba et al[22] only in three out of twelve (minor salivary glands). In the latter

Table 6.2. Detection of cytokine cDNA and mRNA in salivary gland biopsies by polymerase chain reaction (1) and in situ hybridization (2)

Cytokine	Salivary gland biopsies (percent positive)		
	Fox et al (1) (n = 10)	Ogawa et al (1) (n = 17)	Boumba et al (2) (n = 12)
IL-2	90	67	73
INFγ	100	38	25
IL-4	10	20	33
IL-5	10	ND	ND
IL-10	80	25	0
IL-1β	100	25	67
IL-6	100	21	100
TNFα	100	0	58
LT	ND	0	8
TGFβ	ND	100	27

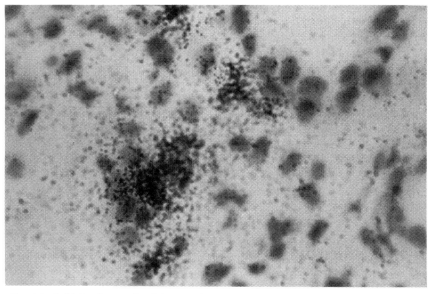

Fig. 6.2. Labial salivary gland biopsy from a patient with primary SS after in situ hybridization with IL-2 antisense 40 mer oligonucleotide probe (magnification x 400). IL-2 producing cells are scattered among lymphocytes in the lesion of the salivary glands of primary SS patients.

three biopsies transforming growth factor β (TGFβ) producing cells were also detected. IFNγ can induce the expression of class II MHC molecules and can be involved in the initiation and perpetuation of the autoimmune process.[23] On the other hand, reduced IFNγ production by T cells in the synovial membrane of inflammatory joints in patients with rheumatoid arthritis, has been considered to be a permissive factor for the progression of the process.[24] It is also known that IFNγ antagonizes the proliferative responses induced by IL-4 and IL-2. Although IFNγ participates in different functions and induces different results in the immune system, its biologic action on the homeostasis of the immune system in vivo are complex. The findings that increased concentrations of this cytokine along with TGFβ are detected locally in the lesion indicate that the fact of its main role in the minor salivary glands of pSS patients does not clarify whether IFNγ is stimulatory or immunosuppresive.

In contrast IL-4, another cytokine produced by activated T cells which induces B cell proliferation, was not detected in labial salivary gland tissue T cells from SS patients. This finding was confirmed using RT-PCR as well as *in situ* hybridization techniques.[20,22] IL-4 was detected only in naïve cells bearing the CD45RA phenotype in small early, periductal lesions.[22] Naïve cells in vitro are not able to produce IL-4 after stimulation[26] whereas they are able to produce IL-2; however these findings were not confirmed in vivo in salivary glands of SS patients.[22] Activation of protein kinase C (PKC) is one of the early biochemical events leading to IL-2 gene expression after antigenic or mitogenic stimulation of T cells.[27] In contrast to IL-2, PKC activation seems to play a dual effect on IL-4 expression, since it has a positive effect during the initial 3 hours of stimulation, and a negative effect after 24 hours of stimulation.[28] Moreover, PKC activation is markedly higher in CD45RO+ than in CD45RA+ cells.[29] These observations could explain the decreased production of IL-4 in the extensive infiltrates of the minor salivary glands of pSS patients in contrast to the production of IL-4 by naïve cells (CD45RA+) in small infiltrates.

The absence of IL-4 in the extensive lymphocytic infiltration of the exocrine glands suggests that there is an immunologic process, leading locally to T helper 1 subset (Th_1) but not to T helper 2 subset (Th_2) cytokine production.[30] Classification of T helper cells has been described in mice, but in humans this classification is less well documented. The subdivision of T helper cells is based on the pattern of cytokines the two subsets secrete after mitogenic or antigenic stimulation. Thus, Th_1 cells secrete IL-2, IFNγ and TNFα, whereas Th_2 cells secrete IL-4, IL-5 and IL-10.[25] The type of cytokine pattern produced by these subsets of T helper cells is determined by different factors such as the nature and concentration of antigen, the type of antigen presenting cell, and the cytokines secreted by other cells in the microenvironment.[31] Thus, the same lymphocytes are able to convert the production of cytokines from one subset to another under different local circumstances and stimuli.[32] Our finding indicates that, whereas the participating cells may produce IL-2 and IL-4 during the initial phase of infiltration, at later stages, when extensive infiltration is found, the participating cells do not produce IL-4.

Using in situ hybridization IL-10 was not detected in the histopathologic lesion of SS patients.[22] In contrast Fox et al[20] using RT-PCR and ELISA described high amounts of IL-10 mRNA and the relevant protein production in the CD4+ T cells of salivary glands and the saliva of SS patients respectively. In humans IL-10 is secreted by the Th_1 and Th_2 helper cells, macrophages and B cells and is inhibitory to macrophage function in antigen presentation and endogenous cytokine secretion, prohibiting the activation of the Th_1 helper cells.[33] As previously discussed the predominant cytokine produced by T cells in the salivary glands of SS patients is IL-2, a Th_1 product. Thus, this observation of IL-10 production seems rather paradoxical. Several possible explanations might be considered: (a) IL-10 may be produced by other cells contaminating the CD4+ cell preparation; (b) the cells may be infected with the Epstein-Barr virus (EBV) genome and express the BCRF1 (open reading frame protein) which has high homology and some of the activities of IL-10.[34] The patients examined may have in situ lymphoma. It is known that IL-10 promotes transformation of normal B cells into EBV transformed B cells to support its proliferation.[35] Additionally Ogawa et al[21] noted in their experiments using RT-PCR that two patients with IL-10 mRNA production in the salivary gland had pseudolymphoma; all of five EBV transformed B cell lines spontaneously established from SS patients also produced IL-10 mRNA.

The above data suggest that B lymphocyte hyperactivity can not be explained only on the grounds of aberrant T lymphocyte function, but perhaps also by an altered B lymphocyte function. In fact, spontaneous development of B cell lines expressing EBV nuclear antigen (EBNA) established from the peripheral blood lymphocytes of SS patients was observed. B cells of SS patients, after 3 days culture, have been shown to secrete multiple cytokines and autocrine B cell growth factors (BCGF).[36]

Proinflammatory Cytokines

Proinflammatory cytokines such as IL-1β and TNFα are produced by cells participating in autoimmune sialadenitis of Sjögren's syndrome.[20,22] Generally, IL-1β and TNFα are produced in abundance by macrophages; T lymphocytes also make TNFα and IL-1α. These cytokines are important mediators in immunologic and inflammatory phenomena and their local production has been implicated in tissue destruction.[37] LT (lymphotoxin), a cytokine produced by T and B lymphocytes, was not present in SS salivary glands.

IL-6 message was detected in cells from all biopsies of pSS patients.[20,22] Both IL-1 and TNFα induce IL-6 production in various tissues from patients with autoimmune diseases.[38] Furthermore viral infections may stimulate IL-6 production from a variety of cells including fibroblasts and monocytes.[39] The triggering factors and the events leading to cytokine expression in salivary glands from pSS had not been addressed by these studies. Recently, Hamano et al[40] examined the expression of cytokine genes during development of autoimmune sialadenitis in MRL/lpr mice. In this study, the authors suggest that the upregulation of the IL-6 gene expression observed in murine salivary glands was due to local production of IL-1 and TNFα since these two cytokines were detected before the expression of IL-6 gene. These findings suggest that local production of IL-1 and TNFα in the salivary glands of these mice may be an important factor for the initiation and induction of IL-6. It is possible that locally produced IL-6 may be involved in the final maturation of B cells and possible B cell neoplasia observed in some of these patients.[38] Therefore, the observation that IL-2 producing cells were not found in autoimmune sialadenitis of MRL/lpr mice in contrast to autoimmune histopathologic lesion of SS, where IL-2 producing cells were detected, suggests that these two lesions may be induced by different pathogenetic mechanisms.

One of the most interesting findings in the studies on cytokines in the labial salivary glands is the production of IL-1β, IL-6 and TNFα by salivary gland epithelial cells[20,22] (Fig. 6.3). These findings, suggest an active role of the salivary gland epithelial cells in the perpetuation of the chronic autoimmune response and emphasizes that these cells are not simply passive targets for autoimmune attack by the infiltrating lymphoid cells. These results extend previous observations that have demonstrated inappropriate MHC class II molecules expression in the surface of the epithelial cells[41] and increased transcription of proto-oncogene *c-myc* by SS salivary gland epithelial cells.[42]

Protective Cytokines

TGFβ is a multifunctional cytokine that plays a role in embryonic development, tumorigenesis, would healing, fibrosis and immunoregulation.[43] Although TGFβ has many biological functions, it appears to have chiefly an immunosuppressive effect in the immune system. For example, TGFβ inhibits human T cell proliferation in vivo through paracrine and autocrine mechanisms,[44] and depresses in vitro the proliferative responses of thymocytes to IL-1, T cells to IL-2 and B cells to B cell growth factors.[45] TGFβ knock-out mice which have a disrupted TGFβ1 gene have been described to develop inflammatory lesions in the salivary and lacrimal glands that resemble an SS lesion, without an apparent infection.[46] TGFβ is produced by normal salivary gland as well as by SS salivary gland.[21,22] It was observed also that TGFβ is produced by ductal epithelial cells in normal as well as SS

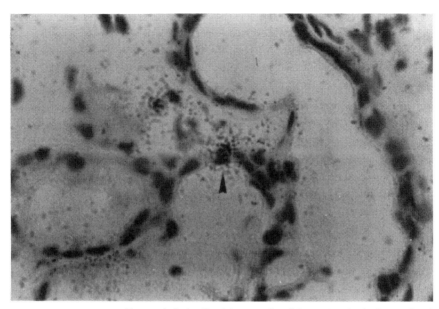

Fig. 6.3. IL-6 is expressed by epithelial cells of the acinal wall (arrow). Labial salivary gland biopsy from a primary SS patient after in situ hybridization with IL-6 antisense 40 mer oligonucleotide probe (magnification x 400).

salivary glands by immunohistochemistry (Talal N, personal communication). Following these observations, it can be speculated that TGFβ operates as a natural immunosuppressive agent in salivary glands. However, it has been found that TGFβ1 promoter is transactivated by human T lymphotropic virus-1 (HTLV-1) p40 (Tax) protein, and longterm ATL cell lines (cells infected by this virus) produce significant amounts of TGFβ.[47] Recently some investigators, using immunohistochemistry, detected the *tax* gene of HTLV-1 in labial salivary glands of SS patients with mild infiltrates.[48] It is possible that the cells in salivary glands express TGF-β mRNA after transactivation by HTLV-1 Tax protein. Compatible with this notion is the observation that *tax* transgenic mice develop a Sjögren's syndrome-like disease.[58]

Interferon α (IFNα) is a regulatory cytokine with multiple biological effects apart from its antiviral actions. It is a highly active intercellular mediator that induces resistance to viruses and inhibits cellular proliferation. An interesting observation was that a large number of patients with autoimmune diseases have increased levels of circulating IFNα.[49] Thus an elevated IFN level has been reported in SLE, rheumatoid arthritis, Sjögren's syndrome, scleroderma, multiple sclerosis, vasculitis and other autoimmune diseases. Interestingly an unusual type of IFNα neutralized by anti-IFNα only, but acid labile (as is IFNγ) seems to be the predominant circulating IFN in SLE and other autoimmune conditions.[50] The same acid-labile IFNα is found in patients with the acquired immune deficiency syndrome (AIDS).[51] In contrast to the raised

IFN levels detected in the sera of patients with various autoimmune diseases, defects in the response of mononuclear cells and especially of NK cells to IFNα in Sjögren's syndrome have been reported.[52,53] Recent studies have shown that IFNα therapy in patients may be complicated by a variety of autoimmune phenomena including thyroid disease, hemolytic anemia and thrombocytopenia.[54] In addition when either IFNα or IFNγ were injected into lupus prone mice, their lifespan was considerably shortened, and the autoantibody levels as well as the severity of immune nephritis were significantly enhanced.[55,56]

On the other hand, treatment of patients with type II mixed cryoglobulinemia with underlying hepatitis C viral infection, using recombinant human leucocyte IFN (IFNα), showed obvious clinical improvement and major reduction in the levels of cryoglobulins. This finding correlated with the reduction of viral RNA in the sera of the patients.[57]

IFN has at least two effects on B lymphocytes: it inhibits both B cell proliferation and infection by Epstein-Barr virus (EBV). However, the mechanism underlying the inhibition of EBV infection and proliferation of EBV-infected B cells by IFNα is not well established. Recently Saito et al[59] reconstituted SCID mice with B cell lines established from SS patients and treated them with subcutaneous injections of IFNα. Treatment with IFNα was shown to be significantly effective in arresting the cell growth of SS B cell lines both in vivo and in vitro. The authors also demonstrated that IFNα reduced the in vitro *c-myc* proto-oncogene expression of SS B cell lines. These results suggest that IFNα may be beneficial for controlling the lymphoproliferation seen in SS patients.

CONCLUDING REMARKS

From the data presented it is apparent that while many studies have been performed to investigate cytokines, both in the peripheral blood and in the local lesion of SS, their role in the pathophysiology of the disorder is not yet clear. It appears that:

1. Th_1 cell cytokines predominate in the focal infiltrates of the exocrine glands while the production of these cytokines by the peripheral blood mononuclear cells seems rather defective. The presence of IFNγ and IL-10 in the local lesions is controversial and needs further clarification.
2. mRNAs for the proinflammatory cytokines arise from both infiltrating lymphocytes and epithelial cells, a phenomenon which suggests that the epithelial cells may be an active counterpart in the autoimmune lesion. It should be noted that LT is not present in the Sjögren's lesion.
3. Increasing levels of circulating soluble IL-2 receptors seem to correlate with the progression of the disease from local to systemic and to malignant lymphoproliferation.

Acknowledgments

This work was supported by the Ministry of Research & Technology, Grant No 91EΔ611.

We wish to thank Dr. Th. Kordossis for his valuable comments and Mrs. P. Papadopoulou for her secretarial assistance.

References

1. Moutsopoulos HM, Chused TM, Mann DL. Sjögren's syndrome (sicca syndrome): current issues. Ann Int Med 1980; 92:212-26.
2. Kassan SS, Thomas T, Moutsopoulos HM et al. Increased risk of lymphoma in Sjögren's syndrome. Ann Intern Med 1978; 89:888-92.
3. Daniels TE, Talal N. Diagnosis and differential diagnosis of Sjögren's syndrome. In: Talal N, Moutsopoulos HM, Kassan SS, eds. Sjögren's syndrome. Clinical and Immunological Aspects. Berlin: Springer 1987:193-99.
4. Moutsopoulos HM. Immunopathology of Sjögren's syndrome: More questions than answers. Lupus 1993; 2:209-11
5. Moutsopoulos HM, Tzioufas AG, Talal N. Sjögren's syndrome: a model to study autoimmunity and lymphoid malignancy. In: Molecular Autoimmunity. N. Talal Ed. Academic Press, San Diego 1991; p. 319-40.
6. Pisa EH, Pisa P, Hang HI et al. High frequency of t (14; 18) translocation in salivary gland lymphoma from Sjögren's syndrome patients. J Exp. Med 1991; 174:1245-50.
7. Hooks JJ, Jordan JW, Cupps T et al. Multiple interferons in the circulation of patients with systemic lupus erythematosus and vasculitis. Arthr Rheum 1982; 25:396-400.
8. Reveille JD, MacLeod MJ, Whittington K et al. Specific amino acid residues in the second hypervariable region of HLA-DQA1 and DQB1 chain genes promote the Ro (SSA)/La(SSB) autoantibody responses. J Immunol 1991; 146:3871-76.
9. Moutsopoulos HM, Papadopoulos GK. Possible viral implication in the pathogenesis of Sjögren's syndrome. Eur J Med 1992; 1:219-23.
10. Moutsopoulos HM, Fauci AS. Immunoregulation in Sjögren's syndrome. Influence of serum factors on T cell subpopulation. J Clin Invest 1980; 65:519-28.
11. Fox RI, Theofilopoulos AN, Altman A. Production of Interleukin-2 (IL-2) by salivary gland lymphocytes in Sjögren's syndrome: detection of reactive cells by using antibody directed to synthetic peptides of IL-2. J Immunol 1985; 135:3109-13.
12. Miyasaka N, Sauvazie B, Pierce D et al. Decreased autologous mixed lymphocyte reaction in Sjögren's syndrome. J Clin Invest 1980; 66:928-33.
13. Miyasaka N, Murota N, Yamaoka K et al. Interleukin 2 defect in the peripheral blood and the lung in patients with Sjögren's syndrome. Clin Exp Immunol 1986; 65:497-505.
14. Gerli R, Bertoto A, Cerneffi C et al. Anti CD3 and anti CD2 induced T cell activation in primary Sjögren's syndrome. Clin Exp Rheumatol 1989; 7 Suppl 3: 129-34.

15. Manoussakis MN, Papadopoulos GK, Drosos AA et al. Soluble interleukin 2 receptor molecules in the serum of patients with autoimmune diseases. Clin Immunol Immunopath 1989; 50:321-32.
16. Flescher E, Vela-Roch N, Escalante A et al. The Oct-1 transcription factor abnormality in Sjögren's (SS) is correctable by dephosphorylation and does not occur in systemic lupus erythematosus (SLE) Abstract. Arthr Rheum 1993; 36: (suppl.9) S43.
17. Fox RI, Adamson TC III, Fong C et al. Characterization of the phenotype and function of lymphocytes infiltrating the salivary gland in patients with primary Sjögren's syndrome. Diagn Immunol 1983; 1:233-39.
18. Dalavanga YA, Drosos AA, Moutsopoulos HM. Labial salivary gland immunopathology in Sjögren's syndrome. Scand J Rheum 1986; 61 (suppl) 67-70.
19. Rowe D, Griffiths M, Stewart J et al. HLA class I and II, interferon, interleukin 2 and the interleukin 2 receptor expression on labial biopsy specimens from patients with Sjögren's syndrome. Ann Rheum Dis 1987; 46:580-6.
20. Fox RI, Kang Ho-Il, Ando D et al. Cytokine mRNA: Expression in salivary biopsies of Sjögren's syndrome. J Immunol 1994; 152:5532-39.
21. Ogawa N, Dang H, Talal N. PCR analysis of cytokines produced in salivary glands of Sjögren's syndrome patients. In: Sjögren's syndrome-State of the Art. Proceedings of the Fourth International Symposium Tokyo. M Homma, S Sugai, Tojo T, Miyasaka N, Akizuki M, eds. Amsterdam: Kugler Publications, 1994:103-10.
22. Boumba D, Skopouli FN, Moutsopoulos HM. Cytokine mRNA expression in the labial salivary gland tissues from patients with primary Sjögren's syndrome. Br J Rheumatol, 1995; 34:326-333.
23. Bottazzo GF, Pujol-Borell R, Hanafusa T et al. Role of aberrant HLA-DR expression and antigen presentation in induction of endocrine autoimmunity. Lancet 1983; 11:1115-8.
24. Jacob CO, McDevitt HO. Interferon gamma and tumor necrosis factor in autoimmune disease models: implications for immunoregulation and genetic susceptibility. In: Talal N, ed. Molecular Autoimmunity. San Diego: Academic Press, 1991:109-26.
25. Fernandez-Botran R, Saunders VM, Mosmann TR et al. Lymphokine mediated regulation of the proliferative response of clones of T helper 1 and T helper 2 cells. J Exp Med 1988; 168:543-48.
26. Salmon M, Kitas GD, Bacon PA. Production of lymphokine mRNA by CD45R+ and CD45R-helper T cells from human peripheral blood and by human CD4+ T cell clones. J Immunol 1989; 143:907-12.
27. Fraser JD, Straus D, Weiss A. Signal transduction events leading to T cell lymphokine gene expression. Immunol Today 1993; 14:357-62.
28. Manoz E, Zubiaga AM, Munoz J et al. Regulation of IL-4 lymphokine gene expression and cellular proliferation in murine T helper type II cells. Cell Regulation 1990; 1:425-9.

CHAPTER 7

CYTOKINES IN SYSTEMIC LUPUS ERYTHEMATOSUS

Josef S. Smolen, Winfried B. Graninger,
Andrea Studnicka-Benke and Günter Steiner

Systemic lupus erythematosus (SLE) is a prototype autoimmune disease characterized by B cell hyperactivity which is manifested by the occurrence of autoantibodies and immune complexes leading to multiple clinical changes commonly involving vital organs. Both autoantibody responses as well as clinical manifestations are broad and heterogeneous.[1]

The etiology of SLE is unknown. In particular, the cause of the significant B cell hyperactivity in SLE is still unresolved. It is polyclonal in nature and the production of autoantibodies appears to be antigen driven.[2,3] Moreover, there is a clearcut genetic predisposition in SLE with an important association with genes of the major histocompatibility complex (MHC).[4] However, a "shared" MHC sequence, which has been reported in populations with different ethnic backgrounds suffering from rheumatoid arthritis (RA),[5] has not been found in patients with SLE. Thus, even more clearly than in RA the class II MHC genes associated with SLE may be seen as high responder genes for reactivity to certain autoantigens rather than as "disease-associated genes". This is supported by the fact that SLE patients have a plethora of autoantibodies, that HLA-DR3 is not only commonly found in SLE, but is also associated with many other autoimmune disorders, and that its presence is particularly related to that of certain autoantibodies.[6]

SLE is also associated with HLA class III genes. This is manifested particularly by complement deficiency[7] which may be responsible for the predisposition to impaired elimination of immune complexes.[8] Interestingly, the TNFα genes are also located within the MHC locus;[9] this may have important implications for the production of

---

Cytokines in Autoimmunity, edited by Fionula M. Brennan and Marc Feldmann.
© 1996 R.G. Landes Company.

cytokines in the context of particular immune responses and thus potentially also for SLE disease expression (see below). Moreover, an MHC association is also seen in murine lupus.[9,10]

In human disease, analyses of other genes, particularly immunoglobulin and T cell receptor genes, have not revealed associations or constitutive abnormalities in contrast to murine lupus.[11,12] However, there may be some skewing of Ig variable gene usage in autoimmunity.[2,13] In any case, family studies[14] and studies in inbred mice[15] have clearly shown that SLE must have a polygenic basis.

If the characteristic B cell hyperactivity of SLE is neither "autonomous" nor "constitutive", which are the mechanisms responsible for it? T cells are, of course, important regulators of B cell function. If B cells are hyperactive by virtue of T cell regulation, it must be assumed that T cells themselves have to be highly activated. And in fact, SLE patients commonly have increased numbers of CD4+ helper-type T cells in peripheral blood, and, on the other hand, there may also be suppressor T cell deficiencies.[16,17] Moreover, SLE T cells commonly express activation markers, such as HLA-DR and IL-2R.[18]

T cell hyperactivity could be partly due to increased longevity of T cells, which could be assumed on the basis that the apoptosis-regulating gene *bcl-2* and its product, the Bcl-2 protein, are overexpressed in SLE T cells.[19] This is in accordance with animal models of Bcl-2 transgenic mice in which overexpression of Bcl-2 leads to lupus-like disease,[20] or with the MRL/lpr mouse model of lupus which is associated with a mutation of the apoptosis-mediating *Fas* gene.[21] Thus, dysregulated or delayed apoptosis could be responsible for some of the T cell hyperactivity. However, it is likely that Bcl-2 over-expression is a consequence of immune activation rather than its underlying cause.[19]

A further indication for T cell hyperactivity comes indirectly from the fine analysis of the well known in vitro hyporesponsiveness to mitogens and other stimuli,[22,23] which reveals "exhaustion" in vivo rather than a real deficiency.[24] (Such overstimulation is also seen with lupus B cells: activation in vitro commonly results in reduced Ig-production which is correctable by preincubation of cells in medium;[25] the significant hyperglobulinemia in SLE as well as the significantly increased spontaneous Ig production of SLE B cells in vitro obviously argue against a genuine B cell deficiency of Ig-synthesis.) Thus lupus T cells apparently not only have an activated phenotype, but seem to be hyperactive in vivo.

Activated T helper cells comprise three putative major functional subsets of cells: Th_1 cells which secrete interleukin-2 (IL-2), interferon gamma (IFNγ), lymphotoxin (LT) but not IL-4 or IL-5, Th_2 cells which produce IL-4, IL-5 and IL-10 (but not IFNγ and TNFβ), Th_0 cells which secrete IL-2, IFNγ, IL-4 and IL-5.[26] IL-4 and IL-10 are potent activators of B lymphocytes,[27,28] but IFNγ can also influence B cell activity,[29] as can IL-6.[30]

In recent years, analysis of cytokines in SLE has attracted particular interest, since these messenger peptides are not only characteristic for certain T cell subpopulations, but are involved in the regulation of the immune and the inflammatory response.[27,31] Many cytokines lead to B or T cell activation or differentiation and many activate macrophages or other nonlymphoid cells which are involved in inflammatory responses. Thus, analyses of cytokines in SLE have been the subjects of several studies.

LYMPHOKINES

The lymphocyte-derived cytokines, such as IL-2, IFNγ, IL-4 or IL-10, have effects upon both lymphoid and nonlymphoid cells[26-28] and are partly produced by different T cell subsets, as stated above.

IL-2 physiologically activates T, B and NK cells and induces their proliferation.[27] One of the earliest studies of cytokines in SLE led to the observation of an in vitro IL-2 deficiency in murine and human lupus: upon stimulation with the mitogen Concanavalin A, lymphocytes were deficient in IL-2 production and IL-2 receptor (IL-2R) expression.[32-35] Consecutive investigations in SLE patients revealed that this defect was correctable by the addition of phorbol esters to the culture: stimulation of SLE lymphocytes with concanavalin A plus phorbol myristic acetate (PMA) led to good proliferative responses as well as good IL-2 production.[31,36] Prompted by these observations, this question was analyzed also in experimental SLE: similar results were clearly seen in murine lupus including the mouse strain with the most significant IL-2-deficiency, MRL/lpr.[37] Moreover, resting of lymphocytes in vitro (e.g., by pre-incubation in medium) before addition of mitogens also led to partial correction of the deficiency,[38,39] an observation which again indicated that T cells from both patients and mice with lupus were hyperactivated in vivo. Such in vivo hyperactivity may explain the observed decreased proliferative activity after mitogenic stimulation in vitro, reflecting an in vivo "exhaustion", i.e., an incapacity to respond to further stimulation by strong stimuli which may revert once cells have rested.

Pre-activation of lymphocytes in vivo can not only be concluded from the increased expression of activation markers, but also from the increased ex vivo expression of cytokine and oncogene mRNA in SLE patients' peripheral blood cells[40] (see also below).

The above findings indicate that IL-2 is overproduced in vivo. The importance of IL-2 overproduction in the pathogenesis of SLE is further bolstered by experiments in which IL-2 hyperexpression after transfection of thymectomized nonautoimmune mice with an IL-2 vaccinia virus construct led to autoantibody production and autoimmune disease.[41] Thus, IL-2 apparently has the capability to restore the response of anergic T cells to (auto)antigenic stimuli. Overproduction of IL-2 in MRL-lpr mice leads to improvement of disease due to the maturation of the abnormal, accumulating T cell population characteristic of this strain.[42] In contrast, application of IL-2 to NZB/W mice does not improve the disease at all;[43] in parallel, transfer of a B/W Th$_1$-cell line specific for a self autoantibody-derived peptide accelerated nephritis and enhanced autoantibody production.[44]

These experimental findings are in line with clinical observations that immunotherapy with cytokines such as IL-2 or IFNα or IFNγ can induce autoimmunity and anti-DNA antibodies.[45,46]

The IFNs represent a family of proteins with antiviral and cell growth regulatory activity. However, only IFNγ is produced exclusively by lymphocytes (Th$_0$ and Th$_1$ cells) and NK cells.[26,27] Its effects are dose and time dependent: thus, IFN may inhibit or augment delayed hypersensitivity reactions depending upon the time of antigen application;[47] IFNγ induces MHC I and II expression on macrophages and many other cell types[48] and thus enhances antigen presentation as well as cytotoxic effects. Moreover, IFNs also induce high affinity Fc receptors[49] and influence B cell activity,[29] including that of SLE B cells.[50] Finally, IFN induces production of other cytokines.

In mice, application of interferon accelerated lupus,[51] while anti-interferon antibodies inhibited the disease and prolonged survival in some[52] but not all studies.[53a]

IFNγ (but also IFNα) blood levels are increased in some SLE patients;[40,53b,54] IFNγ levels usually correlated with disease activity (but not vice versa). Similar to interleukin 2, the IFNγ gene also seems to be activated in some SLE patients in vivo,[40] since increases of IFNγ-mRNA could be demonstrated in peripheral blood mononuclear cells ex vivo (Fig. 7.1). Moreover, in man as in experimental animals interferon can exacerbate pre-existing SLE,[55] and IFN may induce de novo SLE.[46]

Interestingly, similarly to IFNγ, application of another cytokine, IL-12, which upregulates IFNγ production in experimental SLE leads to marked acceleration of disease.[56]

Interleukin 4, a Th$_2$-type cytokine, promotes growth of activated B cells and leads to increased MHC class II expression. In some experimental models and some patients with SLE, autoreactive T cell clones produced IL-4;[57,58] nevertheless, the issue of the T cell types operative in systemic autoimmunity has not yet been finally resolved.[58] Moreover, recent studies have revealed relatively normal or only mildly increased serum levels of IL-4 in SLE.[9,60] In an experimental SLE model, Th$_1$ cytokines, particularly IFNγ, were observed early in the course of disease, while Th$_2$ cytokines, particularly IL-4, predominated at later stages (ref. 61 and E. Mozes, personal communication). Moreover, in another systemic autoimmune disease, rheumatoid arthritis, Th$_1$ clones predominated,[62] although Th$_2$ clones were also found.

In contrast to IL-4, IL-10 production was found to be increased in human SLE. However, IL-10 was not produced by T cells but

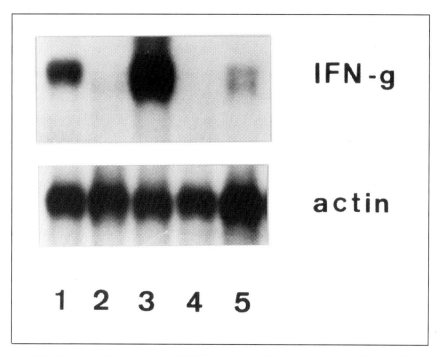

Fig. 7.1. Northern blot analysis of RNA extracted from SLE-PBMC before and after activation with mitogen. Lane 2: healthy control A, before, lane 1: healthy control A, 6 hours after addition of anti-CD3; lanes 4 and 3: healthy control B, otherwise as lanes 2 and 1; lane 5: active SLE patient prior to anti-CD3-stimulation.

rather by the non-T cell populations.[63] IL-10 not only activates B cells, but is also a potent inhibitor of (Th$_1$) cytokine production. It is interesting to note that treatment of NZB/W mice with monoclonal anti-IL-10 antibody resulted in significant suppression of disease,[64] which was accompanied by increased levels of TNFα. Thus, the situation in human as well as experimental SLE is quite complex, and is in some contrast to the cytokine pattern in rheumatoid arthritis (see chapter 2).

Thus, different mechanisms may be operative during disease induction and disease perpetuation. Alternatively, since in the relevant experimental models cytokines or anticytokines are administered already at an early age, maturation of pathogenic cells may be influenced in different ways by these procedures.

Taken together, SLE T cells seem to be activated in vivo which is also indicated by the high degree of oncogene activation observed.[65,40] Moreover, such pre-activation is also compatible with the *bcl-2* gene activation mentioned above,[19,20] since pro-longed activity (or hyperactivity) of T cells is to be expected if pathways of apoptosis are impaired. This is also supported by the observation of upregulation of the apoptosis-1/Fas protein, particularly on CD29-positive (i.e., activated) T cells.[66]

Our own data both on cytokine levels in sera of SLE patients as well as cytokine gene activation in resting and activated cells from SLE patients[40] together with the interpretation of the published findings discussed above are indicative of a Th_0 (or Th_1) predominance in SLE (Table 7.1). Although this issue may not yet have been fully resolved,[58] the subtle increase in IL-4 and the high production of IL-10 (by macrophages, not by T cells!) may be interpreted either as an attempt to counterbalance Th_0/Th_1 hyperactivation (thus being a protective event) or as a secondary pathogenetic mechanism occurring at later stages of disease. The finding of IL-4 producing T cell clones would then not be surprising at all, particularly since such clones have usually been obtained from established rather than early disease.

Thus, the currently available data indicate that T cells are activated and hyperactive in SLE, that they probably belong to the Th_0 or Th_1 rather than the Th_2 population, and that particularly IL-2 and IFNγ may contribute significantly to the pathogenesis.

MONOKINES

Among the major proinflammatory monokines, TNFα constitutes the top of the 'hierarchy', since it induces expression of IL-1 and consequently of IL-6.[67]

In NZB/W mice, a genetic polymorphism of an allele of the TNFα gene was shown to correlate with decreased TNFα production and the presence of nephritis.[68] Effects of TNFα application to experimental animals with lupus appeared to be dose-dependent: in low doses, TNFα led to deterioration of nephritis in NZB/W;[69] in high doses, it improved survival.[70]

Table 7.1. Cytokines and related molecules in SLE

Cytokine	Changes	Remarks
TNFα	++	Important genetic polymorphism?
IL-1	+/-	Exp. LE: high, SLE: low or normal
IL-6	++	Correlation to CRP?
TNF-R55	++	
TNF-R75	+++	Correlation to TNF, IL-6, disease activity
IL-2	+	
IFNγ	++	
IL-4	+/-	
IL-2R	+++	Correlation to disease activity
IL-10	++	Monocyte derived

+, ++, +++, increased by different degrees; +/-, probably normal

High TNFα production may be associated with the B8/DR3 haplotype[68] and among these patients there seems to be a lack of predisposition to develop nephritis. In fact, a base change in the promotor region of TNFα has been found associated with the HLA-A1, B8, DR3 haplotype,[71] which is seen in 40% of SLE patients.[4,6] Cell lines of this haplotype produce higher amounts of TNFα than other cell lines.[72] The particular TNFα allele has also been found associated particularly with the presence of anti-Ro and anti-La antibodies;[68] these autoantibodies have been also found associated with the B8, DR3 haplotype.[6]

In SLE patients serum TNFα levels are commonly increased[73,74] and correlate well with disease activity in our hands.[75] TNF-receptor (TNF-R) levels are also increased and highly correlated to TNFα.[75] Thus, TNF-R also correlates well with disease activity, anti-DNA levels and acute phase responses (Figs. 7.2, 7.3, 7.4). Others have reported that some patients may have reduced TNFα levels in association with the DR2/DQw1 haplotype,[71] and that these patients may be particularly prone to develop nephritis. We have not been able to confirm the association of low TNFα levels with nephritis. Rather TNFα levels in our hands correlated with disease activity and thus were often observed to be high in nephritis patients.[75,76] Nevertheless, polymorphism at the TNFα (and β) locus as well as TNFα production may be involved in the etiology and/or pathogenesis of the disease. Whether as

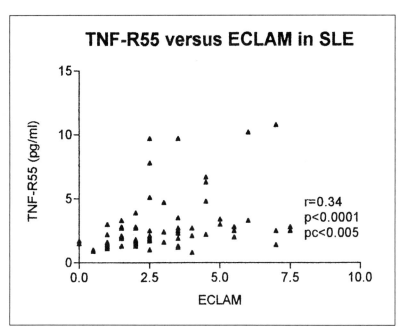

Fig. 7.2. Correlation of TNF-R55 with disease activity according to the ECLAM score.[96] (Pc:P-value corrected for the number of comparisons in the whole study).

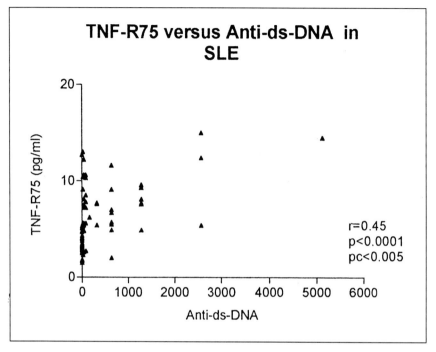

Fig. 7.3. Correlation of TNF-R75 with anti-DNA antibody levels by RIA (in IU/ml).

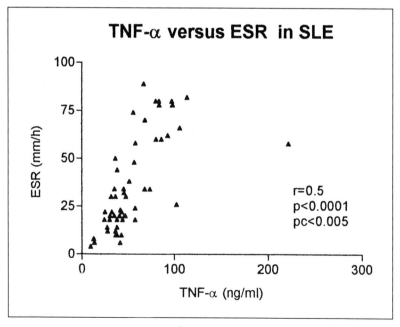

Fig. 7.4. Correlation of TNFα with ESR.

suggested by anti-TNFα therapy, TNFα plays a different role in SLE than in RA,[77] where it is a major therapeutic target, will remain to be proven by future investigations.

The monokines interleukin-1 and interleukin-6 are elevated in murine SLE.[78,79] In contrast, IL-1 has not been found to be increased in human SLE.[31,80,81] However, there may be an association of SLE, particularly discoid lupus and photosensitivity, with a particular allele of the polymorphic IL-1 receptor antagonist gene which is located in the IL-1 gene cluster on chromosome 2.[82]

In addition to TNFα and IL-1, at least in mice, IL-6 levels may also be increased in SLE lupus.[31,83,84] Application of IL-6 to NZB/W mice enhanced the manifestations of this experimental lupus model,[85] whereas anti-IL-6 antibodies suppressed disease in this lupus-prone mouse strain,[86] as did blockade of IL-6-receptors (in MRL/lpr mice) by specific monoclonal antibodies.[87] These studies indicate an important pathogenetic role of IL-6 in SLE.

In the context of SLE, it is of interest that IL-6 is not only a differentiation factor for B and T cells,[30] but also induces proliferation of glomerular mesangial cells.[88] On the other hand, since IL-6, in particular, is a potent inducer of acute phase responses, the observation of increased IL-6 levels in SLE was surprising, since acute phase proteins are rarely increased to a degree[89] that would relate to the increased IL-6 levels observed. Nevertheless, in our patients IL-6 levels correlated with

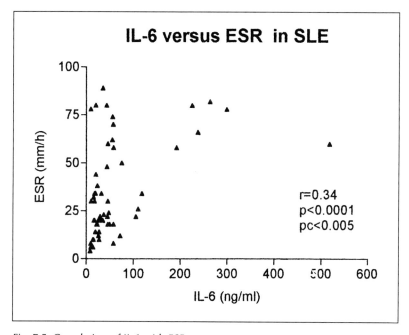

Fig. 7.5. Correlation of IL-6 with ESR.

the acute phase response (Fig. 7.5). However, whether IL-6 levels correlate with the disease course or not remains an issue of debate.

Increased IL-6 levels could explain, at least in part, the increase in B cell precursors readily observed in bone marrow of NZB mice. IL-6 promotes differentiation of B cells into antibody-producing cells and also enhances T cell activation and proliferation;[30] both increased antibody production as well as hyperactive T cells are characteristic of SLE, and, therefore, IL-6 may be of major importance for disease pathogenesis. Its increase in SLE could be involved in the B cell hyperactivity of the disease, potentially even in an autostimulatory manner.[90] In fact, spontaneous IgG production in SLE B lymphocytes is enhanced by addition of IL-6 in vitro,[81] and similar findings have been made in experimental animals even for autoantibodies.[91] Moreover, increased IL-6 levels were not only found in sera, but also in cerebrospinal fluids and kidneys from SLE patients.[92,93] B cells from SLE patients had increased numbers of IL-6-receptors and could be activated in an autocrine manner.[90,94]

The above findings may constitute primary phenomena, but could well represent secondary events due to increased amounts of immune complexes and tissue damage.[84] Tissue damage would include liberation of nucleosomes which may be capable of inducing cytokine production[95] and thus may be one of the potential driving antigenic/activating forces in SLE.

Taken together, the investigations on cytokines in SLE published hitherto have led to several consistent and only a few contradictory observations. These studies have improved our understanding of some of the immunoregulatory abnormalities in SLE. Nevertheless, they do not permit the conclusion that the phenomena observed are primary and not secondary ones. Despite this caveat we can be almost convinced that cytokines do play a major role in the pathogenic events of the disease, even if, maybe, only later in the disease course, perpetuating and augmenting the pathologic events. Moreover, their study has advanced SLE research from one residing at the level of corpuscular-cellular communication less than a decade ago to one involving the molecules responsible for such communication, and it is likely that this research will yield new therapeutic approaches.

Acknowledgment

This study was supported in part by the Austrian Ministry of Health and Consumer Protection.

References

1. Smolen JS. Clinical and serologic features: incidence and diagnostic approach. In: Smolen, Zielinski, eds. Systemic lupus erythematosus—clinical and experimental aspects. Berlin-Heidelberg-New York: Springer Verlag, 1987:170-196.

2. Diamond B, Katz JB, Paul E et al. The role of somatic mutation in the pathogenic anti-DNA response. Ann Rev Immunol 1992; 10:731.
3. Van Venrooij WJ, van Gelder CWG. B cell epitopes on nuclear autoantigens—what can they tell us? Arthritis Rheum 1994; 37:608-616.
4. Reinertsen JL, Klippel JH, Johnson AH et al. B lymphocyte alloantigens associated with systemic lupus erythematosus. N Engl J Med 1978; 299:515-518.
5. Gregersen PK, Silver J, Winchester RJ. The shared epitope hypothesis: an approach to understanding the molecular genetics of susceptibility to rheumatoid arthritis. Arthritis Rheum 1987; 30:1205-1213.
6. Smolen JS, Klippel JH, Penner E et al. HLA-DR antigens in systemic lupus erythematosus: association with specificity of autoantibody responses to nuclear antigens. Ann Rheum Dis 1987; 46:457-462.
7. Carroll MC, Belt KT, Palsdottir A et al. Molecular genetics of the fourth component of human complement and steroid 21-hydroxylase. Immunol Rev 1985; 87:39-60.
8. Frank MM, Hamburger MI, Lawley TJ et al. Defective reticuloendothelial system Fc receptor function in systemic lupus erythematosus. N Engl J Med 1979; 300:518-523.
9. Jacob CO, McDevitt HO. Tumor necrosis factor alpha in murine autoimmune 'lupus' nephritis. Nature 1988; 331:356.
10. Babcock SK, Appel VB, Schiff M et al. Genetic analysis of the imperfect association of H-2 haplotype with lupus-like autoimmune disease. Proc Natl Acad Sci USA 1989; 86:7552.
11. Kofler R, Dixon FJ, Theofilopoulos AN. The genetic origin of autoantibodies. Immunol today 1987; 80:374.
12. Mountz JD, Smith TM, Toth KS. Altered expression of self-reactive T cell receptor Vβ regions in autoimmune mice. J Immunol 1990; 144:2159.
13. Singer PA, Theofilopoulos AN. T cell receptor Vβ repertoire expression in murine models of SLE. Immunol Rev 1990; 118:103.
14. Arnett FC, Reveille JD, Wilson RW et al. Systemic lupus erythematosus: current state of the genetic hypothesis. Semin Arthritis Rheum 1984; 14:24-35.
15. Raveche ES, Novotny EA, Hansen CT et al. Genetic studies in NZB mice: V. Recombinant inbred lines demonstrate that separate genes control autoimmune phenotype. J Exp Med 1981; 153:1187-1197.
16. Smolen JS, Chused TM, Leiserson WM et al. Heterogeneity of immunoregulatory T cell subsets. Correlation with clinical features. Am J Med 1982; 72:783-790.
17. Sakane T, Steinberg AD, Green I. Studies of immune functions of patients with SLE: I. Dysfunction of suppressor T cells related to impaired generation of, rather than response to, suppressor cells. Arthritis Rheum 1978; 21:657-664.
18. Yu DTY, Winchester RJ, Fu SM. Peripheral blood Ia positive T cells: increases in certain diseases and after immunizaion. J Exp Med 1980; 151:91-100.

19. Aringer M, Wintersberger W, Steiner CW et al. Circulating T- but not B-cells contain high levels of bcl-2 protein in systemic lupus erythematosus. Arthritis Rheum 1994; 37:1423-1430.
20. Strasser H, Whittingham S, Vaux DL et al. Enforced bcl-2 expression in B-lymphoid cells prolongs antibody responses and elicits autoimmune diseases. Proc Natl Acad Sci USA 1991; 88:8661-8665.
21. Watanabe-Fukunaga R, Brannan CI, Copeland NG et al. Lymphoproliferative disorder in mice explained by defects in Fas antigen that mediates apoptosis. Nature 1992; 356:314-317.
22. Tsokos GC. Overview of cellular immune function in systemic lupus erythematosus. In: Lahita G, ed. Systemic lupus erythematosus. 2nd ed. New York: Churchill Livingston, 1992:13-48.
23. Sakane TA, Steinberg AD, Green I. Failure of autologous mixed lymphocyte reactions between T and non-T cells in patients with systemic lupus erythematosus. Proc Natl Acad Sci USA 1978; 75:135-142.
24. Huang YP, Perrin LH, Miescher PA et al. Correlation of T and B cell activities in vitro and serum IL-2 levels in systemic lupus erythematosus. J Immunol 1988; 141:827.
25. Beale MG, Nash GS, Bertovich MJ et al. Similar disturbance in B cell activity and regulatory T cell function in Henoch-Schönlein purpura and systemic lupus erythematosus. J Immunol 1982; 28:486-491.
26. Romagnani S. Human Th_1 and Th_2 subsets: doubt no more. Immunol today 1991; 12:256.
27. Oppenheim JJ, Rossio J, Gearing AJH. Clinical applications of cytokines: role in diagnosis, pathogenesis and therapy. Oxford Univeristy Press, 1993.
28. Biere F, Servet-Deprat C, Bridon JM et al. Human interleukin 10 induces naive surface immunoglobulin D+ (sIgD+) B cells to secrete IgG1 and IgG3. J Exp Med 1994; 179:757-762.
29. Sonnenfeld G. Modulation of immunity by interferon. In: Pick E, ed. Lymphokine Reports, Vol 1. New York: Academic Press, 113-131.
30. Van Snick J. Interleukin 6: an overview. Annu Rev Immunol 1990; 8:253.
31. Luger TA, Smolen JS. The role of lymphokines in the pathogenesis of systemic lupus erythematosus. In: Smolen JS, Zielinski CC, eds. Systemic lupus erythematosus—clinical and experimental aspects. Berlin-Heidelberg-New York: Springer Verlag, 1987:145-167.
32. Wofsy D, Murphy ED, Rothe JB et al. Deficient Interleukin 2 activity in MRL/Mp and C57BL/6J mice bearing the lpr gene. J Exp Med 1981; 154:1671-1680.
33. Altman A, Theofilopoulos AN, Weiner R et al. Analysis of T cell function in autoimmune murine strains. J Exp Med. 1981; 154:791-808.
34. Alcocer Varela J, Alarcon Segovia D. Decreased production of and response to interleukin-2 by cultured lymphocytes from patients with systemic lupus erythematosus. J Clin Invest 1983; 69:1388-1392.
35. Murakawa Y, Takada S, Ueda Y et al. Characterization of T lymphocyte subpopulations responsible for deficient interleukin 2 activity in patients with systemic lupus erythematosus. J Immunol 1985; 134:187-195.

36. Smolen JS, Luger TA (unpublished observations).
37. Santoro TJ, Luger TA, Ravache ES et al. In vitro correction of the interleukin 2 defect of autoimmune mice. Eur J Immunol 1983; 13:601-604.
38. Santoro TJ, Malek TR, Rosenberg YJ et al. Signals required for activation and growth of autoimmune T lymphocytes. J Mol Cell Immunol 1984; 1:347-356.
39. Huang YP, Miescher PA, Zubler RH. The interleukin 2 secretion defect in vitro in systemic lupus erythematosus is reversible in rested cultured T cells. J Immunol 1986; 137:3515.
40. Graninger W, Graninger P, Aschauer B et al. Oncogene and cytokine gene expression in peripheral blood of patients with connective tissue diseases (abstr.) Clin Rheumatol 1989; 8:36.
41. Andreu-Sanchez JL, Alboran IM, Mareos MAR et al. Interleukin 2 abrogates the nonresponsive state of T cells expressing forbidden T cell receptor repertoire and induces autoimmune disease in neonatally thymectomized mice. J Exp Med 1991; 173:1323.
42. Gutierrez-Ramos JC, Andreu JL, Revilla Y et al. Recovery from autoimmunity of MRL/lpr mice after infection with an interleukin-2/vaccinia recombinant virus. Nature 1990; 346:271-274.
43. Owen KL, Shibata T, Izui S et al. Recombinant interleukin-2 therapy of systemic lupus erythematosus in the New Zealand black/New Zealand white mouse. J Biol Response Mod 1989; 8:366-374.
44. Singh RR, Ebling FM, Sercarz EE et al. Self autoantibody-derived T cell determinants upregulate autoimmunity in murine SLE (abstr.). Lupus 1995; 4:48.
45. Atkins MB, Mier JW, Parkinson DR et al. Hypothyroidism after treatment with interleukin 2 and lymphokine activated killer cells. New Engl J Med 1988; 318:1557-561.
46. Graninger WB, Hassfeld W, Pesau BB et al. Induction of systemic lupus erythematosus by interferon-gamma in a patient with rheumatoid arthritis. J Rheumatol 1991; 18:1621-1622.
47. De Maeyer E, De Maeyer-Guignard J. Effects of interferon on sensitization and expression of delayed hypersensitivity in the mouse. In: De Weck AL, ed. Biochemical characterization of lymphokines. New York: Academic Press, 1980:383-391.
48. Sztein MB, Steeg PS, Johnson HM et al. Regulation of human peripheral blood monocyte DR antigen expression by lymphokines and recombinant interferons. J Clin Invest 1984; 73:556-565.
49. Fridman WH, Gesser I, Bandu MT et al. Interferon enhances the expression of Fc-receptors. J Immunol 1980; 124:2436-2441.
50. Funauchi M, Sugishima H, Minoda M et al. Effect of interferon-gamma on B lymphocytes of patients with systemic lupus erythematosus. J Rheumatol 1991; 18:368-372.
51. Adam C, Thoua Y, Ronco P et al. The effect of exogenous interferon: acceleration of autoimmune and renal disease in NZB/W F1 mice. Clin Exp Immunol 1980; 40:373-382.

52. Gresser I, Morel-Maroger L, Verroust P. Anti-interferon inhibits the development of glomerulonephritis in mice infected at birth with lymphocytic choriomeningitis virus. Proc Natl Acad Sci USA 1978; 75:3413-3416.
53a. Jacob CO, van der Meide PH, McDevitt HO. In vivo treatment of (NZBxNZW)F1 lupus-like nephritis with monoclonal antibody to γ interferon. J Exp Med 1987; 166:798-809.
53b. Hooks JJ, Jordan GW, Cupps T et al. Multiple interferons in systemic lupus erythematosus and vasculitis. Arthritis Rheum 1982; 25:396-400.
54. Kim T, Kanayama Y, Negoro N et al. Serum levels of interferons in patients with systemic lupus erythematosus. Clin Exp Immunol 1987; 70:562-569.
55. Machold, KP, Smolen JS. Interferon-γ induced exacerbation of systemic lupus erythematosus. J Rheumatol 1990; 17:831-832.
56. Mittleman BB, Shearer GM, Payne S, Wolf S, Mozes E. Treatment of experimental LE with recombinant murine IL-12 (abstr.). Lupus 1995; 4:7.
57. Ando DG, Sercarz EE, Hahn BH. Mechanisms of T and B cell collaboration in the in vitro production of anti-DNA antibodies in the NZB/NZW F1 murine SLE model. J Immunol 1987; 138:3185.
58. Romagnani S. Lymphokine production by human T cells in disease states. Annu Rev Immunol 1994; 12:227-257.
59. Al Janadi M, Al Wabel A, Raziuddin S. Soluble CD23 and interleukin-4 levels in autoimmune chronic active hepatitis and systemic lupus erythematosus. Clin Immunol Immunopathol 1994; 71:33-37.
60. Al Janadi M, Raziuddin S. B cell hyperactivity is a function of T cell derived cytokines in systemic lupus erythematosus. J Rheumatol 1993; 20:1885-189.
61. Segal R, Dayan M, Zinger H et al. Methotrexate treatment in murine experimental SLE. Clinical benefits associated with cytokine manipulation (abstr.). Lupus 1995; 4:69.
62. Quayle AJ, Chomarat P, Miossec P et al. Rheumatoid inflammatory T-cell clones express mostly Th_1 but also Th_2 and mixed (Th_0-like) cytokine patterns. Scand J Immunol 1993; 38:75-82.
63. Llorente L, Richaud-Patin Y, Fior R et al. In vivo production of interleukin-10 by nonTcells in rheumatoid arthritis, Sjögren's syndrome and systemic lupus erythematosus. Arthritis Rheum 1994; 37:1647-1655.
64. Ishida H, Muchamuel T, Sakaguchi S et al. Continuous administration of anti-interleukin 10 antibodies delays onset of autoimmunity in NZB/W F1 mice. J Exp Med 1994; 179:305-315.
65. Mountz JD, Mushinski JF, Mark GE et al. Oncogene expression in autoimmune mice. J Mol Cell Immunol 1985; 2:121-131.
66. Mysler E, Bini P, Drappa J et al. The apoptosis-1/Fas protein in human systemic lupus erythematosus. J Clin Invest 1994; 93:1029-1034.
67. Dinarello CA, Cannon JG, Wolff SM et al. Tumor necrosis factor (cachectin) is an endogeneous pyrogen and induces production of interleukin 1. J Exp Med 1986; 163:1433.

68. Jacob CO, Lewis GD, McDevitt HO. MHC class II-associated variation in the production of tumor necrosis factor in mice and humans: relevance to the pathogenesis of autoimmune diseases. Immunol Res 1991; 10:156.
69. Brennan DC, Yui MA, Wuthrich RP et al. Tumor necrosis factor and IL-1 in New Zealand Black/White mice. J Immunol 1989; 143:34-40.
70. Jacob CO, Mc Devitt HO. Tumour necrosis factor-α in murine autoimmune 'lupus' nephritis. Nature 1988; 331:356-358.
71. Jacob CO, Fronek Z, Lewis GD et al. Heritable major histocompatibility complex class II-associated differences in production of tumor necrosis factor α: relevance to genetic predisposition of systemic lupus erythematosus. Proc Natl Acad Sci USA 1990; 87:1233.
72. Jongeneel CV, Briant L, Udalova IA et al. Extensive genetic polymorphism in the human tumor necrosis factor region and relation to extended HLA haplotypes. Proc Natl Acad Sci USA 1991; 88:9717.
73. Maury CPJ, Teppo A-M. Tumor necrosis factor in the serum of patients with systemic lupus erythematosus. Arthritis Rheum 1989; 32:146-150.
74. Meijer C, Huysen V, Smeenk RT et al. Profiles of cytokines (TNF alpha and IL-6) and acute phase proteins (CRP and alpha1 AG) related to the disease course in patients with systemic lupus erythematosus. Lupus 1993; 2:359-365.
75. Studnicka-Benke A, Steiner G, Höfler E et al. Cytokines in SLE: levels of IL-6, IFN-γ, TNFα and TNF-receptor (TNF-R) fluctuate in the course of disease (abstr.). Arthritis Rheum 1993; 36:S196.
76. Studnicka-Benke A, Steiner G, Petera P et al. TNFα and its soluble 55kD and 75kD receptors parallel clinical disease and autoimmune activity in systemic lupus erythematosus. (Submitted).
77. Maini RN, Elliott MJ, Charles PJ et al. Immunological intervention reveals reciprocal roles for tumor necrosis factor-α and interleukin-10 in rheumatoid arthritis and systemic lupus erythematosus. Springer Semin Immunopathol 1994; 16:327-336.
78. Brennan DC, Yui MA, Wutrich RP et al. Tumor necrosis factor and IL-1 in New Zealand Black/White mice—enhanced expression and acceleration of renal injury. J Immunol 1989; 143:3470.
79. Boswell JM, Yui MA, Endress S et al. Novel and enhanced IL-1 gene expression in autoimmune mice with lupus. J Immunol 1988; 141:118.
80. Alcocer-Varela J, Alarcon Segovia D. Defective monocyte production of, and T lymphocyte response to, interleukin-1 in the peripheral blood of patients with systemic lupus erythematosus. Clin Exp Immunol 1983; 54:125-132.
81. Linker-Israeli M, Bakke AC, Kitridou RC et al. Defective production of interleukin 1 and interleukin 2 in patients with systemic lupus erythematosus (SLE). J Immunol 1983; 130:2651-2655.
82. Blakemore AIF, Tarlow JK, Cork MJ et al. Interleukin-1 receptor antagonist gene polymorphism as a disease severity factor in systemic lupus erythematosus. Arthritis Rheum 1994; 37:1380-1385.

83. Linker-Israeli M, Deans RJ, Wallace DJ et al. Elevated levels of endogenous IL-6 in systemic lupus erythematosus: a putative role in pathogenesis. J Immunol 1991; 147:117-123.
84. Spronk PE, Borg EJ, Limburg PC et al. Plasma concentration of IL-6 in systemic lupus erythematosus; an indicator of disease activity? Clin Exp Immunol 1992; 90:106-110.
85. Ryffel B, Car BD, Gunn H et al. Interleukin-6 exacerbates glomerulonephritis in (NZBxNZW)F1 mice. Am J Pathol 1994; 144:927-937.
86. Finck BK, Chan B, Wofsy D. Interleukin 6 promotes murine lupus in NZB/NZW F1 mice. J Clin Invest 1994; 94:585-591.
87. Kiberd BA. Interleukin-6 receptor blockade ameliorates murine lupus nephritis. J Am Soc Nephrol 1993; 4:58-61.
88. Horii Y, Muraguchi A, Iwano M et al. Involvement of IL-6 in mesangial proliferative glomerulonephritis. J Immunol 1989; 143:3949.
89. Becker GJ, Waldburger M, Hughes GRV et al. Value of C-reactive protein measurements in the investigation of fever in systemic lupus erythematosus. Ann Rheum Dis 1980; 39:50-52.
90. Kitani A, Hara M, Hirose T et al. Autostimulatory effects of IL-6 on excessive B cell differentiation in patients with systemic lupus erythematosus: analysis of IL-6 production and IL-6R expression. Clin Exp Immunol 1992; 88:75-83.
91. Alarcon-Riquelme ME, Möller G, Fernandez C. Age-dependent responsiveness to interleukin-6 in B lymphocytes from a systemic lupus erythematosus-prone (NZBxNZW)F1 hybrid. Clin Immunol Immunopathol 1992; 62:264-269.
92. Hirohata S, Miyamoto T. Elevated levels of interleukin-6 in cerberospinal fluid from patients with systemic lupus erythematosus and central nervous system involvement. Arthritis Rheum 1989; 33:644-649.
93. Alcoder-Varela J, Aleman-Joey D, Alarcon Segovia D. Interleukin-1 and interleukin-6 activities are increased in the cerebrospinal fluid of patients with CNS lupus erythematosus and correlate with local late T-cell activation markers. Lupus 1992; 1:111-117.
94. Nagafuchi H, Suzuki N, Mizushima Y et al. Constitutive expression of IL-6 receptors and their role in the excessive B cell function in patients with systemic lupus erythematosus. J Immunol 1993; 151:6525-6534.
95. Hefeneider SH, Cornell KA, Brown LE et al. Nucleosomes and DNA bind to specific cell-surface molecules on murine cells and induce cytokine production. Clin Immunol Immunopathol 1992; 63:245-251.
96. Vitali C, Bencivelli W, Isenberg DA et al. Identification of the variables indicative of disease activity and their use in the development of an activity score. Clin Exp Rheumatol 1992; 10:541-548.

CHAPTER 8

SCLERODERMA

Carol M. Black and Christopher P. Denton

INTRODUCTION

Systemic sclerosis (scleroderma; SSc) is a clinically heterogeneous connective tissue disease with a variety of clinical subtypes. The systemic form of the disorder is uncommon, with a prevalence of approximately 10 cases per million in the United Kingdom and has a female predisposition.[1] There are pathological similarities between SSc and localized scleroderma disorders. The most widely used classification of the scleroderma spectrum disorders is shown in Table 8.1.[2] Clinical discrimination between the limited and diffuse cutaneous subtypes (lcSSc and dcSSc respectively) is by the extent of skin sclerosis. In the diffuse form of the disease, skin involvement extends widely over the limbs and trunk whereas in lcSSc involvement is generally confined to the extremities, face and neck. Other clinical manifestations also vary between these different forms of disease; for example vascular abnormalities and Raynaud's phenomenon are often more prominent in lcSSc, whereas severe renal involvement or pulmonary fibrosis are typically seen in the more severe cases of dcSSc.[3] Also, the clinical course of lcSSc is generally more protracted than dcSSc, often with Raynaud's symptoms preceding skin disease by many years. Whether the pathogenetic processes in these different forms are similar is uncertain but the pathological hallmarks of tissue fibrosis, immunological abnormalities and endothelial cell activation and damage are common to both subsets.[4] Some of the autoantibodies occurring in SSc are specific for different disease subsets, for example anti-topoisomerase-1 (Scl-70) and anti-RNA polymerase antibodies are typically associated with diffuse cutaneous SSc. In contrast, anti-centromere antibody occurs in localized cutaneous SSc,[5] previously termed CREST syndrome.

Crosstalk between cells is likely to be central to SSc pathogenesis in view of the range of pathological features involving different cell types; consequently most hypotheses of etiopathogenesis focus on the interplay between early immunological and inflammatory events and the later

---

Cytokines in Autoimmunity, edited by Fionula M. Brennan and Marc Feldmann.
© 1996 R.G. Landes Company.

Table 8.1. Classification of the systemic sclerosis subsets

1. **"Pre-Scleroderma"**
   Raynaud's phenomenon plus nailfold capillary changes, disease specific circulating antinuclear autoantibodies, (antitopoisomerase-I, anticentromere (ACA), or nucleolar), and digital ischemic changes.

2. **Diffuse cutaneous SSc (dcSSc)**
   Onset of skin changes (puffy or hidebound) within 1 year of onset of Raynaud's
   Truncal and acral skin involvement
   Presence of tendon friction rubs
   Early and significant incidence of interstitial lung disease, oliguric renal failure, diffuse gastrointestinal disease, and myocardial involvement
   Nailfold capillary dilatation and drop out
   Anti-topoisomerase-I (Scl-70) antibodies (30% of patients)

3. **Limited cutaneous SSc (lcSSc)**
   Raynaud's for years (occasionally decades)
   Skin involvement limited to hands, face, feet and forearms (acral)
   A significant (10-15 %) late incidence of pulmonary hypertension, with or without interstitial lung disease, skin calcification, telangiectasiae and gastrointestinal involvement
   A high incidence of ACA (70-80%)
   Dilated nailfold capillary loops, usually without capillary dropout.

4. **Scleroderma sine scleroderma**
   Raynaud's +/-
   No skin involvement
   Presentation with pulmonary fibrosis, scleroderma renal crisis, cardiac or gastrointestinal disease
   Antinuclear antibodies may be present (Scl70, ACA, nucleolar)

generation of a population of activated fibrogenic fibroblasts, which are generally regarded as the effector cells in the disease.[6] There is considerable evidence that the vascular and endothelial (EC) changes precede other disease features. Firstly endothelial damage has been observed in early skin disease;[7] also in the lung, bowel and kidney in SSc there is ultrastructural EC damage early in disease before abnormalities can be detected by light microscopy.[8-10] Moreover, recent studies of endothelial cell phenotype in SSc have demonstrated an increase in EC surface expression of adhesion molecules including E-selectin, VCAM-1 and ICAM-1 in clinically "yet to be involved" skin suggesting that EC activation is one of the earliest disease events.[11] Immunological abnormalities in SSc include an early inflammatory infiltrate of mononuclear cells in affected tissues. The majority of these cells express differentiation markers of activated T lymphocytes, including CD3, CD4, CD45, HLA-DR and LFA-1.[12] Also notable in SSc is the occurrence of a range of autoantibodies including many directed against chromatin components including anti-topoisomerase-1, anti-RNA polymerase and anti-centromere antibodies. The role, if any, of these antibodies in disease pathogenesis is still debated,[13] although they do appear to correlate with certain clinical features as outlined above. Further clues to immune processes operating in SSc are the reportedly increased T cell reactivity against collagen antigens in vitro and the elevated serum levels of the immunologically active lymphocyte products IL-2 and IL-4 in some SSc patients.[14]

Much research effort has been directed towards elucidating fibroblast properties in SSc in view of the apparently pivotal role of this cell in fibrotic processes. Early reports of enhanced production of extracellular matrix components by dermal SSc fibroblasts in vitro, including collagen types I and III,[15] have been widely confirmed.[16-18] One of the intriguing properties of such cells, which are summarized in Table 8.2, is the persistence of their abnormal phenotype over several passages in conventional tissue culture.[19] Ultimately dermal fibroblasts in SSc appear to revert to a more typical phenotype and this has led to the hypothesis that cells in vivo and early passage in vitro are exposed to stimuli which are absent from later cultures.[20]

Cellular interactions in SSc are likely to include paracrine and autocrine pathways between the cell types listed in Table 8.3. Also important in regulating cell properties are their interactions with the extracellular matrix (ECM). It has been shown that extracellular matrix interactions influence cytokine responsiveness and that in turn ECM interactions can be themselves modulated by exogenous cytokines and growth factors.[21] Thus, it seems increasingly likely that a number of cytokines and growth factors are central to SSc pathogenesis and that they might also be future possible targets for therapeutic attack in this potentially lethal condition. With these points in mind some aspects of cytokine biology relevant to SSc will now be considered, followed by a review of the current evidence implicating individual mediators in scleroderma pathogenesis.

CELLULAR SOURCES FOR CYTOKINES IN THE PATHOGENESIS OF SSC

The case for cytokines and other paracrine factors being important in SSc pathogenesis has been strengthened considerably in recent

Table 8.2. Characteristic properties of SSc dermal fibroblasts in tissue culture

Property	References
Increased:	
collagen I and III production mRNA and protein	15, 16
proteoglycan synthesis	4
prolyl and lysyl hydroxylase enzyme activity	20
PDGF receptor expression	59, 66
cytokine production (see Table 8.4)	20, 26, 35, 38
serum independent proliferation	30
Reduced:	
collagen (I) mRNA downregulation in collagen gel matrix culture	23
collagenase production	97

years by the realization that most of the cell types implicated in disease development, including the endothelial cell (EC) and the fibroblast are, when appropriately activated, capable of producing a range of such factors as outlined in Table 8.3. Previously it had been assumed that inflammatory cells and lymphocytes were the major source of paracrine factors in this disease. The ability of fibroblasts and endothelial cells to produce and release cytokines or to mobilize growth factors such as bFGF from the extracellular matrix[22] raises the possibility of reciprocal paracrine interactions between these cell types which might be central to disease pathogenesis. It is hypothesized that autocrine or paracrine loops of cytokines may be responsible for the generation and/or persistence of the abnormal SSc fibroblast phenotype. Some of the possible interactions between these cell types are illustrated in Figure 8.1. Different loops may operate at different stages of the disease or in its various clinical subsets. A number of research groups are currently investigating such processes in SSc in a variety of culture systems.[23,24]

CYTOKINE MEDIATED MODULATION OF CELL-CELL CONTACT IN SSC

Another potentially important role of cytokines in SSc, in addition to their direct cellular effects and influences on fibroblast-ECM interactions is through their ability to modulate cell-cell interaction. The role of proinflammatory cytokines such as IL-1 and TNFα in enhancing leucocyte adhesion to EC and subsequent extravasation has been clearly shown,[25] and the presence of activated EC in SSc lesions[26] is indirect evidence of the relevance to such factors to the disease. Studies by Abraham and others[27] have demonstrated that SSc fibroblasts bind lymphocytes in vitro and have suggested that this system can be used as a model for cellular interaction in vitro. ICAM-1, a cytokine inducible member of the immunoglobulin superfamily of adhesion molecules has been identified as the major ligand responsible for the enhanced lymphocyte binding by such fibroblasts through its interaction with the LFA-1 counter-receptor.[28] Recently IL-1, TNFα and IFNγ have been shown to augment the expression of ICAM-1 by SSc fibroblasts.[29]

Table 8.3. Potential cellular sources for cytokines implicated in SSc pathogenesis

Cell Type	Major Cytokine Products
Immune cells/inflammatory	
monocyte/macrophage	IL-1, TNFα
lymphocytes	IL-2,-4,-6,-8
mast cells/neutrophils/eosinophils	bFGF
Endothelial cells	
activated/damaged	IL-1, IL-6, IL-8, IGF-1, PDGF, TGF, ET-1, bFGF
Fibroblasts	
SSc fibroblasts	TNFα, IL-1, IL-6, PDGF, TGF

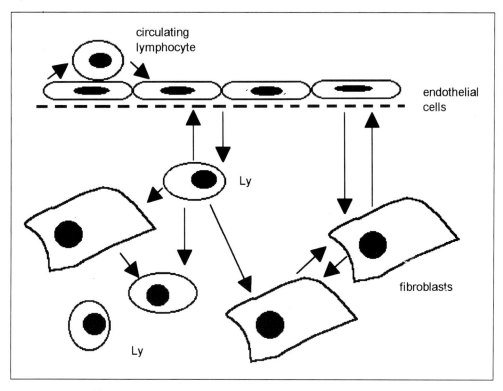

Fig. 8.1. Potential loops of paracrine interaction between cells involved in scleroderma pathogenesis Activated cells of the immune system (Ly), endothelial cells and fibroblasts are all capable of releasing cytokines and growth factors which might exert a paracrine or autocrine influence on other cells. This could in turn modulate celluar properties and induce production of the same or other factors. Thus, there is the potential for local cytokine loops to initiate and perpetuate the immunological, vascular and fibrotic components of scleroderma pathology. Candidate mediators are listed in Table 8.3 and potential autocrine mechanisms for fibroblast stimulation described in more detail in Figure 8.2.

DIRECT EVIDENCE FOR THE ROLE OF CYTOKINES IN THE INITIATION OR MAINTENANCE OF THE SSC FIBROBLAST PHENOTYPE

Many groups have investigated the possible paracrine factors which might initiate or maintain the typical SSc fibroblast phenotype. Early work by LeRoy and others[30] focused on the inherent ability of SSc cells to grow well in low serum environments and their reduced responsiveness to exogenous PDGF. These findings were rationalized by the demonstration that SSc fibroblasts themselves secrete PDGF, thereby rendering them less sensitive to the exogenous growth factors.[31] Interestingly this group and other workers have shown that there is considerable enhancement of the fibroblast mitogenic response to other mediators including PDGF, IL-6 and endothelin-1, a vasoactive peptide product of endothelial cells by TGFβ.[32] The marked matrix stimulatory properties of the transforming growth factors, particularly TGFβ, have fueled interest in these factors as candidate cytokines in SSc. TGFβ can be readily demonstrated immunohistochemically in involved skin in SSc in early but not late disease.[33] However, attempts to induce long term enhancement of collagen I production by fibroblasts by regular pulsed exposure to TGFβ have failed,[34] as have attempts to demonstrate coordinate regulation of collagen I and TGFβ by SSc fibroblasts. More recently interest has been directed to the production and regulation of the cytokines IL-6 and IL-1 by SSc fibroblasts. Feghali and others have shown that SSc cells produce much more IL-6 than controls and that this constitutes one of the soluble mitogenic factors transferable in culture medium derived from such cells.[35,36] Enhancement of IL-6 production occurs through the binding of nucleoproteins to the promoter region of the IL-6 gene.[37] IL-1α is also produced excessively by SSc fibroblasts at the mRNA and protein level[38] and has been proposed to act as a autocrine or paracrine stimulus, contributing to their abnormal properties in culture. It seems likely that interplay between a number of cytokines and growth factors will be found to underly pathogenesis in SSc, perhaps acting sequentially at different stages of the disease.[39] Some possible autocrine networks are illustrated in Figure 8.2.

CIRCULATING CYTOKINES AND ADHESION MOLECULES IN SSC

Increased levels of circulating IL-1, IL-2, IL-2R, IL-4, IL-8, TNFα and interferon have been found in scleroderma and antibodies to IL-6 and IL-8 reported.[40,41] Although it is now generally accepted that investigation of cytokine levels can provide useful additional information about the pathogenesis of disease, the presence of a cytokine at high level does not necessarily indicate a pathogenic role: in addition, it has become clear that interpretation of these studies is dependent upon the assay used (bio- or immunoassay) and a realization of the many factors which interfere within each system. Immunoassays for example are particularly limited, in that they give little information regarding levels of biologically active protein, whereas bioassays are not cytokine specific, cytokine inhibitors may interfere with cytokine bioactivity and the assays are labor intensive and lack reproducibility. Bearing in mind these reservations, the short half-lifes of many of the cytokines and the discrepancies between some of the studies, the increased levels of the various cytokines supports a cellular immune mechanism in scleroderma, and an ongoing expansion of T cells and the secreted products, by their well-defined actions, may modulate fibrosis or promote vascular damage. The presence of antibodies to some of the cytokines may add a further dimension, for not only may they inhibit the biological function of the molecule, but paradoxically they might enhance cytokine function, prolong its half-life and deliver the cytokine to its target cell. Again, it is pertinent to remember that because the effect of any given cytokine will be influenced by other cytokines present in the micro-environment, the pattern of cytokines may be more important than any individual member,

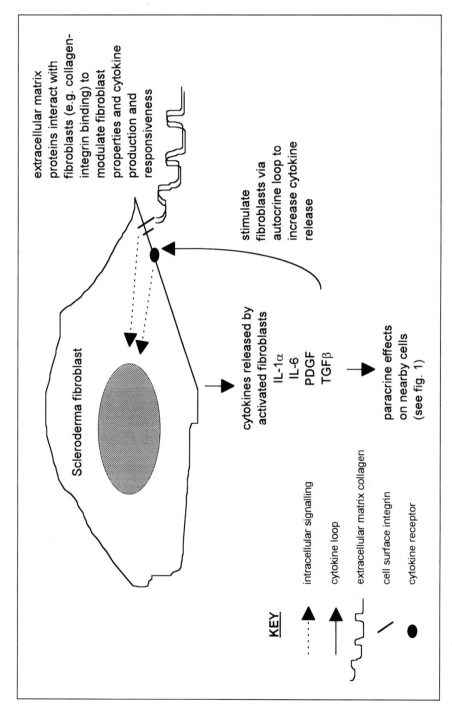

Fig. 8.2. Schematic representation of potential autocrine regulatory loops modulating fibroblast properties
There is considerable evidence (see text) supporting the hypothesis that fibroblast properties are regulated by events at the cell surface, involving both soluble cytokines (through receptor-ligand interactions) and the interaction between fibroblasts and extracellular matrix components (e.g. collagen I engagement by β1 integrins). Since activated fibroblasts produce increased amounts of cytokines (e.g. IL-1, IL-6) and matrix components, and may also up-regulate a number of cell surface receptor molecules, there is considerable potential for autocrine stimulation of fibroblast properties. Interplay between these regulatory events is likely to occur within the complex intracellular signalling pathways linking cell surface events with regulation of gene transcription, but these processes remain poorly understood.

and it must be borne in mind that the soluble cytokines are not exclusive to systemic sclerosis. However, their presence and known interactions may provide clues to the correct cell types and relevant tissues involved in disease development.

Cell surface adhesion molecules including ICAM-1, VCAM-1 and E-selectin are upregulated by cytokines and are present in soluble forms in serum and biological fluids.[42] Elevated levels of circulating adhesins sICAM-1, sVCAM-1 and sE-selectin have been observed in SSc and other inflammatory conditions.[43,44] Their precise significance is uncertain, as is any possible in vivo role[45] but in vitro studies suggest that they might correlate with cytokine induced activation of cell types expressing these molecules. It is hoped that such adhesins may be useful surrogate markers of disease processes in SSc and the results of preliminary studies are encouraging.[46]

THERAPEUTIC IMPLICATIONS

There is currently no curative treatment for SSc, although new potential therapies are currently being evaluated and many agents are already being used, based on largely anecdotal information regarding their efficacy. These include the antifibrotic drugs such as D-penicillamine and interferon-α and immunosuppressive agents such as cyclophosphamide, cyclosporin or methotrexate. Vasoactive drugs such as prostacyclin and prostaglandin infusions are also used to treat vasospasm associated with SSc. Different pathogenetic factors are likely to be important at different stages of the disease; also, different subsets may involve different mechanisms. Targeted attack on relevant cytokines would be appealing and might perhaps be most appropriate during the early inflammatory stage of diffuse SSc, but is likely to be difficult because:

1. No single mediator central to pathogenesis which might be targeted has yet been identified.
2. Diagnosis of dcSSc is late, often after the first 18 months of disease when such targeted treatment is likely to be most effective.
3. Cascades of mediators with redundant or duplicated pathways probably exist and so effective, prolonged cytokine antagonism may be difficult to achieve.

Agents which suppress cytokine production, including some of the newer immunosuppressive drugs, are probably more likely to be effective than antibody treatments because of the problems of high antibody doses for neutralization, the potential for anticytokine antibodies to potentiate cytokine activities and potential problems with excessive cytokine removal (e.g., infection). Also, the progressive nature of established SSc suggests that prolonged inhibition of effector pathways would be essential to success. In diffuse SSc the reported benefits from treatment with antithymocyte globulin[47] support the view that immunosuppression, with the consequent reduction in lymphocyte derived cytokines, may be helpful. New, more specific, anticytokine agents are eagerly awaited by those engaged in the management of patients suffering from this difficult connective tissue disease.

SUMMARY OF THE EVIDENCE FOR A ROLE OF INDIVIDUAL CYTOKINES IN SSC

TGFβ

Of the cytokines capable of regulating the synthesis of the extracellular matrix and affecting endothelial cell function, TGFβ has undoubtedly received the most attention in SSc. Its theoretical potential in this disease is considerable, but despite this, studies of skin biopsies, bronchoalveolar lavage (BAL) and blood samples for measurement of TGFβ mRNA and protein have yielded inconsistent and conflicting results. This may be because these studies have used different SSc populations: both patients with diffuse and limited disease have been included. Biopsies have been taken at different times of the disease—lesional and nonlesional skin have been used from various sites of the body and the rate of progression of the condition has been yet another variable. There may also be methodological or reagent differences. These several factors make exact comparison of results very difficult. It is still not known whether the growth factor acts at a very early stage of the disease and loses its effect with chronicity, (although the literature would support this concept), whether its effects vary in extent from organ to organ and whether it acts alone, or more likely, in concert with other cytokines. In addition, and most importantly, its role not only in the acquisition, but also maintenance of the SSc phenotype has not been determined.

There are studies on both the circulating levels of TGFβ and its tissue distribution. Falanga and Julien[48] failed to find elevated circulating plasma TGFβ in SSc samples compared to controls; a finding confirmed in our own work.[33] Keystone et al[49] found elevated TGFβ1 in the serum of patients with both diffuse and limited SSc, although they do not comment on the higher levels of systemic TGFβ in the early phase of the disease. Gay was one of the first to show TGFβ immunoreactivity in lesional skin of SSc patients;[50] others soon followed and the emphasis in these reports was on the early inflammatory lesions before dense fibrosis had occurred.[51,52]

Our own work has shown maximal extracellular TGFβ1 immunoreactivity in the nonlesional skin taken from SSc patients with minimal staining in the lesional areas.[33] The same biopsies show a reverse pattern with respect to pro-collagen type III reactivity, implying that TGFβ activity is an early event. Such a concept is supported by the work of Gabrielli et al,[53] who have demonstrated extracellular TGFβ not only in the papillary dermis of SSc patients but also in patients with primary Raynaud's (antibody and capillary status undefined). In addition, he showed both intra- and extracellular TGFβ in endothelial cells in skin biopsies from primary Raynaud's phenomenon (PRP) and scleroderma patients. All control biopsies were negative. These data suggest that TGFβ may be one of the cytokines involved in the early stages of pathogenesis of SSc and that endothelial cells in SSc and PRP be a source and/or target of TGFβ. TGFβ per se does not seem to be sufficient, however, since many PRP patients do not develop SSc and since SLE patients also studied in these experiments displayed TGFβ throughout the dermal connective tissue and such patients do not develop a fibrotic disease. In situ hybridization experiments have not helped to clarify the picture. Peltonen et al[54] using this technique found no elevation of TGFβ mRNA in biopsy samples from SSc patients in contrast to patients with eosinophilic fasciitis and morphea, where the TGFβ probes were hybridized to regions with inflammatory infiltrates. In contrast, Gruschwitz et al[52] found elevated TGFβ1 and TGFβ2 message levels in perivascular inflammatory foci, as well as within dermal and epidermal keratinocytes. Patients with other connective tissue disorders such as SLE also showed this elevated signal and they considered the TGFβ elevation to be more a reflection of inflammation rather than specific to the disease. Kulozik et al also found elevated TGFβ2 and type I collagen mRNA levels in proximity to inflammatory infiltrates in SSc biopsy samples.[51]

Needleman[56] failed to show any direct involvement of TGFβ after demonstrating that there was no difference in the levels of the total TGFβ in the supernatants of SSc fibroblasts, compared to normal controls and in series of extensive experiments we have endeavored to pursue the contribution of TGF to the scleroderma phenotype. Our studies have demonstrated that SSc fibroblasts are not characterized by elevated TGFβ synthesis. The ability of fibroblasts (SSc and normal) to activate exogenous latent forms of TGFβ was tested and SSc fibroblasts were found to have an impaired ability to activate the small latent complex of TGFβ. There was also no evidence of coordinate regulation of TGFβ and collagen over passage number as the cells aged in culture, suggesting that collagen is not under autocrine control by TGFβ in SSc fibroblasts. Furthermore, repeated pulses of TGFβ did not significantly induce sustained procollagen α1(I) mRNA synthesis in normal fibroblasts and this treatment did not significantly alter collagen regulation by normal fibroblasts, in a collagen gel. Collagen and TGFβ-type II receptor mRNA were also found to be inducible by TGFβ in both SSc and control cells, indicating that the lack of a sustained elevation in collagen synthesis is not due to lack of responsiveness by the fibroblasts but is rather a reflection of the transient nature of TGFβ-induced fibrogenesis (maximum at 12 hours). Therefore, our data gives no support to the hypothesis that TGFβ alone maintains the SSc phenotype in vitro, or that it is able to induce this phenotype.[55] The possibility of cytokine interactions being important in the pathogenesis of the disease is implied in several papers, and TGFβ may play an important role by such interactions. Gay et al[50] found TGFβ immunoreactivity and elevated PDGF in lesional skin of SSc patients. Kikuchi et al[57] showed that the mitogenic response of SSc fibroblasts to basic FGF was impaired after pre-incubation with TGFβ and SSc fibroblasts, unlike normal ones, do not exhibit a normal augmented adhesion to ECM components in the presence of TGFβ.[58] TGFβ is also an indirect mitogen for fibroblasts acting via PDGFα receptors.

Yamakage et al demonstrated that fibroblasts from SSc patients, in contrast to normal adult and newborn foreskin fibroblasts, express increased numbers of PDGF-β receptors on their surface in response to TGFβ1, and that there is a corresponding increase in PDGF-β receptor protein and messenger RNA.[59] TGFβ was able to increase mitogenic responses to PDGF-AA which binds only to the β receptor, in contrast to PDGF-B which binds to both the α and β receptors for scleroderma cells. PDGF-AA was found immunohistochemically in SSc dermis near blood vessels and hair follicles. It was absent from normal dermis.[53] These results suggest that the increased expression of fibroblast populations in SSc may be due in part to activation of the PDGF-AA ligand/α receptor pathway, induced by TGFβ.

All the above studies have been performed with either skin or dermal fibroblasts, as this is the easiest tissue to obtain from an SSc patient. It is, however, clinically apparent that internal organ involvement which is responsible for the increased mortality in SSc is qualitatively and sometimes quantitatively different from dermal disease. Diseases of the lung are now the major cause of death in this disorder and studies of cytokine function in this organ are critically important. Duguchi, using a nuclear run-on assay, demonstrated increased TGFβ transcription in bronchoalveolar mononuclear cells from patients with scleroderma lung fibrosis in comparison with controls, and also showed increased spontaneous TGFβ synthesis by cultured mononuclear cells.[60] However, in a study by Moreland and co-workers,[61] bronchoalveolar lavage cells from patients with SSc were shown to contain similar amounts of mRNA to cells from normal individuals, and epithelial lining fluid TGFβ concentrations were found to be lower in the disease population. Methodological differences may explain the variable results. Deguchi was studying the dynamic situation whereas Moreland's study involved measurement of steady state mRNA levels and concentrations of epithelial lining fluid protein. It is also possible that such discordant data were due to patients being studied at different stages of the disease. As with skin biopsies, immunohistochemical studies of open lung biopsy samples from patients with SSc have shown immunoreactivity with TGFβ antibodies. As in the skin, this reactivity does not appear to be exclusive to SSc since it is seen not only in biopsies taken from SSc patients with fibrosing lung disease, but also patients with cryptogenic fibrosing alveolitis or cystic fibrosis.[62]

PDGF

Although PDGF has no direct collagen-stimulatory effect,[30,63-65] it is a potent mitogen and chemoattractant for normal fibroblasts, thus causing elevated total collagen synthetic rates as a consequence of cell growth; it also has the potential, as discussed above, to act in concert with other cytokines in the creation of the scleroderma fibroblast phenotype. Gay et al[50] had detected PDGF in the endothelial lining of early scleroderma lesions in mononuclear cell infiltrates and in the dermis of old lesions. Klareskog et al[66] using immunohistochemical techniques have shown increased expression of PDGF type β receptors in the skin of 13 out of 14 patients with SSc. Receptor expression was specifically elevated in the smooth muscle cells of the dermal vessels and in adjacent fibroblasts and was often accompanied by an inflammatory infiltrate. The notable correlation of PDGF receptor expression with disease lasting from 1-25 years, and the fact that the patient showing the shortest disease duration (0.5 years) was the only negative biopsy, suggest that PDGF may play an active role in disease perpetuation. Evidence from the wound healing literature suggests that PDGF-BB applied to linear incisions at the time of wounding can cause marked prolonged collagen deposition, much more than when TGFβ is applied in the same manner.

The potential interplay of cytokines in scleroderma is exceedingly complex, and PDGF may be important in the reduced epidermal growth factor affinity seen in SSc fibroblasts,[67] as PDGF is known to decrease the affinity of such receptors. Because EGF can decrease the rate of transcription of *pro-α1(I)* and *pro-α2(I)* genes in human skin fibroblasts, it is possible that the decrease in EGF binding ability of SSc fibroblasts may be related to collagen overexpression. All these studies reiterate the necessity of recognizing the evolving nature of scleroderma. It is possible that an early transient expression of a cytokine such as TGFβ initiates a cascade of chemotactic, proliferative and differentiated events mediated by PDGF, EGF or bFGF. PDGF is a mediator capable of increasing the rate of transcription of bFGF in normal fibroblasts; in scleroderma it is deposited close to PDGF in a perivascular distribution in the lower dermis of early lesions, suggesting that these growth factors may be related to endothelial injury in scleroderma.[68] PDGF has been shown to regulate expression of genes that are important in the mitogenic response and Gay et al found increased *ras* oncogene product in early lesional skin in association with vascular endothelium and mononuclear cells. Other studies have established that fibroblasts expressing the *ras* oncogene produce increased levels of bFGF, suggesting that bFGF may play an autocrine role leading to growth stimulation.[69]

PDGF has been well investigated in cryptogenic fibrosing alveolitis, and found to play an important role, perhaps through its potent fibroblast mitogenicity. Interestingly, there are few studies in fibrosing alveolitis associated with SSc (FASSc) and they are conflicting; one group[70] has shown that alveolar mononuclear cells secrete increased amounts of PDGF in comparison with normal individuals. Cells with features of myofibroblasts were cultured from lung lavage samples, and they showed an increased proliferative response to stimulation with PDGF and TGFβ.[70] On the contrary, Harrison et al showed that the mitogenic property of bronchoalveolar lavage fluid from FASSc patients was not due to PDGF but rather to IGF-1, a cytokine of interest which has, to date, been inadequately investigated in SSc.[71] The cytokine responses seen in the lung and skin may vary because of the different cellular content of the particular organ. The inflammatory response in the skin is mainly lymphocytic, with fewer neutrophils and macrophages, whereas the lung has an abundance of mononuclear macrophages which produce large amounts of IL-8, a highly potent neutrophil chemo-attractant, probably responsible for the large number of neutrophils seen in FASSc. Macrophages from patients with systemic sclerosis contain mRNA for IL-8, and IL-8 is also found in epithelial lining fluid from patients with systemic sclerosis.[72,73] Importantly, enhanced IL-8 expression is found mainly in patients with FASSc with much less being present in the lungs of patients without evidence of diffuse parenchymal disease identified by thin section computed tomography. IL-8 has potential importance in the dermal changes in SSc and increased levels of this cytokine and an autoantibody to IL-8 have been found in SSc sera.[41] The biological significance of anticytokine autoantibodies is not clear (they are found in normal individuals also) but their presence, plus the evidence emerging from pulmonary studies, implies that IL-8 might be particularly important to the development of SSc lung disease.[74]

TNFα

Attributing a role to TNFα in scleroderma is complicated by the fact that it may have both positive and negative effects on fibroblasts. Produced by monocytes, macrophages and T cells, it stimulates fibroblast replication, but depending on the culture conditions, it may either promote or inhibit collagen production. It also increases collagenase production. Results to date in SSc are sparse. There is a report by Takeda of lymphotoxin (LT) inhibiting collagen production and reducing collagen I and III mRNA levels whilst increasing collagenase activity and collagenase mRNA levels in SSc fibroblasts,[97] a study in which the circulating levels of soluble TNFα receptors[75] are increased in SSc and a report that TNFα is produced spontaneously by alveolar macrophages from patients with FASSc in increased amounts by comparison with normal individuals or patient with sarcoidosis.[76]

This cytokine may, in addition, play an important role in inflammatory recruitment in the dermis and lung by increasing the expression on vascular endothelium of the adhesion molecules ICAM-1, E-selectin and VCAM-1. The finding of soluble E-selectin, VCAM-1 and ICAM-1 in the sera and lavage of SSc patients and the expression of these molecules in the dermis and lung tissue, supports the concept of adhesion molecule up-regulation within such tissues.[77,78] Lung TNFα mRNA levels also rise following bleomycin-induced pulmonary fibrosis in mice and TNFα antiserum reduces collagen deposition.[79] Bleomycin may also produce a scleroderma-like illness in humans.[1]

INTERFERON

Reduced interferon production in scleroderma in vitro has been reported by all investigators who have studied this family of mediators,[80] and yet there is well-documented expression of HLA class II on skin fibroblasts in scleroderma. As interferon is the most potent inducer of HLA class II, either a different peptide is responsible for in vivo HLA-DR expression, or there is a difference between the in vitro and in vivo environments.

The findings in patients with pulmonary SSc are similar. Serum levels of interferon are reduced in patients with scleroderma-related fibrosing alveolitis (FASSc) but elevated in patients with sarcoidosis.[80] The levels in the lavage fluid were not notable. Lack of spontaneous production by mononuclear cells and an impairment of T cell synthesis of interferon after mitogen stimulation in vitro in patients with FASSc and FA, but not in sarcoidosis, suggests that in patients with fibrosing alveolitis there is a defect in T cell production of interferon gamma. Because interferon can suppress synthesis of collagen by fibroblasts in vitro, decreased production may enhance tissue fibrosis and be one of the mechanisms by which fibrosis develops in patients with scleroderma. These interactions yet again indicate the highly complex nature of the cytokine pathways in SSc. There may be important differences between the different IFN types in SSc pathology, but there is good preliminary evidence suggesting that IFNα is a useful antifibrotic agent for diffuse SSc.[81]

IL-1

Interleukin-1 (IL-1) is a pleiotropic proinflammatory cytokine first identified as a product of cells of monocyte/macrophage lineage but now known to be produced by many cell types. Of relevance to SSc is its production by endothelial cells[82] and activated fibroblasts[83] as well as mononuclear cells of the immune system. Two distinct forms coded by separate genes have been characterized IL-1α and IL-1β. Though distinct molecules, these appear to act via the same cell surface receptors and exert similar biological effects. The pattern of release of α or β isoforms varies between different cell types; for example IL-1 α is the main fibroblast product whereas IL-1 β predominates for macrophages.[84] Several studies have demonstrated that presence of both mRNA species does not always correspond to production of the protein. IL-1 has been shown to induce both proliferation and collagen production in normal fibroblasts.[84] It also induces fibroblasts to produce many GFs and cytokines including IL-1, IL-6, IL-8, TNFα and PDGF. SSc fibroblasts have elevated surface expression of IL-1 type I receptors at transcriptional, protein and cell surface levels, spontaneously produce greater amounts of IL-1 inducible proteins (such as IL-6 and PDGF) than normal cells and most recently that they actively produce IL-1α in much larger amounts than control fibroblasts.[38] Upregulation of IL-1 receptors has also been shown and correlated with increased functional responsiveness to IL-1β.[85] Recently, increased responses by SSc fibroblasts have been shown, assessed by sophisticated methods including IL-6 production and IL-1β mRNA synthesis.[38] The ubiquitous presence of IL-1 in many pathological states makes a specific role in the pathogenesis of SSc unlikely, but it may be an important factor through its proinflammatory properties acting in concert with other factors and contributing to the endothelial cell, fibroblast and immune cell activation in the disease. IL-1 is produced by EC, fibroblasts and mononuclear cells, all of which are activated in SSc; it is therefore certainly present in the SSc microenvironment and its effects on fibroblasts may be relevant, e.g., mitogenicity and enhancement of collagen production. The regulation of IL-1 is complex and may involve alteration in cell surface receptor expression. Both types I and II IL-1 receptor possess a transmembrane domain, but only type I signals. The type II receptor is the main source of production of soluble IL-1 receptor, which retains IL-1 binding capacity and can neutralize the activities of IL-1 in vitro. The IL-1 receptor antagonist, a 17-25 kDa molecular weight polypeptide, is produced by many cell types and inhibits the activity of endogenous IL-1.[86]

IL-6

This cytokine, like IL-1, is produced by fibroblasts as well as many other cell types including endothelial cells and lymphocytes. Interest in this cytokine in SSc was stimulated by reports of elevated circulating levels in the disease by Needleman[40] and by subsequent reports that SSc fibroblasts constitutively produce elevated levels of IL-6, and that this is in part responsible for the mitogenic activity of SSc fibroblast conditioned media.[35,36] It has been suggested that cytokines such as IL-1 are important through their induction of IL-6 synthesis. Interestingly, IL-6 production by normal fibroblasts is increased 13-fold[87] when grown in three dimensional collagen gels, emphasizing the importance of the extracellular matrix in modulation of fibroblast properties and perhaps relevant to the excessive matrix deposition in SSc.

Recent studies by Feghali have shown that production of IL-6 by SSc fibroblasts is thirty times greater than controls, and clarified some of the regulatory mechanisms involved in this overproduction. Molecular biological studies confirm increased production at the transcriptional level[37] via the binding of nuclear factors to the IL-6 promoter, thereby raising steady-state levels of IL-6 mRNA. Mobility shift assays of sequence specific DNA binding proteins suggest different factors are involved in constitutive compared with induced IL-6 production. It is possible that some of the effects of IL-1 in SSc are actually a consequence of secondary induction of IL-6. Immunologically active cytokine may be responsible for some of the constitutional features of

SSc and lymphocyte activation. Induction of high affinity IL-2 receptors on lymphocytes is one property of IL-6, and this may cause the greater proliferative response of SSc lymphocytes to IL-2.[88]

In addition to raised serum levels of circulating cytokine, anti-IL-6 antibodies have also been demonstrated in SSc. Their functional effects are complex both in vivo and within assay systems where different assays may produce conflicting results.[89] The presence of such antibodies and antibody/IL-6 complexes may explain the differences in reported circulating levels of IL-6 in SSc sera when measured by bioassay compared with immunoassay.[90] It has recently been shown that a significant part of the IL-6 activity in SSc serum is associated with IL-6-antibody complexes, which retain approximately 60% of their biological activity and are able to bind to recombinant IL-6R.[89] Interestingly, the prevalence of anti-IL-6 antibodies was significantly greater in patients with lcSSc than those with the diffuse form and normal individuals; it has been suggested that this may be related to disease duration at sampling.[91]

bFGF

The fibroblast growth factor family is becoming better understood although there is little direct evidence to support a role for these cytokine in SSc pathogenesis. Nine separate members of this family have now been identified[92] but the best characterized are types I and II, also termed acidic and basic FGF (aFGF, bFGF) respectively. Both have affinity for heparin and other proteoglycans which stabilize the growth factors from proteolytic degradation[93] and increase their activity.[94] At the cell surface heparan sulphate appears to operate as a low affinity receptor for bFGF in addition to the specific high affinity receptors, which are tyrosine kinases.

FGF-I (bFGF) is an 18 kDa cationic protein produced by many cell types including endothelial cells. Takehara et al report reduced responsiveness to bFGF by SSc fibroblasts in both the proliferating and confluent stages.[67] The mechanism of release of this factor by cells is unclear since the polypeptide chain lacks a leader sequence generally required for active secretion. It has been suggested that FGF-1 is released by cells in response to mechanical damage or death, perhaps by apoptosis. It is apparently sequestered, bound to extracellular matrix proteoglycan[95] from which it can later be released, perhaps proteolytically.

In addition to its profound mitogenic activity for a variety of cell types including fibroblasts, Tan et al have shown that bFGF is a potent downregulator of collagen (I) gene transcription.[96] This makes a prime role as an effector cytokine in SSc unlikely but it may be important as a member of a cytokine network. It appears to be a potent stimulus to endothelial cells in the process of angiogenesis and current research is directed towards elucidating the importance of these growth factors in SSc pathogenesis. Recent work suggests a potential interaction between TGFβ and bFGF, the former being able to restore bFGF responsiveness in SSc fibroblasts via the induction of high affinity bFGF receptor.[63]

In conclusion, there is increasing evidence that cytokines are intimately involved in the pathogenesis of the various forms of scleroderma. However, there is no clear cut therapeutic target, although TGFβ and PDGF, the cytokines most extensively studied, are the closest to potential candidates. Further work is needed to understand the complex cytokine interactions in this disease.

REFERENCES

1. Black CM, Stephens CO. Scleroderma—systemic sclerosis. In: PJ Maddison, DA Isenberg, P Woo, DN Glass, eds. Oxford Textbook of Rheumatology. Oxford: Oxford University Press, 1993:771-789.
2. LeRoy EC, Black CM, Fleischmajer R et al. Scleroderma (Systemic Sclerosis): Classification, Subsets and Pathogenesis. J Rheumatol 1988; 15:202-5.
3. Black CM. Scleroderma—clinical aspects. J Int Med 1993; 243:115-8.
4. Fleischmajer R. The pathophysiology of scleroderma. Int J Dermatol 1977; 16:310.
5. Tan EM. Antinuclear antibodies: diagnostic markers for autoimmune diseases and probes for cell biology. Advances in Immunology 1989; 44:93-151.
6. Kahari VM. Activation of dermal connective tissue in scleroderma. Ann Int Medicine 1994; 25:511-518.
7. Prescott RJ, Freemont AJ, Jones CJ et al. Sequential dermal microvascular and perivascular changes in the development of scleroderma. J Path 1992; 166:255-63.
8. Kaye SA, Seifalian AM, Lim SF et al. Ischemia of the small intestine in patients with SSc: Raynaoud's phenomenon or chronic vasculopathy. Q J Med (1994) 87:495-500.
9. Harrison NK, Myers AR, Corrin B et al. Structural features of interstitial lung disease in systemic sclerosis. Am Rev Respir Dis 1991; 144:706-713.
10. Kovalchik MT Guggenheim SJ, Robertson JS et al. The kidney in progressive systemic sclerosis: a prospective study. Ann Int Med 1978; 89:881-7.
11. Claman HN, Giorgio RC, Seibold JR. Endothelial and fibroblastic activation in scleroderma: "the myth of uninvolved skin". Arthritis Rheum 1991; 834:1495-1501.
12. Fleischmajer R, Perlish JS, Reeves JRT. Cellular Infiltrates in scleroderma. Arthritis Rheum 1977; 20:975-984.
13. Kahaleh B. Immunological Aspects of SSc. Current Opinions in Rheum 1993; 5:760-765.
14. Needleman BW. Immunologic aspects of scleroderma. Current Opinions in Rheum 1992; 4:862-868.
15. LeRoy EC. Increased collagen synthesis by scleroderma skin fibroblasts in vitro. A possible defect in regulation or activation of scleroderma fibroblasts. J Clin Invest 1974; 54:880-9.
16. Jimenez S, Feldmenn G, Bashey R et al. Co-ordinate increase in the expression of type I and type III collagen genes in progressive systemic sclerosis fibroblasts. Bioch J 1986; 237:837-43.

17. Kreig T, Perlish JS, Fleischmajer R. Collagen synthesis by scleroderma fibroblasts. Ann NY Acad Sci 1986; 460:375-386.
18. Kreig T, Perlish JS, Fleismajer R et al. Collagen synthesis in scleroderma: selection of fibroblast populations during subcultures. Arch Dermatol Res 1978; 263:171-178.
19. Mauch C, Eckes B, Hunzelman N et al. Control of fibrosis in systemic scleroderma. J Invest Dermatol 1993; 100:92S-96S.
20. Smith EA. Connective tissue metabolism including cytokines in scleroderma. Current Opinions in Rheum 1992; 4:869-77.
21. Tan EML, Hoffren J, Rouda S et al. Decorin, Versican, and Biglycan gene expression by keloid and normal fibroblasts: differential regulation by bFGF. Exp Cell Res 1993; 209:200-207.
22. Bashkin P, Doctrow S, Klagsbrum M et al. bFGF binds to subendothlial matrix and is released by heparinase and heparin-like molecules. Biochemistry 1989; 28:1737-1743.
23. Ivarsson M, McWhirter A, Black CM et al. Impaired regulation of collagen pro-α1(I) mRNA and change in pattern of collagen binding integrins on scleroderma fibroblasts. J Invest Dermatol 1993; 101:216-221.
24. Denton CP, Shiwen Xu, Welsh K I et al. Modulation of scleroderma and control fibroblast phenotype by co-culture with human endothelial cells. Arthritis Rheum 1994; 37:S264 [abstract].
25. Haskard DO. Adhesion molecules induced by cytokines on vascular endothelial cells. In: Growth factors of the vascular and nervous systems. Basel, Karger 1992:56-62.
26. Koch AE, Kronfield-Harrington LB, Szechnecz A et al. In situ expression of cytokines and cellular adhesion molecules in the skin of patients with systemic sclerosis. Pathobiology 1993; 61:239-246.
27. Abraham D, Lupoli S, McWhirter A et al. Expression and function of surface antigens on scleroderma fibroblasts. Arthritis Rheum 1991; 34:1164-1172.
28. Needleman BW. Increased expression of intercellular adhesion molecule-1 on the fibroblasts of scleroderma patients. Arthritis Rheum 1990; 33:1847-1851.
29. Shiwen X, Panesar M, Vancheeswaran R et al. Expression and shedding of ICAM-1 and LFA-3 by normal and scleroderma fibroblasts. Arthritis Rheum 1994; 37:89-97.
30. LeRoy EC, Mercurio S, Sherer GK. Replication and phenotypic expression of control and scleroderma human fibroblasts: responses to growth factors. Proc Natl Acad Sci USA 1982; 79:1286-1290.
31. LeRoy EC, Smith EA, Kahaleh MB et al. A strategy for determining the pathogenesis of systemic sclerosis: Is transforming growth factor β the answer? Arthritis Rheum 1989; 32:817-829.
32. Hamilton JA, Butler DM, Stanton H. Cytokine interactions promoting DNA synthesis in human synovial fibroblasts. Journal of Rheumat 1994; 21:797-803.
33. Higley H, Persichitte K, Chu S et al. Immunocytochemical localisation and serological detection of transfoming growth factor-β1: association with

type-I procollagen and inflammatory markers in diffuse and limited systemic sclerosis, morphea and Raynaud's phenomenon. Arthritis Rheum 1994; 37:278-288.
34. McWhirter A, Colosetti, Rubin K et al. TGFβ1 as a modulator of collagen regulation in scleroderma. Lab Invest [in press, 1994]
35. Feghali CA, Bost KL et al. Mechanisms of pathogenesis of scleroderma I. Overproduction of IL-6 by fibroblasts cultured from affected skin sites of patients with scleroderma. J Rheum (1992). 19(8): 1207-1211.
36. Feghali CA, Boulware DW, Levy, Laura S. Mechanisms of pathogenesis in scleroderma II. Effects of serum and conditioned culture medium on fibroblast function in scleroderma. J Rheum 1992; 19:1212-9.
37. Feghali CA, Bost KL, Boulware DW et al. Control of IL-6 expression and response in fibroblasts from patients with systemic sclerosis. Autoimmunity 1994; 17:309-318.
38. Kawaguchi Y. IL-1α gene expression and protein production by fibroblasts from patients with systemic sclerosis. Clinical & Experimental Immunology 1994; 97:445-50.
39. Black C M. The aetiopathogenesis of systemic sclerosis. J Internal Med 1993; 234:3-8.
40. Needleman BW, Wigley FM, Stair RW. IL-1, IL-2, IL-4, IL-6, TNFα and IFNγ levels in sera from patients with scleroderma. Arthritis Rheum 1992; 35:67-72.
41. Reitamo S, Remitz A, Varga J et al. Demonstration of IL-8 and autoantibodies to IL-8 in the serum of patients with systemic sclerosis. Arch Dermatol 1993; 129:189-92.
42. Gearing AJH, Newman W. Circulating adhesion molecules in disease. Immunol Today 1993; 14:506-512.
43. Carson CW, Beall LD, Hunder GG et al. Serum ELAM-1 is increased in vasculitis, scleroderma, and systemic lupus erythematosus. J Rheumatol 1993; 20:809-14.
44. Sinclair HD, Vancheeswaran R, Kapaphi P et al. Circulating cell adhesion molecules in systemic sclerosis, primary Raynaud's disease and morphea. Arthritis Rheum 1992; 35:S151 [abstract].
45. Gorski A. The role of cell adhesion molecules in immunopathology. Immunology Today 1994; 15:251-5.
46. Denton CP, Bickerstaff MCM, Shiwen X et al. Serial levels of VCAM-1 and E-selectin correlate with the extent of renal and lung disease in systemic sclerosis. Arthritis Rheum 1994; 37: S220 [abstract].
47. Tarkowski A, Andersson-Gare B, Aurell M. Use of anti-thymocyte globulin in the management of refractory systemic autoimmune diseases. Scandinavian Journal of Rheumatology 1993; 22:261-6.
48. Falanga V, Julien J. Observations in the potential role of TGF-β in cutaneous fibrosis: systemic sclerosis. In: Piez K and Sporn M, eds. Transforming Growth Factor β's; Chemistry, Biology and Therapeutics. NY Acad Sci 1990; 593:161-171.
49. Keystone E, Lok C, Appleton B et al. Elevated serum levels of TGF-β in patients with scleroderma. Arthritis Rheum (suppl) 1992; 35: S206 [abstract].

50. Gay S, Jones R, Huang G et al. Immunohistologic demonstration of platelet derived growth factor (PDGF) and sis-oncogene expression in scleroderma. J Invest Dermatol 1989; 92:301-303.
51. Kulozik M, Hogg A, Lankat-Buttgereit B et al. Co-localization of transforming growth factor beta 2 with α1(I) procollagen mRNA in tissue sections of patients with systemic sclerosis. J Clinical Invest 1990; 86:917-22.
52. Gruschwitz M, Muller PU, Sepp N et al. Transcription and expression of transforming growth factor type β in the skin of progressive systemic sclerosis: a mediator of fibrosis? J Invest Dermatol 1990; 94:197-203.
53. Gabrielli A, De Loreto C, Taborro R et al. Immunohistochemical localisation of intracellular and extracellular associated TGF-β in the skin of patients with systemic sclerosis (scleroderma) and primary Raynaud's phenomenon. Clin Immunol Immunopathol 1993; 63:340-349.
54. Peltonen J, Kahari L, Jaakkola S et al. Evaluation of TGF-β and type-I procollagen gene expression in fibrotic diseases by in situ hybridisation. J Invest Dermatol 1990; 94:365-371.
55. McWhirter A, Colosetti P, Rubin K et al. Collagen type-I is not under autocrine control by TGF-β1 in normal and scleroderma fibroblasts. Lab Invest 1994; (in press).
56. Needleman BW, Choi J, Burrows-Mezu A et al. Secretion and binding of transforming growth factor-β by scleroderma and normal fibroblasts. Arthritis Rheum 1990; 33:650-656.
57. Kikuchi K, Yamakage A, Smith E et al. Differential modulation of bFGF receptors by TGF-β in adult skin, scleroderma skin and newborn foreskin fibroblasts. J Invest Dermatol 1992; 99:201-205.
58. Majewski S, Hunzelmann N, Schirren C et al. Increased adhesion of fibroblasts from patients with scleroderma to extracellular matrix components: in vitro modulation by interferon-γ but not by TGF-β. J Invest Dermatol 1992; 98:86-91.
59. Yamakage A, Kikuchi K, Smith E et al. Selective up-regulation of PDGF-A receptors by TGF-β in scleroderma fibroblasts. J Exp Med 1992; 175:1227-1234.
60. Deguchi Y. Spontaneous increase in TGF-β production by bronchalveolar mononuclear cells of patients with systemic autoimmune diseases affecting the lung. Ann Rheum Dis 1992; 51:362-365.
61. Moreland LW, Goldsmith KT, Russell WJ et al. TGFβ within fibrotic scleroderma lungs. Am J Med 1992; 93:628-636.
62. Corrin B, Butcher D, McNulty BJ et al. Immunohistochemical localisation of TGFβ1 in the lungs of patients with systemic sclerosis, cryptogenic fibrosing alveolitis and other lung diseases. Histopathology 1994; 24:145-50.
63. LeRoy EC. The control of fibrosis in systemic sclerosis: a strategy involving extracellular matrix, cytokines and growth factors. Journal of Dermatology 1994; 21:1-4.
64. Allen-Hoffmann BL, Schlosser SJ, Brondyk WH et al. Fibronectin levels are enhanced in human fibroblasts over expressing the c-sis protooncogene. Journal of Biological Chemistry 1990; 265:5219-25.

65. LeRoy EC, Trojanowska MI, Smith EA. Cytokines and human fibrosis. [Review] European Cytokine Network 1990; 1:215-9.
66. Klareskog L, Gustafsson R, Schneyiu A et al. Increased expression of PDGF B receptors in the skin of patients with scleroderma. Arthritis Rheum 1990; 33:1534-1541.
67. Takehara K, Soma Y, Igarashi A et al. Response of scleroderma fibroblasts to various growth factors. Archives of Dermatological Research 1991; 283:461-4.
68. Gay S, Trabandt A, Moreland LW et al. Growth factors, extracellular matrix, and oncogenes in scleroderma.[Review] Arthritis Rheum 1992; 35:304-10.
69. Thornton SC, Robbins JM, Penny R et al. Fibroblast growth factors in connective tissue disease associated interstitial lung disease. Clin Exp Immunol 1992; 90:447-452.
70. Ludwicka A, Trojanowska M, Smith EA et al. Growth and characterisation of fibroblasts obtained from bronchoalveolar lavage of patients with scleroderma. J Rheumatol 1992; 19:1716-1723.
71. Harrison NK, Cambrey AD, Myers AR et al. Insulin-like growth factor-1 is partially responsible for fibroblast proliferation induced by broncho-alveolar lavage fluid from patients with systemic sclerosis. Clin Sci (1993, in press) [abstract].
72. Carre PC, Mortensen RL, King TEJ et al. Increased expression of the IL-8 gene by alveolar macrophages in idiopathic pulmonary fibrosis. J Clin Invest 1991; 88:1802-1810.
73. Southcott AM, Jones KP, Pantelidis P et al. IL-8 is associated with the presence of pulmonary fibrosis in systemic sclerosis. Am Rev Resp Dis 1993; 147:A755.
74. Zwahlen R, Walz A, Rot A. In vitro and in vivo activity and pathophysiology of human interleukin-8 and related peptides. [Review] Int Rev Exp Path 1993; 34:27-42.
75. Heilig B, Fiehn C, Brockhaus M et al. Evaluation of soluble tumor necrosis factor (TNF) receptors and TNF receptor antibodies in patients with systemic lupus erythematosus, progressive systemic sclerosis, and mixed connective tissue disease. J Clin Immunology 1993; 13:321-8.
76. Pantelidis P, Southcott AM, du Bois RM. Alveolar macrohages from fibrosing alveolitis patients secrete more TNFα than patients with sarcoidosis and normal individuals. Thorax (1994, in press) [abstract].
77. Du Bois RM, Hellewell PG, Hemingway I et al. Soluble cell adhesion molecules ICAM-1, VCAM-1 and E-selectin are present in epithelial lining fluid in patients with interstitial lung disease. Am Rev Resp Dis 1992; 145: A190 [abstract].
78. Sinclair HD, Vancheeswaran R, Kapaphi P et al. Circulating cell adhesion molecules in systemic sclerosis, primary Raynaud's disease and morphea. Arthritis Rheum 1992; 35: S151 [abstract].
79. Piguet PF, Collart MA, Grau GE et al. Tunour necrosis factor/cachectin plays a key role in bleomycin induced pneumopathy and fibrosis. J Exp Med 1989; 170:655-63.

80. Prior C, Haslam PL. In vivo levels and in vitro production of interferon-γ in fibrosing interstitial lung diseases. Clin Exp Immunology 1992; 88:280-7.
81. Stevens W, Vancheeswaran R, Black CM. Alpha interferon-2a (Roferon-A) in the treatment of diffuse cutaneous systemic sclerosis: a pilot study. UK Systemic Sclerosis Study Group. British J Rheum 1992; 31:683-9.
82. Miossec P, Cavender D, Ziff M. Production of IL-1 by human endothelial cells. J Immunol 1986; 136:2486-91.
83. Dinarello CA, Wolff SM. The role of IL-1 in disease. N Eng J Med 1992; 328:106-113.
84. Kovacs EJ. Fibrogenic cytokines: the role of immune mediators in the development of scar tissue. Immunology Today 1991; 12:17-21.
85. Yasushi KG, Masagushi H et al. Interleukin 1 receptors on fibroblasts from systemic sclerosis patients induce excessive functional responses to IL-1b. Biochem Biophys Res Comm 1993; 190:154-61.
86. Arend WP. IL-1 receptor antagonist: a new member of the IL-1 family. J Clin Invest 1991; 88:1445-51.
87. Eckes B, Hunzelmen N, Zeigler-Heitbrock HW et al. IL-6 expression by fibroblasts grown in three dimensional cultures. FEBS 298:229-32.
88. Kahaleh MB, Yin T. Enhanced expression of high-affinity IL-2 receptors in scleroderma: a possible role for IL-6. Clin Immunol Immunopath 1992; 62:97-102.
89. Suzuki H, Takemura H, Yoshizaki K et al. IL-6-Anti-IL-6 autoantibody complexes in sera from some patients with systemic sclerosis. J Immunol 1994; 152:935-41.
90. Crilly A, Madhok R. IL-6 in scleroderma [letter]. Arthritis Rheum (1992); 35:1402.
91. Takemara H, Suzuki H, Yoshizaki K et al. Anti-IL-6 autoantibodies in rheumatic diseases. Arthritis Rheum 1991; 35:940-43.
92. Mason IJ. The Ins and Outs of fibroblast growth factors. Cell 1994; 78:547-552.
93. Arakawa T, Wen J, Philo JS. Stoichiometry of heparin binding to basic fibroblast growth factor. Arch Biochem Biophys 1994; 308:267-73.
94. Coltrini D, Rusnati M, Zoppetti G et al. Different effects of mucosal, bovine lung and chemically modified heparin on selected biological properties of bFGF. Biochem J 1994; 303:583-590.
95. Roghani M, Mansukhani A, Dell'Era P et al. Heparin increases the affinity of basic fibroblast growth factor for its receptor but is not required for binding. Journal of Biological Chemistry 1994; 269:3976-84.
96. Tan EM, Rouda S, Greenbaum SS et al. Acidic and basic FGF down-regulate collagen gene expression in keloid fibroblasts. Am J Path 1993; 142:463-470.
97. Takeda K, Hatamochi A, Ueki H et al. Decreased collagenase expression in cultured systemic sclerosis fibroblasts. J Invest Dermatol; 103:359-63.

CHAPTER 9

PSORIASIS

Stephen M. Breathnach and William G. Phillips

Dysregulation of the skin immune system, comprising skin-homing T lymphocytes, resident antigen presenting cells, dermal vascular endothelium, and keratinocyte-derived cytokines, is thought to be fundamental to the pathogenesis of psoriasis, a common genetically determined inflammatory and proliferative skin disorder. The clinical efficacy of cyclosporin A treatment is one of the main arguments for this concept, since the drug inhibits epidermal antigen-presenting cell function, T cell activation and lymphokine release, and results in clearing of immunocompetent cells from the skin before clinical effects are evident. Abnormalities in all of the elements of the skin immune system have been documented in psoriasis. Here we review the role of cytokines in the pathogenesis of psoriasis, and the potential for manipulation of the skin cytokine system in the therapy of this common economically important and distressing condition which is the cause of considerable patient morbidity.

INTRODUCTION

CLINICAL FEATURES

The typical patient with psoriasis presents with chronic well-demarcated dull-red scaly plaques on the elbows, knees and scalp and elsewhere (Fig. 9.1). Other variants include guttate psoriasis, in which widespread small lesions appear acutely scattered over the trunk and limbs following an upper respiratory tract infection, localized pustular psoriasis of the palms and soles, and more severe forms such as erythrodermic or generalized pustular psoriasis. Cutaneous lesions may be accompanied by a rheumatoid factor negative peripheral and/or spinal arthropathy. The population prevalence of cutaneous psoriasis is between 1.5% and 3%, and that of psoriatic arthritis has been estimated at between 0.02% and 0.1%.[1]

IMMUNOGENETICS

There is a genetic predisposition to psoriasis, given that about 30% of patients have affected first-degree relatives, and that there is a high concordance rate of 65% to 72% in monozygotic twins compared with 15% to 30% in dizygotic twins.[1,2] Psoriasis is associated with the major histocompatibility complex (MHC) antigens HLA-B13, -B17, -B37, and HLA-DR7, and there is a stronger association with HLA Cw6 (relative risk up to 24).[2] HLA-A26, -B38 and -DR4 are increased in psoriatic arthritis, HLA-DR3 in erosive arthritis, and HLA-B27 in spondylitis and sacroiliitis. Type 1 psoriasis, characterized by early onset (mean age 16 to 20 years) and a positive family history, is associated with HLA-Cw6,

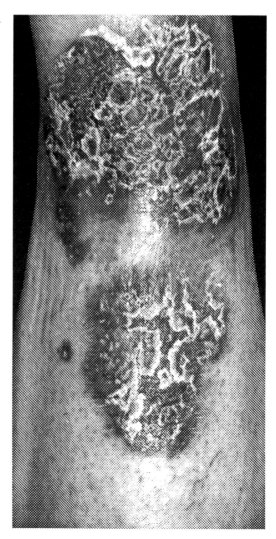

Fig. 9.1. Scaly red plaques of psoriasis on the shin.

-B13, -Bw57, as well as with HLA-DRB1*0701/2, -DQA1*0201, -DQB1*0303, whereas type 2 psoriasis, which has a later onset, and is more likely to be sporadic and nonfamilial, has a weaker association with HLA-Cw2 and -B27.[3,4] The importance of the genetic linkage in psoriasis may lie in the determination of the nature of the immunological response to certain endogenous or exogenous antigens. Alternatively, the HLA haplotypes associated with psoriasis may be in linkage disequilibrium with other as yet unidentified genes concerned with the regulation of inflammatory and immune responses, which include those encoding for cytokines, such as tumor necrosis factor α (TNFα).

HISTOPATHOLOGY

Amongst the earliest changes seen in developing skin lesions of psoriasis are dilatation and tortuosity of superficial dermal blood vessels, and perivascular infiltration by lymphocytes, monocyte-macrophages and neutrophil leukocytes (Figs. 9.2 to 9.4). Epidermal hyperplasia, hyperkeratosis, and parakeratosis, and leukocyte invasion of the lower epidermis with formation of sterile spongioform pustules containing neutrophils, are features of established lesions.[1,5] Increased numbers of proliferating basal epidermal stem cells, and a marked decrease in the epidermal turnover time, have been demonstrated in cellular kinetic studies.[1] There is much current interest in the potential role of cytokines, derived either from keratinocytes or from infiltrating inflammatory cells, in promoting the development and maintenance of the above histological and cell kinetic abnormalities.

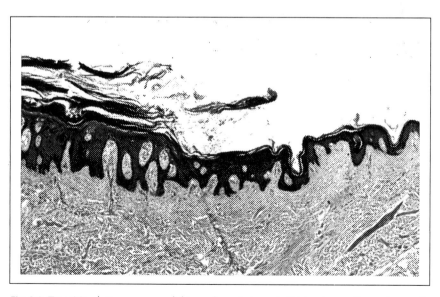

Fig. 9.2. Transition between normal skin and psoriasis: note thickening and hyperkeratosis of involved skin. (Hematoxylin & Eosin).

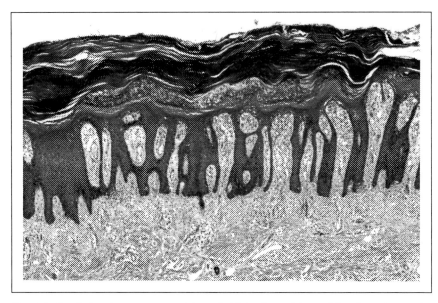

Fig. 9.3. Psoriatic plaque: note epidermal thickening and overlying hyperkeratosis. (Hematoxylin & Eosin).

Although it is now well accepted that psoriasis has an immunogenetic basis, the fact that concordance amongst monozygotic twins for psoriasis is not complete points to the additional importance of environmental factors. Psoriasis may be exacerbated or precipitated by infection, especially upper respiratory tract infection by *Streptococcus sp*, trauma, treatment with certain drugs,[6] and perhaps also by stress. Our current concept of the etiology of psoriasis is that one or other of the above factors, in a genetically susceptible individual, triggers dysregulation of the skin immune system and autoreactivity, resulting in the characteristic clinical features.[7-15] In order to appreciate the role of cytokines in psoriasis, it is necessary first to outline the structure and function of the normal skin immune system; we will then review the abnormalities in cytokines reported in psoriasis and how these may account for the pathology, and discuss the effects of current and potential treatments for psoriasis on these abnormalities.

THE SKIN IMMUNE SYSTEM

The skin may be regarded as the most peripheral outpost of the immune system. The skin immune system[16] comprises recirculating lymphocytes which home to the skin,[17] antigen-presenting $CD1^+$ $HLA-DR^+$ Langerhans cells,[18] which circulate between the epidermis and the regional lymph nodes, dermal antigen-presenting cells (including perivascular factor $XIIIa^+$ dermal dendritic cells and $CD1a^+$ Langerhans-like cells),[19-22] keratinocytes which produce a wide range of immunoregulatory and growth regulatory cytokines,[23,24] and vascular endothelium. The adhesion molecules intercellular adhesion molecule 1 (ICAM-1), vascular cell adhesion molecule 1 (VCAM-1), and endothelial-leukocyte adhesion molecule-1 (E-selectin) are expressed only at a low level on dermal endothelial cells in normal skin. ICAM-1 is the ligand for lymphocyte function associated molecule-1, a molecule expressed by all leukocytes. E-selectin, initially identified as an endothelial adhesion molecule for neutrophil leukocytes, is also the ligand for cutaneous lymphocyte associated antigen (defined by the antibody HECA 451) present on the surface of a subset of circulating memory T cells which preferentially home to sites of cutaneous inflammation.[25-27] Upregulation of these adhesion molecules on dermal microvascular endothelium facilitates leucocyte adherence and is critical to the recruitment of inflammatory cells into the skin.[28-31]

KERATINOCYTE-DERIVED CYTOKINES

Keratinocytes are the source of a large array of cytokines, listed in Table 9.1, which may modulate inflammatory reactions in the skin and/or affect cell proliferation.[16-19,23,24,31,32] Interleukin 10 has been reported to be produced by murine keratinocytes, but it has not proved

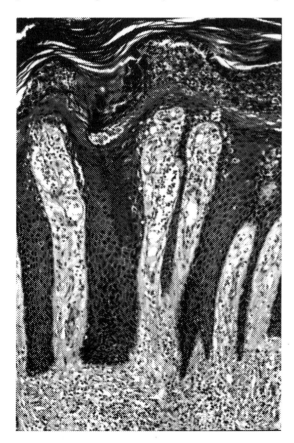

Fig. 9.4. Higher power view of psoriatic plaque, showing downward elongation of epidermal rete ridge, hyperkeratosis, parakeratosis, neutrophil accumulation in the stratum corneum, and dermal lymphohistiocytic infiltration with dilated capillaries. (Hematoxylin & Eosin).

possible to demonstrate IL-10 production by human keratinocytes. Keratinocyte-derived cytokines are especially released following insult to the epidermis. IL-1 induces inflammation when injected into human dermis.[33] IL-1 bioactivity in the skin is predominantly cell-associated, and is confined to IL-1α in extracts of cultured keratinocytes and keratome biopsies of normal skin.[34] IL-1β is present only as a 31 kD latent peptide, as keratinocytes lack IL-1 convertase which is required to cleave latent IL-1β peptide into the 17 kD active form.[35] Keratinocytes also make the intracellular form of a specific antagonist of IL-1α and IL-1β, termed interleukin 1 receptor antagonist (IL-1ra), which is not normally secreted but is released on disruption of keratinocyte membranes.[36-38] Although IL-1ra, IL-1α and IL-1β have a similar affinity for type I and type II IL-1 receptors, IL-1ra must be present in excess to block signal transduction following exposure to IL-1, as only a small number of the target cell IL-1 receptors need to bind ligand to elicit a maximal response.[39] Thus the net effect of the IL-1 cytokine network in diseased or damaged skin reflects the balance between the concentrations of IL-1α, its receptors, and IL-1ra. IL-1, IL-6, IL-7, IL-8, and TNFα are in general proinflammatory, while TGF-β, α-MSH and IL-1ra tend to downregulate cutaneous inflammation. IL-1 stimulates B and T cells,[40] promotes (with GM-CSF) Langerhans cell maturation into potent immunostimulatory dendritic cells,[41,42] and induces genes for a large number of immunoregulatory

Table 9.1. Keratinocyte derived cytokines

Cytokine	Abbreviation
Interleukin 1α	IL-1α
Interleukin 1β	IL-1β
Interleukin 1 receptor antagonist	IL-1ra
Interleukin 3	IL-3
Interleukin 6	IL-6
Interleukin 7	IL-7
Interleukin 8	IL-8
Melanoma growth stimulatory activity	MGSA/groα
Tumor necrosis factor α	TNFα
Transforming growth factor α	TGFα
Transforming growth factor β	TGFβ
Granulocyte/macrophage colony stimulating factor	GM-CSF
Granulocyte colony stimulating factor	G-CSF
Macrophage colony stimulating factor	M-CSF
Basic fibroblast growth factor	bFGF
Platelet derived growth factor	PDGF
Pro-opiomelanocortin	POMC
α melanocyte stimulating hormone	α-MSH
Vascular endothelial growth factor	VEGF

cytokines,[40] including that for the chemotactic cytokine IL-8.[43,44] IL-1, with other keratinocyte-derived cytokines such as GM-CSF, IL-6, and TGFα, stimulates keratinocyte proliferation.[45-50] IL-1 and TNFα upregulate expression of ICAM-1, VCAM-1, and E-selectin on dermal endothelial cells.[51-53] TNFα has been reported to enhance adhesiveness of cultured porcine dermal microvascular endothelial cells for peripheral blood mononuclear cells,[54] promote preferential attachment of memory T cells from peripheral blood to cultured human umbilical vein endothelial cells,[55] and (like IL-1α) increase IL-8 production by keratinocytes, dermal fibroblasts and endothelial cells.[43,56,57] TNFα also increases the rate of secretion of IL-1 and IL-6 by cultured human keratinocytes.[58] IL-7 promotes T cell proliferation.[59] IL-8 and the related proteins MGSA/GROα (originally characterized as an autocrine growth factor for melanoma cells) and MCP-1/MCAF have chemotactic properties for neutrophils and/or mononuclear cells.[44] Colony stimulating factors stimulate migration of leukocytes into the skin in inflammation, and enhance their function.[60]

TGF-β appears to have an important regulatory role in the cytokine system.[61] TGF-β has immunosuppressive actions on T and B lymphocytes and may inhibit Langerhans cell antigen-presenting function.[62,63] TGF-β also decreases dermal microvascular endothelial cell adhesiveness for circulating lymphocytes, monocytes and neutrophils and thus downregulates inflammatory cell infiltration of the skin induced by TNFα and IL-1,[54] and induces production of IL-1ra.[64] Moreover, TGF-β antagonizes the growth-promoting properties of TGF-α on keratinocytes.[65] α-MSH acts as an antagonist of IL-1.[66] Another compound with immunosuppressive properties present in the epidermis is the neuropeptide calcitonin gene related peptide (CGRP). CGRP-containing nerve fibers have recently been reported in intimate association with epidermal Langerhans cells, and CGRP inhibits Langerhans cell antigen presentation.[67] This observation provides one mechanism for interaction between the skin immune system and the nervous system. Vascular permeability factor (vascular endothelial growth factor) stimulates angiogenesis, and may play an important role in wound healing.[68]

In view of the large repertoire of cytokines released following keratinocyte injury, it has been proposed that perturbation of the epidermal barrier leads directly to antigen-independent initiation of cutaneous inflammation; antigen-dependent mechanisms of amplification and persistence of inflammation, involving T cell-Langerhans cell or -dermal macrophage interactions, may then take over at a later stage.[31,69] Keratinocytes express ICAM-1 in many inflammatory dermatoses, probably as a result of exposure to interferon γ (IFNγ) secreted by infiltrating T cells.[70-72] Keratinocyte ICAM-1 expression promotes mononuclear cell adherence to keratinocytes, and may therefore be important in determining the exocytosis of leukocytes into the epidermis.[71]

THE SKIN IMMUNE SYSTEM AND PSORIASIS

Abnormalities in all the elements of the skin immune system have been implicated in psoriasis. These will be reviewed in turn, and the way in which cytokines may be involved will be discussed. Reports on the levels of individual cytokines in psoriatic lesional skin will also be reviewed.

T Lymphocytes

The dermal infiltrate in psoriatic lesional skin consists mainly of T lymphocytes and macrophages; the T cells are mostly CD4+ with fewer CD8+ cells.[7-12,14,15] Lesional and uninvolved psoriasis skin also contains more CD4+ T cells than CD8+ T cells, and cell lines derived from psoriasis skin are predominantly CD4+.[73] T cells proliferating in the dermis in patients with psoriasis are primarily recall antigen-reactive helper T cells.[74] Cloned T cells propagated from psoriatic lesions secrete lymphokines capable of inducing keratinocyte ICAM-1 and HLA-DR expression,[75] and are of the T helper 1 (Th_1) subset, since they produce IFNγ and high amounts of IL-2.[76] Activated T cells, and keratinocytes expressing ICAM-1, occur primarily in the suprapapillary regions of psoriatic lesions nearest the dermal capillaries. mRNA for Th_1 cytokines IFNγ and TNFα, but not for the Th_2 cytokines IL-4, IL-5 or IL-10, was detected in psoriatic lesional biopsies by polymerase chain reaction.[76,77] Similarly, only mRNA for IFNγ, and not for IL-4, was produced by synovial fluid mononuclear cells in patients with psoriatic arthritis.[76] T lymphocytes cloned from psoriatic lesional skin produce growth factors of uncertain nature which induce keratinocyte proliferation.[78]

Persistent T cell stimulation in psoriasis might occur as a result of autoreactivity.[9,11,14] Cell lines from psoriatic lesional skin demonstrated autoreactivity, with possible specificity directed against minor HLA antigens in one study.[73] T cell clones propagated from lesional skin were activated by autologous epidermal cells from involved skin, and by autologous peripheral blood mononuclear cells, in another study.[12] Seventy-five percent of the T cells in lesional skin, but only 20% of psoriatic peripheral blood cells, bind anti-UM4D4 monoclonal antibody, which recognizes the surface molecule UM4D4 (CDw60), capable of direct activation of T cells via an antigen-independent mechanism.[12,75] It has been proposed that streptococcal infection may initiate an ongoing autoimmune reaction in genetically susceptible individuals, since there is cross-reactivity between normal keratinocyte components and streptococcal antigens.[79,80] Group A streptococcal antigen-specific T cells lines are isolated more consistently from skin lesions of guttate psoriasis than other inflammatory dermatoses.[81]

Superantigens and Psoriasis

An alternative possible explanation for the association between psoriasis and streptococci, particularly between acute guttate psoriasis and group A β-hemolytic streptococcal infection, is that streptococcal M proteins and toxins may act as superantigens capable of selectively activating T cells expressing particular T cell receptor β-chain variable gene segment (Vβ) families, and whose presentation is not restricted by MHC class II antigens.[82-85] Thus these particular Vβ genes might be disproportionately represented in patients with psoriasis.[14] Support for this hypothesis has come from recent studies reporting a marked over-representation of Vβ2+ T lymphocytes in the dermis and epidermis, and a less marked dermal increase in Vβ5.1+ T lymphocytes, in patients with both guttate and chronic plaque psoriasis compared with the peripheral blood,[86] and expansion of certain Vβ subsets in the skin but not blood of two patients.[87] Another study has documented persistently increased expression of Vβ3 and/or Vβ13.1 messages in CD8+, but not CD4+, T cells in most psoriatic lesional skin biopsies.[88] Clonality of the Vβ sequence data indicated that the cells were recruited and expanded locally in the skin. A further possible role for superantigens in psoriasis has emerged. While under normal circumstances keratinocytes induced to express class II MHC antigen by IFNγ cannot present nominal antigens to resting T cells, and favor induction of tolerance,[89,90] MHC class II+ keratinocytes have been shown to activate T cells in the presence of staphylococcal enterotoxin B.[91-94] Moreover, staphylococcal enterotoxin B stimulated keratinocytes to produce TNFα.[93]

ANTIGEN PRESENTING CELLS

The number and function of antigen-presenting cells capable of activating autologous T cells, including epidermal and dermal Langerhans cells, as well as CD1-DR+ non-Langerhans antigen-presenting cells, such as lymph node-based RFD-1+ interdigitating reticulum cells and factor XIIIa+ perivascular dendritic cells, are increased in lesional psoriasis skin.[20,95,96] Epidermal antigen presenting cells from psoriatic lesional skin resemble lymphoid dendritic cells rather than freshly isolated normal Langerhans cells, in that they are able to induce vigorous stimulation of autologous T cells,[95,96] and respond differently to treatment with TGF-β and chloroquine.[63,97] It has therefore been proposed that psoriasis involves inappropriate T cell activation in the epidermis due to abnormal Langerhans cell function. In this regard, it is of interest that 20% of epidermal T cells in psoriatic lesions express activation markers, compared with only 5% of dermal T cells, implying that entry into the epidermis is associated with activation.[98] CD36+CD11b- macrophage-like cells capable of triggering stimulation of immunoregulatory T cells in the absence of antigen are present in psoriatic lesional skin.[12]

VASCULAR ENDOTHELIUM AND EXPRESSION OF ADHESION MOLECULES

Cytokines which stimulate endothelial cell adhesiveness for lymphocytes, such as IL-1, TNFα, and IFNγ, may be upregulated in psoriasis.[31,100-103] In psoriatic skin, superficial dermal postcapillary venules are strongly ICAM-1+, and endothelial cells of these and of the intrapapillary capillary loop also express E-selectin and VCAM-1.[31,104] Cytokine responsiveness of microvascular endothelial cells is altered in psoriasis.[103,104] TGF-β normally inhibits baseline, and IL-1- and TNFα-induced increases in, lymphocyte adherence to cultured normal dermal microvascular endothelial cells. Psoriatic dermal microvascular endothelial cells show specific unresponsiveness to the effects of TGF-β.[105] Lymphocytes from psoriasis patients also demonstrate specific cytokine-independent augmented binding to cultured human umbilical vein endothelial cells.[106] Thus abnormalities in both lymphocytes and endothelial cells may be involved in the prominent cutaneous inflammation characteristic of psoriatic skin lesions.

CYTOKINE AND CYTOKINE RECEPTOR LEVELS IN PSORIASIS

Cytokines released from activated keratinocytes, or activated leukocytes, are now thought to play a major role in the immunopathogenesis of psoriasis.[100-103] Increased levels of soluble IL-2 receptor, indicative of T cell activation, have been detected in the serum of psoriasis patients[103] and in suction blister fluids from psoriatic skin.[107] Keratinocytes, which lie in close proximity to the endothelial cells of the upper dermal vasculature in the region of the tips of the dermal papillae, may orchestrate inflammatory events in the dermis. In addition, T cell activation is potentiated by cytokines released by lesional psoriatic, but not normal, epidermis.[108] Therefore, a large number of studies have attempted to quantify cytokine expression in psoriatic lesional skin compared with uninvolved and normal skin.

IL-1

IL-1 has been the subject of particular interest, in view of its proinflammatory action in vivo, and its capacity to potentiate T cell activation, stimulate eicosanoid metabolism, induce fibroblast proliferation, upregulate endothelial cell adhesion molecule expression, and stimulate keratinocyte proliferation, all of which are features of psoriatic skin. However, although some authors have reported elevated levels of IL-1 in psoriatic lesions,[109] this has not been confirmed by the majority of authors.[37,38,110-113] Levels of bioactive IL-1 are markedly reduced in lesional psoriatic skin, although levels of nonfunctional IL-1β are increased.[37,110-113] We and others have found the levels of IL-1ra to be decreased in lesional psoriatic skin.[37,38] Despite this, the ratio of IL-1ra to IL-1α, which is central to the net proinflammatory effect of IL-1, is greatly increased in stable psoriatic plaques.[37]

TNFα

Several studies have failed to show elevated levels of TNFα on either the in situ mRNA or protein level in psoriatic lesions,[111,114] while another study showed prominent TNFα mRNA expression using polymerase chain reaction methodology.[77] TNFα was reported to be expressed mainly by papillary dermal dendrocytes, and to a lesser extent by Langerhans cells and keratinocytes.[115] We found upregulation of TNFα and of its receptors on dermal endothelium and perivascular infiltrating cells in psoriasis in an immunohistochemical study; TNFα immunostaining was distributed throughout the epidermis in lesional skin.[116] TNFα immunoreactivity and biological activity, and concentrations of soluble TNF receptors (especially p55 TNF receptor) were reported to be increased in aqueous extracts of stratum corneum from lesional compared with uninvolved psoriatic skin.[117] TNFα immunoreactivity was increased in suction blister fluid from involved psoriatic skin.[118]

TGFα

TGFα, a potent autocrine growth factor for keratinocytes, is overexpressed in psoriatic epidermis,[101,119,120] as is TGFα mRNA.[102] In addition, there is upregulation of TGFα/epidermal growth factor receptors in psoriatic lesional skin.[120]

IL-6

IL-6, another growth factor for keratinocytes, is expressed at high levels in skin, monocytes and serum in psoriasis patients; this finding is relatively specific, since it is not found in atopic dermatitis patients.[118,121-124] IL-6 production by human dermal microvascular endothelial cells is upregulated by IL-1β and TNFα.[125]

IL-8 AND RELATED CHEMOTACTIC COMPOUNDS

Levels of IL-8, which is chemotactic for neutrophil polymorphs and for T lymphocytes, have been reported to be increased in psoriatic lesional skin.[111,114,115,126-130] mRNA for IL-8 has been localized to the upper or suprabasal layers of the epidermis, which may account for why neutrophil polymorphs migrate through the epidermis.[102,114] IL-8 receptor expression has also been found to be elevated in psoriasis.[131] Monocyte chemotactic protein 1/monocyte activation factor (MCP-1/MCAF) mRNA was localized to the region of proliferating basal keratinocytes of the tips of the rete ridges, and to a lesser extent of cells in the dermal papillae.[132] This distribution may account for the sub-basal distribution of macrophages characteristic of the histology of psoriasis. GRO-α mRNA and protein is overexpressed in psoriatic lesional skin.[133,134]

TGFβ

TGFβ1 and TGFβ3 mRNA levels in psoriatic lesional skin were reported as not different from nonlesional skin.[102] Similarly, no difference in the steady-state level of TGFβ1 mRNA in the epidermis of normal or psoriatic skin was detected in another study.[119] An immunohistochemical investigation found an extracellular form of TGFβ1 present within the epidermis of psoriatic plaques, in addition to an intracellular form found in both plaque and uninvolved psoriatic epidermis.[135]

GM-CSF
GM-CSF mRNA is increased in lesional psoriatic skin,[77] and GM-CSF could be detected in psoriatic scale.[136]

INTERFERONS
IFN activity was detected in suction blister fluid from psoriatic skin,[137] and IFNγ[138] and IFNγ mRNA[139] was found in psoriatic plaques. Raised serum IFNγ levels have been reported in psoriasis.[140] Moreover, the IFNγ-induced protein IP-10 is detectable in psoriatic lesions.[141] However, receptors for IFNγ are reportedly reduced in the upper part of psoriatic epidermis,[142] and neither IFNγ nor IFNα2 had any effect on DNA-synthesis in psoriatic epidermis following intralesional injection.[143]

THE EFFECT OF EXOGENOUS CYTOKINES ON PSORIASIS
There have been relatively few reports on the effects of exogenously administered cytokines on the evolution of psoriasis, as follows:

INTERFERON
IFNα used in the treatment of disseminated carcinoma,[144,145] or intralesionally for viral warts,[146] has been reported to exacerbate or trigger onset of psoriasis; psoriatic arthritis was also triggered in one case.[147] Psoriasis appeared at the site of subcutaneous injection of recombinant IFNγ in patients with psoriatic arthritis,[148] and at the site of intralesional injection in a patient receiving recombinant interferon beta for a basal cell carcinoma.[149]

TNFα
Surprisingly in view of a proposed proinflammatory role for TNFα in psoriasis, beneficial effects on clinical psoriasis have been reported in a few patients, following systemic administration of this cytokine.[150,151]

GM-CSF
GM-CSF has been reported to improve psoriasis in a patient with aplastic anaemia,[152] but to cause an exacerbation of psoriasis in a patient with myelodysplasia.[153]

THE EFFECTS OF THERAPIES FOR PSORIASIS ON CYTOKINES
Available treatments for psoriasis range from relatively nontoxic topical agents, to systemic drugs with major side effects; many of these have immunoregulatory properties including effects on cytokines.

TOPICAL CORTICOSTEROIDS

The mode of action of topical corticosteroids in psoriasis involves at least in part effects on the skin immune system.[154] Steroids inhibit mitogen-stimulated, alloantigen-stimulated, and antigen-specific, T lymphocyte proliferation, perhaps by inhibiting interleukin 2 production.[155,156] Hydrocortisone inhibits human monocyte antigen presentation and antagonizes the effect of IL-1.[157] Topical corticosteroids cause a dose-related reversible decrease in Langerhans cell surface markers (including membrane ATPase, Fc and C3 receptors, class II major histocompatibility complex antigen, and CD1a antigen), and antigen presenting capacity.[154]

DITHRANOL

Dithranol, an anthrocene compound, is a standard treatment for patients with psoriasis. Dithranol prevents keratinocyte proliferation by inhibiting DNA synthesis and repair. Dithranol also has immunosuppressive properties, in that it inhibits mitogen-stimulated lymphocyte proliferation.[158] Therapeutic concentrations of dithranol downregulate keratinocyte receptors for epidermal growth factor,[159] and decrease TGFα expression and EFG-receptor binding in vitro,[160] which may contribute to its antipsoriatic action.

CALCIPOTRIOL

Calcipotriol, used as an alternative therapy to topical corticosteroids in the management of stable plaque psoriasis, is a synthetic analogue of vitamin D. The vitamin D receptor is expressed by keratinocytes as well as by approximately 50% of Langerhans cells, monocytes and T cells in normal skin.[161] Naturally occurring $1,25(OH)_2 D_3$ regulates transcription of TGFβ1 and c-myc, and expression of epidermal growth factor receptor (EGF-R), with resultant inhibition of keratinocyte proliferation and increased morphological and biochemical differentiation.[162] $1,25(OH)_2 D_3$ inhibits proliferation of activated T lymphocytes, IL-2 release by mitogen-stimulated leukocytes,[163] IL-8 release by keratinocytes and IL-1-stimulated leukocytes,[164] and IFNγ release by lymphocytes.[165] Calcipotriol is an analogue of $1,24(OH)_2 D_3$ which is rapidly transformed to inactive metabolites, and is therefore much less potent in inducing hypercalcemia than $1,25(OH)_2 D_3$, but equally potent in its affinity for the vitamin D receptor and in its other effects.

ULTRAVIOLET LIGHT PHOTOTHERAPY

Natural sunlight, ultraviolet B phototherapy (UV-B), and psoralen plus ultraviolet A phototherapy (PUVA) are all used in the management of psoriasis. UV-B and PUVA irradiation may cause suppression of delayed type hypersensitivity reactions in the skin, mediated in part by effects on Langerhans cells and T cells.[167-169] The immunosuppressive effects of phototherapy on Langerhans cells may involve light-induced generation of cis-urocanic acid within the epidermis, which in turn causes local release of TNFα, and prevents migration of Langerhans cells to the regional lymph nodes.[170a] UV-B-induced suppression of delayed type hypersensitivity in the skin is associated with functional inactivation of Th$_1$ cells, in that levels of IFNγ and IL-2 are markedly reduced.[170b] PUVA therapy suppresses keratinocyte DNA synthesis and cell division. Reported effects of PUVA on lymphocytes include inhibition of in vitro alloantigen-stimulated and mitogen-induced lymphocyte proliferation in some but not all studies, perhaps as a result of impaired IL-2 production.[171]

CYCLOSPORIN A

The efficacy of cyclosporin in psoriasis[172] is one of the most powerful arguments for an immunological basis for the condition. Cyclosporin is a potent inhibitor, particularly of CD4+ helper-inducer and cytotoxic T cells, which inhibits IL-2 production and prevents secondary release of the T cell-derived cytokines IFNγ, GM-CSF, and macrophage migration inhibition factor, and thus causes reversible blockade of cellular immune reactivity. Cyclosporin therapy of psorasis results in a reduction in epidermal and dermal CD4+ and CD8+ T cells, HLA-DR+CD1− dendritic cells in the epidermis, keratinocyte expression of HLA-DR, ICAM-1, IL-1β and IL-8, and dermal papillary endothelial expression of ICAM-1,[173-175] as well as of GRO-α mRNA in the epidermis.[133] The concentration of soluble IL-2 receptor in the serum is also decreased.

MONOCLONAL ANTIBODIES TO CD4 ANTIGEN

Monoclonal anti-CD4 antibodies have been reported to induce temporary remission in patients with severe types of psoriasis.[176-178] This provides further strong evidence for the role of CD4+ T cells in the immunopathogenesis of the condition.

CONCLUSION

Whether or not abnormalities in cytokine secretion are of primary significance in causing the hyperproliferation and cutaneous inflammation seen in psoriasis, they are involved in the dysregulation of the skin immune system which underlies the pathogenesis of this condition. Many of the currently available therapies for psoriasis have effects on the skin immune system, and on cytokines in particular. Future advances in the management of psoriasis may come from application of information on cytokine abnormalities in psoriasis, by targeting specific cytokines using cytokine antagonists, including nonpeptidic antagonists, soluble receptors, and anticytokine antibodies.[179] However, soluble receptors and anticytokine antibodies may also in certain circumstances agonize cytokine activity, so that their use may be something of a 'double-edged sword'.[179] It will be fascinating to see how this field develops.

REFERENCES

1. Camp RDR. Psoriasis. In: Champion R, Burton J, Ebling FGJ, eds. Textbook of Dermatology, 5th ed. Oxford: Blackwell Scientific Publications, 1991:1391-1457.
2. Elder JT, Nair RP, Voorhees JJ. Epidemiology and the genetics of psoriasis. J Invest Dermatol 1994; 102:24S-27S.
3. Henseler T, Christopher E. Psoriasis of early and late onset: characterization of two types of psoriasis vulgaris. J Am Acad Dermatol 1985; 13:450-6.
4. Schmitt-Egenolf M, Boehncke W-H, Ständer M et al. Oligonucleotide typing reveals association of type I psoriasis with the HLA-DRB1*0701/2, -DQA1*0201, -DQB1*0303 extended haplotype. J Invest Dermatol 1993; 100:749-52.
5. Lever WF, Schaumburg-Lever G. Histopathology of the Skin, 7th ed. Philadelphia: JB Lippincott Company, 1990.
6. Breathnach SM, Hintner H. In: Adverse Drug Reactions and the Skin. Oxford: Blackwell Scientific Publications, 1992.
7. Valdimarsson H, Baker BS, Jonsdottir I, Fry L. Psoriasis: a disease of abnormal keratinocyte proliferation induced by T lymphocytes. Immunol Today 1986; 7:256-9.
8. Fry L. Psoriasis. Br J Dermatol 1988; 119:445-61.
9. Bos JD. The pathomechanisms of psoriasis; the skin immune system and cyclosporin. Br J Dermatol 1988; 118:141-55.
10. Streilein JW. Speculations on the immunopathogenesis of psoriasis: T-cell violation of a keratinocyte sphere of influence. J Invest Dermatol 1990; 95:20S-21S.
11. Baadsgaard O, Fisher G, Voorhees JJ et al. The role of the immune system in the pathogenesis of psoriasis. J Invest Dermatol 1990; 95:32S-34S.
12. Cooper KD. Psoriasis: leukocytes and cytokines. In: Sauder DN, ed. Immunodermatology. Dermatologic Clinics 1990; 8(4):737-45.
13. Barker JNWN. The pathophysiology of psoriasis. Lancet 1991; 338:227-30.
14. Baker BS, Fry L. The immunology of psoriasis. Br J Dermatol 1992; 126:1-9.
15. Breathnach SM. The skin immune system and psoriasis. Clin Exp Immunol 1993; 91:343-5.
16. Bos JD, ed. Skin immune system (SIS). Boca Raton, Florida: CRC Press, Inc., 1990.
17. Bos JD, Zonneveld I, Das PK et al. The skin immune system: Distribution and immunophenotype of lymphocyte populations in normal human skin. J Invest Dermatol 1989; 92:190-5.
18. Schuler G, ed. Epidermal Langerhans Cells. Boca Raton, Florida: CRC Press, Inc., 1991.
19. Nickoloff BJ, ed. Dermal Immune System. Boca Raton, Florida: CRC Press, Inc., 1993.

20. Cerio R, Griffiths CEM, Cooper KD et al. Characterization of factor XIIIa positive dermal dendritic cells in normal and inflamed skin. Br J Dermatol 1989; 121:421-31.
21. Meunier L, Gonzalez-Ramos A, Cooper KD. Heterogeneous populations of class II MHC⁺ cells in human dermal cell suspensions. Identification of a small subset responsible for potent dermal antigen-presenting cell activity with features analogous to Langerhans cells. J Immunol 1993; 151:1-14.
22. Sepulveda-Merrill C, Mayall S, Hamblin AS, Breathnach SM. Antigen presenting capacity in normal human dermis is mainly subserved by CD1a⁺ cells. Br J Dermatol 1994; 131:15-22.
23. Schwarz T, Luger TA. Pharmacology of cytokines in the skin. In: Muhktar H, ed. Pharmacology of the Skin. Boca Raton, Florida: CRC Press, 1992:283-313.
24. Luger TA, Schwarz T, eds. Epidermal Growth Factors and Cytokines. New York: Marcel Dekker, Inc., 1994.
25. Picker LJ, Kishimoto TK, Smith CW et al. ELAM-1 is an adhesion molecule for skin-homing T-cells. Nature 1991; 349:796-9.
26. Mackay CR. Skin-seeking memory T cells. Nature 1991; 349:737-8.
27. Picker LJ, Treer JR, Ferfuson-Darnell B et al. Control of lymphocyte recirculation in man. Differential regulation of the cutaneous lymphocyte-associated antigen, a tissue-selective homing receptor for skin-homing T cells. J Immunol 1993; 150:1122-36.
28. Lisby S, Ralfkiaer E, Rothlein R et al. Intercellular adhesion molecule-1 (ICAM-1) expression correlated to inflammation. Br J Dermatol 1989; 120:479-84.
29. Groves RW, Allen MH, Barker JNWN et al. Endothelial leucocyte adhesion molecule-1 (ELAM-1) expression in cutaneous inflammation. Br J Dermatol 1991; 124:117-23.
30. Norris P, Poston RN, Thomas DS et al. The expression of endothelial leukocyte adhesion molecule 1 (ELAM-1), intercellular adhesion molecule 1 (ICAM-1) and vascular cell adhesion molecule-1 (VCAM-1) in experimental cutaneous inflammation: a comparison of ultraviolet B erythema and delayed hypersensitivity. J Invest Dermatol 1991; 96:763-70.
31. Barker JNWN, Mitra RS, Griffiths CEM et al. Keratinocytes as initiators of inflammation. Lancet 1991; 337:211-4.
32. Schauer E, Trautinger F, Kock A et al. Proopiomelanocortin-derived peptides are synthesized and released by human keratinocytes. J Clin Invest 1994; 93:2258-62.
33. Dowd PM, Camp RDR, Greaves MW. Human recombinant interleukin-1 alpha is pro-inflammatory in normal human skin. Skin Pharmacol 1988; 1:30-7.
34. Cooper KD, Hammerberg C, Baadsgaard O et al. IL-1 activity is reduced in psoriatic skin: decreased IL-1 alpha and increased non-functional IL-1 beta. J Immunol 1990; 144:4593-603.

35. Mizutani H, Black R, Kupper TS. Human keratinocytes produce but do not process pro-interleukin-1 (IL-1)β. Different strategies of IL-1 production and processing in monocytes and keratinocytes. J Clin Invest 1991; 87:1066-71.
36. Bigler CF, Norris DA, Weston WL et al. Interleukin-1 receptor antagonist production by human keratinocytes. J Invest Dermatol 1992; 98:38-44.
37. Hammerberg C, Arend WP, Fisher GJ et al. Interleukin-1 receptor antagonist in normal and psoriatic epidermis. J Clin Invest 1992; 90:571-83.
38. Kristensen M, Deleuran B, Eedy DJ et al. Distribution of interleukin 1 receptor antagonist protein (IRAP), interleukin 1 receptor, and interleukin 1α in normal and psoriatic skin. Decreased expression of IRAP in psoriatic lesional epidermis. Br J Dermatol 1992; 127:305-11.
39. Arend WP, Welgus HG, Thompson RC et al. Biological properties of recombinant human monocyte-derived interleukin 1 receptor antagonist. J Clin Invest 1990; 85:1694-7.
40. Cork MJ, Duff GW. Interleukin 1. In: Luger TA, Schwarz T, eds. Epidermal Growth Factors and Cytokines. New York: Marcel Dekker, Inc., 1994:19-48.
41. Heufler C, Koch F, Schuler G. Granulocyte/macrophage colony-stimulating factor and interleukin 1 mediate the maturation of murine epidermal Langerhans cells into potent immunostimulatory dendritic cells. J Exp Med 1988; 167:700-5.
42. Romani N, Heufler C, Koch F et al. Cytokines and Langerhans cells. In: Luger TA, Schwarz T, eds. Epidermal Growth Factors and Cytokines. New York: Marcel Dekker, Inc., 1994:345-63.
43. Matsushima K, Morishita K, Yoshimura T et al. Molecular cloning of a human monocyte-derived neutrophil chemotactic factor (MDNCF) and the induction of MDNCF mRNA by interleukin 1 and tumour necrosis factor. J Exp Med 1988; 167:1883-93.
44. Schröder J-M, Sticherling M, Smid P et al. Interleukin 8 and structurally related cytokines. In: Luger TA, Schwarz T, eds. Epidermal Growth Factors and Cytokines. New York: Marcel Dekker, Inc., 1994:89-112.
45. Ristow H-J. A major factor contributing to epidermal proliferation in inflammatory skin disease appears to be interleukin 1 or a related protein. Proc Natl Acad Sci USA 1987; 84:1940-4.
46. Hancock GE, Kaplan F, Cohn ZA. Keratinocyte growth regulation by the products of immune cells. J Exp Med 1988; 168:1395-402.
47. Braunstein S, Kaplan G, Gottlieb AB et al. GM-CSF activates regenerative epidermal growth and stimulates keratinocyte proliferation in human skin in vivo. J Invest Dermatol 1994; 103:601-4.
48. Yoshizaki K, Kishimoto T. Interleukin 6. In: Luger TA, Schwarz T, eds. Epidermal Growth Factors and Cytokines. New York: Marcel Dekker, Inc., 1994:49-62.
49. Klein SB, Fisher GJ, Jensen TC et al. Regulation of TGF alpha expression in human keratinocytes: PKC-dependent and -independent pathways. J Cell Physiol 1992; 151:326-36.

50. Elder JT. Transforming growth factor-α and related growth factors. In: Luger TA, Schwarz T, eds. Epidermal Growth Factors and Cytokines. New York: Marcel Dekker, Inc., 1994:205-40.
51. Detmar M, Tenorio S, Hettmannsperger U et al. Cytokine regulation of proliferation and ICAM-1 expression of human dermal microvascular endothelial cells in vitro. J Invest Dermatol 1992; 98:147-53.
52. Groves RW, Ross E, Barker JNWN et al. Effect of in vivo interleukin-1 on adhesion molecule expression in normal human skin. J Invest Dermatol 1992; 98:384-7.
53. Swerlick RA, Garcia-Gonzalez E, Kubota Y et al. Studies of the modulation of MHC antigen and cell adhesion molecule expression on human dermal microvascular endothelial cells. J Invest Dermatol 1991; 97:190-6.
54. Cai JP, Falanga V, Chin YH. Transforming growth factor-beta regulates the adhesive interactions between mononuclear cells and microvascular endothelium. J Invest Dermatol 1991; 97:169-74.
55. Ikuta S, Kirby JA, Shenton BK et al. Human endothelial cells: effect of TNF-alpha on peripheral blood mononuclear cell adhesion. Immunology 1991; 73:71-6.
56. Larsen CG, Anderson AO, Oppenheim J et al. Production of interleukin-8 by dermal fibroblasts and keratinocytes in response to interleukin-1 and tumor necrosis factor. Immunology 1989; 68:31-6.
57. Strieter RM, Kunkel SL, Showell HJ et al. Endothelial cell gene expression of a neutrophil chemotactic factor by TNFα, LPS, and IL-1α. Science 1989; 43:1467-9.
58. Partridge M, Chantry D, Turner M et al. Production of interleukin-1 and interleukin-6 by human keratinocytes and squamous cell carcinoma lines. J Invest Dermatol 1991; 96:771-6.
59. Dalloul A, Laroche L, Bagot M et al. Interleukin-7 is a growth factor for Sézary lymphoma cells. J Clin Invest 1992; 90:1054-60.
60. Schrader JW. Colony-stimulating factors and the skin. In: Luger TA, Schwarz T, eds. Epidermal Growth Factors and Cytokines. New York: Marcel Dekker, Inc., 1994:147-62.
61. Chantry D et al. Modulation of cytokine production by transforming growth factor β. J Immunol 1989; 142:4295-4300.
62. Wahl SM. Regulation of tissue inflammation, repair, and fibrosis by transforming growth factor beta. In: Luger TA, Schwarz T, eds. Epidermal Growth Factors and Cytokines. New York: Marcel Dekker, Inc., 1994:241-52.
63. Demidem A, Taylor JR, Grammer SF et al. Comparison of effects of transforming growth factor-beta and cyclosporin A on antigen-presenting cells of blood and epidermis. J Invest Dermatol 1991; 96:401-7.
64. Turner M, Chantry D, Katsikis P et al. Induction of the IL-1 receptor antagonist protein, by transforming growth factor beta. Eur J Immunol 1991; 21:1635-1639.

65. Partridge M et al. Production of TGF-α and TGF-β by cultured keratinocytes, skin and oral squamous cell carcinomas—potential autocrine regulation of normal and malignant epithelial cell proliferation. Br J Cancer 1989; 60:542-8.
66. Becher D, Knop J. Epidermal cell-derived cytokines and delayed-type hypersensitivity. In: Luger TA, Schwarz T, eds. Epidermal Growth Factors and Cytokines. New York: Marcel Dekker, Inc., 1994:365-76.
67. Hosoi J, Murphy GF, Egan CL et al. Regulation of Langerhans cell function by nerves containing calcitonin gene-related peptide. Nature 1993; 363:159-63.
68. Brown LF, Yeo KT, Berse B et al. Expression of vascular permeability factor (vascular endothelial cell growth factor) by epidermal keratinocytes during wound healing. J Exp Med 1992; 176:1375-9.
69. Nickoloff BJ, Naidu Y. Perturbation of epidermal barrier function correlates with initiation of cytokine cascade in human skin. J Am Acad Dermatol 1994; 30:535-46.
70. Griffiths CE, Voorhees JJ, Nickoloff BJ. Characterization of intercellular adhesion molecule-1 and HLA-DR expression in normal and inflamed skin: Modulation by recombinant gamma interferon and tumor necrosis factor. J Am Acad Dermatol 1989; 20:617-29.
71. Nickoloff BJ, Griffiths CEM. T lymphocytes and monocytes bind to keratinocytes in frozen sections of biopsy specimens of normal skin treated with gamma interferon. J Am Acad Dermatol 1989; 20:736-43.
72. Boyera N, Cavey D, Delamadeleine F et al. A novel in vitro model for the study of human keratinoctye/leukocyte interactions under autologous conditions. Br J Dermatol 1993; 129:521-9.
73. Nikaein A, Phillips C, Gilber SC et al. Characterization of skin-infiltrating lymphocytes in patients with psoriasis. J Invest Dermatol 1991; 96:3-9.
74. Morganroth GS, Chan LS, Weinstein GD et al. Proliferating cells in psoriatic dermis are comprised primarily of T cells, endothelial cells, and factor XIIIa+ perivascular dendritic cells. J Invest Dermatol 1991; 96:333-40.
75. Baadsgaard O, Tong P, Elder JT et al. UM4D4+ (CDw60) T-cells are compartmentalized into psoriatic skin and release lymphokines that induce a keratinocyte phenotype expressed in psoriatic lesions. J Invest Dermatol 1990; 95:275-82.
76. Schlaak JF, Buslau M, Jochum W et al. T cells involved in psoriasis vulgaris belong to the Th_1 subset. J Invest Dermatol 1994; 102:145-9.
77. Uyemura K, Yamamura M, Fivenson DF et al. The cytokine network in lesional and lesion-free psoriatic skin is characterized by a T-helper type 1 cell-mediated response. J Invest Dermatol 1993; 101:701-5.
78. Strange P, Cooper KD, Hansen ER et al. T-lymphocyte clones initiated from lesional psoriatic skin release growth factors that induce keratinocyte proliferation. J Invest Dermatol 1993; 101:695-700.

79. Swerlick RA, Cunningham MW, Hall NK. Monoclonal antibodies cross-reactive with group A streptococci and normal and psoriatic human skin. J Invest Dermatol 1986; 87:367-71.
80. McFadden JP, Valdimarsson H, Fry L. Cross-reactivity between streptococcal M surface antigen and human skin. Br J Dermatol 1991; 125:443-7.
81. Baker BS, Bokth S, Powles AV et al. Group A streptococcal antigen-specific T lymphocytes in guttate psoriatic lesions. Br J Dermatol 1993; 128:493-9.
82. Tomai MA, Aelion JA, Dockter ME et al. T cell receptor V gene usage by human T cells stimulated with the superantigen streptococcal M protein. J Exp Med 1991; 174:285-8.
83. Tomai MA, Schlievert PM, Kotb M. Distinct T-cell receptor Vβ gene usage by human T lymphocytes stimulated with the streptococcal pyrogenic exotoxins and pep M5 protein. Infect Immun 1992; 60:701-5.
84. Hermann A, Kappler JW, Marrack P et al. Superantigens: mechanism of T-cell stimulations and role in immune responses. Annu Rev Immunol 1991; 9:745-2.
85. Möller G. Superantigens. Immunol Rev 1993; 131:1-200.
86. Lewis HM, Baker BS, Bokth S et al. Restricted T-cell receptor Vβ usage in the skin of patients with guttate and chronic plaque psoriasis. Br J Dermatol 1993; 129:514-20.
87. Leung DYM, Walsh P, Giorno R et al. A potential role for superantigens in the pathogenesis of psoriasis. J Invest Dermatol 1993; 100:225-8.
88. Chang JCC, Smith LR, Froning KJ et al. CD8+ T cells in psoriatic lesions preferentially use T-cell receptor $V_\beta 3$ and/or $V_\beta 13.1$ genes. Proc Natl Acad Sci USA 1994; 91:9282-6.
89. Gaspari AA, Jenkins MK, Katz SI. Class II MHC-bearing keratinocytes induce antigen-specific unresponsiveness in hapten-specific Th_1 clones. J Immunol 1988; 141:2216-20.
90. Bal V, McIndoe A, Denton G et al. Antigen presentation by keratinocytes induces tolerance in human T cells. Eur J Immunol 1990; 20:1893-7.
91. Strange P, Skov L, Baadsgaard O. Interferon gamma-treated keratinocytes activate T cells in the presence of superantigens: involvement of major histocompatibility complex class II molecules. J Invest Dermatol 1994; 102:155-9.
92. Nickoloff BJ, Mitra RS, Green J et al. Activated keratinocytes present bacterial-derived superantigens to T lymphocytes: relevance to psoriasis. J Dermatol Sci 1993; 6:127-33.
93. Tokura Y, Yagi J, O'Malley M et al. Superantigenic staphylococcal exotoxins induce T-cell proliferation in the presence of Langherhans cells or class II-bearing keratinocytes and stimulate keratinocytes to produce T-cell activating cytokines. J Invest Dermatol 1994; 102:31-8.
94. Nickoloff BJ, Turka LA. Immunological functions of non-professional antigen-presenting cells: new insights from studies of T-cell interactions with keratinocytes. Immunol Today 1994; 15:464-9.

95. Schopf RE, Hoffmann A, Jung M et al. Stimulation of T cells by autologous mononuclear leukocytes and epidermal cells in psoriasis. Arch Dermatol Res 1986; 279:89-94.
96. Baadsgaard O, Gupta AK, Taylor RS et al. Psoriatic epidermal cells demonstrate increased numbers and function of non-Langerhans antigen-presenting cells. J Invest Dermatol 1989; 92:190-5.
97. Demidem A, Taylor JR, Grammer S et al. Effects of chloroquine on antigen-presenting functions of epidermal cells from normal and psoriatic skin. J Invest Dermatol 1992; 98:181-6.
98. Nickoloff BJ, Griffiths CEM. Lymphocyte trafficking in psoriasis: a new perspective emphasizing the dermal dendrocyte with active dermal recruitment mediated via endothelial cells followed by intra-epidermal T-cell activation. J Invest Dermatol 1990; 95:35S-37S.
99. Chin Y-H, Falanga V, Cai J-P. Lymphocyte adhesion to psoriatic dermal endothelium: mechanism and modulation. J Invest Dermatol 1990; 95:29S-31S.
100. Krueger JG, Krane JF, Carter DM et al. Role of growth factors, cytokines, and their receptors in the pathogenesis of psoriasis. J Invest Dermatol 1990; 94:135S-40S.
101. Elder JT, Klein SB, Tavakkol A et al. Growth factor and proto-oncogene expression in psoriasis. J Invest Dermatol 1990; 95:7S-9S.
102. Schmid P, Cox D, McMaster GK et al. In situ hybridization analysis of cytokine, proto-oncogene and tumour suppressor gene expression in psoriasis. Arch Dermatol Res 1993; 285:334-40.
103. Kapp A. The role of cytokines in the psoriatic inflammation. J Dermatol Sci 1993; 5:133-42.
104. Petzelbauer P, Pober JS, Keh A et al. Inducibility and expression of microvascular endothelial adhesion molecules in lesional, perilesional, and uninvolved skin of psoriatic patients. J Invest Dermatol 1994; 103:300-5.
105. Cai J-P, Falanga V, Taylor JR, Chin Y-H. Transforming growth factor-beta differentially regulates the adhesiveness of normal and psoriatic dermal microvascular endothelial cells for peripheral blood mononuclear cells. J Invest Dermatol 1992; 98:405-9.
106. Lee ML, To SST, Cooper A et al. Augmented lymphocyte binding to cultured endothelium in psoriasis. Clin Exp Immunol 1993; 91:346-50.
107. Takematsu H, Tagami H. Interleukin 2, soluble interleukin 2 receptor, and interferon-gamma in the suction blister fluids from psoriatic skin. Arch Dermatol Res 1990; 282:149-52.
108. Chang EY, Hammerberg C, Fisher G et al. T-cell activation is potentiated by cytokines released by lesional psoriatic, but not normal, epidermis. Arch Dermatol 1992; 128:1479-85.
109. Romero LI, Ikejima T, Pincus SH. In situ localization of interleukin-1 in normal and psoriatic skin. J Invest Dermatol 1989; 93:518-22.
110. Takematsu H, Suzuki R, Tagami H et al. Inteleukin-1-like activity in horny layer extracts: decreased activity in scale extracts of psoriasis and sterile pustular dermatoses. Dermatologica 1986; 172:236-40.

111. Gearing AJ, Fincham NJ, Bird CR et al. Cytokines in the skin lesions of psoriasis. Cytokine 1990; 2:68-75.
112. Cooper KD, Hammerberg C, Baadsgaard O et al. IL-1 activity is reduced in psoriatic skin. Decreased IL1α and increased non-functional IL-1β. J Immunol 1990; 144:4593-603.
113. Cooper KD, Hammerberg C, Baadsgaard O et al. Interleukin-1 in human skin: dysregulation in psoriasis. J Invest Dermatol 1990; 95:24S-26S.
114. Gillitzer R, Berger R, Mielke V et al. Upper keratinocytes of psoriatic skin lesions express high levels of NAP-1/IL-8 mRNA in situ. J Invest Dermatol 1991; 97:73-9.
115. Nickoloff BJ, Karabin GD, Barker JNWN et al. Localization of IL-8 and its inducer TNFα in psoriasis. Am J Pathol 1991; 138:129-40.
116. Kristensen M, Chu CQ, Eedy DJ et al. Localization of tumour necrosis factor-alpha (TNFα) and its receptors in normal and psoriatic skin: epidermal cells express the 55-kD but not the 75-kD TNF receptor. Clin Exp Immunol 1993; 94:354-62.
117. Ettehadi P, Greaves MW, Wallach D et al. Elevated tumour necrosis factor -alpha (TNFα) biological activity in psoriatic skin lesions. Clin Exp Immunol 1994; 96:146-51.
118. Bonifati C, Carducci M, Cordiali Fei P et al. Correlated increases of tumour necrosis factor-α, interleukin-6 and granulocyte monocyte-colony stimulating factor levels in suction blister fluids and sera of psoriatic patients—relationships with disease severity. Clin Exp Dermatol 1994; 19:383-7.
119. Elder JT, Fisher GJ, Lindquist PB et al. Overexpression of transforming growth factor α in psoriatic epidermis. Science 1989; 243:811-14.
120. King LE Jr, Gates RE, Stoscheck CM et al. Epidermal growth factor/ transforming growth factor alpha receptors and psoriasis. J Invest Dermatol 1990; 95:10S-12S.
121. Grossman RM, Krueger J, Yourish D et al. Interleukin 6 is expressed in high levels in psoriatic skin and stimulates proliferation of cultured human keratinocytes. Proc Natl Acad Sci USA 1989; 86:6367-71.
122. Neuner P, Urbanski A, Trautinger F et al. Increased IL-6 production by monocytes and keratinocytes in patients with psoriasis. J Invest Dermatol 1991; 97:27-33.
123. Nakamura T, Oishi M, Johno M et al. Serum levels of interleukin 6 in patients with pustulosis palmaris et plantaris. J Dermatol 1993; 20:763-6.
124. Ohta Y, Katayama I, Funato T et al. In situ expression of messenger RNA of interleukin-1 and interleukin-6 in psoriasis: interleukin-6 involved in formation of psoriatic lesions. Arch Dermatol Res 1991; 283:351-6.
125. Hettmannsperger U, Detmar M, Owsianowki M et al. Cytokine-stimulated human dermal microvascular endothelial cells produce interleukin 6—inhibition by hydrocortisone, dexamethasone, and calcitriol. J Invest Dermatol 1992; 99:531-7.

126. Schröder JM, Christophers E. Identification of C5a$_{desarg}$ and an anionic neutrophil-activating peptide (ANAP) in psoriatic scales. J Invest Dermatol 1986; 87:53-8.
127. Takematsu H, Terui T, Ohkochi K et al. Presence of chemotactic peptides other than C5a in scales of psoriasis and sterile pustular psoriasis. Acta Derm Venereol (Stockh) 1986; 66:93-7.
128. Schröder JM. Biochemical and biological characterization of NAP/IL-8-related cytokines in lesional psoriatic scale. Adv Exp Med Biol 1991; 305:97-107.
129. Sticherling M, Bornscheuer E, Schröder J-M, Christophers E. Localization of neutrophil-activating peptide-1/interleukin-8-immunoreactivity in normal and psoriatic skin. J Invest Dermatol 1991; 96:26-30.
130. Schröder JM, Gregory H, Young J et al. Neutrophil-activating proteins in psoriasis. J Invest Dermatol 1992; 98:241-7.
131. Schulz BS, Michel G, Wagner S et al. Increased expression of epidermal IL-8 receptor in psoriasis. Down-regulation by FK-506 in vitro. J Immunol 1993; 151:4399-406.
132. Gillitzer R, Wolff K, Tong D et al. MCP-1 mRNA expression in basal keratinocytes of psoriatic lesions. J Invest Dermatol 1993; 101:127-31.
133. Kojima T, Cromie MA, Fisher GJ et al. GRO-α mRNA is selectively overexpressed in psoriatic epidermis and is reduced by cyclosporin A in vivo, but not in cultured keratinocytes. J Invest Dermatol 1993; 101:767-72.
134. Tettelbach W, Nanney L, Ellis D et al. Localization of MGSA/GRO protein in cutaneous lesions. J Cutan Pathol 1993; 20:259-66.
135. Kane CJM, Knapp AM, Mansbridge JN, Hanawalt PC. Transforming growth factor-β1 localization in normal and psoriatic epidermal keratinocytes in situ. J Cell Physiol 1990; 144:144-50.
136. Takematsu H, Tagami H. Granulocyte-macrophage colony-stimulating factor in psoriasis. Dermatologica 1990; 181:16-20.
137. Livden JK, Bjercke JR, Degre M, Matre R. The effect of Goeckerman therapy on inteferon in serum and suction blister fluid from patients with psoriasis. Br J Dermatol 1986; 114:217-25.
138. Livden JK, Nilsen R, Bjerke JR, Matre R. In situ localization of interferons in psoriatic lesions. Arch Dermatol Res 1989; 281:392-7.
139. Barker JNWN, Karabin G, Stoof T et al. Detection of gamma interferon mRNA in psoriatic epidermis by polymerase chain reaction. J Dermatol Sci 1991; 2:106-11.
140. Gomi T, Shiohara T, Munakata T et al. Interleukin 1 alpha, tumor necrosis factor alpha, and interferon gamma in psoriasis. Arch Dermatol 1991; 127:827-30.
141. Gottlieb AB, Luster AD, Posnett DN, Carter DM. Detection of a gamma interferon-induced protein IP-10 in psoriatic plaques. J Exp Med 1988; 168:941-8.

142. Scheynius A, Fransson J, Johansson C et al. Expression of interferon-gamma receptors in normal and psoriatic skin. J Invest Dermatol 1992; 98:255-8.
143. Schulze JH, Mahrle G. Effect of interferons (rIFN,-alpha 2, rIFN-gamma) on DNA synthesis and HLA-DR expression in psoriasis. Arch Dermatol Res 1986; 278:416-8.
144. Quesada JR, Gutterman JU. Psoriasis and alpha-interferon. Lancet 1986; i:1466-8.
145. Hartmann F, von Wussow P, Deicher H. Psoriasis—Exacerbation bei Therapie mit alpha-Interferon. Dtsch Med Wochenschr 1989; 114:96-8.
146. Shiohara T, Kobayashi M, Abe K, Nagashima M. Psoriasis occurring predominantly on warts. Possible involvement of interferon alpha. Arch Dermatol 1988; 124:1816-21.
147. Jucgla A, Marcoval J, Curco N, Servitje O. Psoriasis with articular involvement induced by interferon alpha. Arch Dermatol 1991;127:910-1.
148. Fierlbeck G, Rassner G, Müller C. Psoriasis induced at the injection site of recombinant interferon gamma. Arch Dermatol 1990; 126:351-5.
149. Kowalzick L, Weyer U. Psoriasis induced at the injection site of recombinant interferons. Arch Dermatol 1990; 126:1515-16.
150. Takematsu H, Ozawa H, Yoshimura T et al. Systemic TNF administration in psoriatic patients: a promising therapeutic modality for severe psoriasis. Br J Dermatol 1991; 124:209-10.
151. Creaven PJ, Stoll HL. Response to tumor necrosis factor in two cases of psoriasis. J Am Acad Dermatol 1991; 24:735-7.
152. Raychaudhuri SP. Granulocyte-macrophage colony stimulating factor and psoriasis. J Am Acad Dermatol 1994; 30:144-5.
153. Kelly RI, Marsden RA. Granulocyte-macrophage colony stimulating factor and psoriasis. J Am Acad Dermatol 1994; 30:144.
154. Ashworth J, Booker J, Breathnach SM. Effects of topical corticosteroid therapy on Langerhans cell antigen presenting function in human skin. Br J Dermatol 1988; 118:457-70.
155. Hirschberg H, Hirschberg T, Nousiainen H et al. The effects of corticosteroids on the antigen presenting properties of human monocytes and endothelial cells. Clin Immunol Immunopathol 1982; 23:577-85.
156. Larsson E-L. Cyclosporin A and dexamethasone suppress T cell responses by selectively acting at distinct sites of the triggering process. J Immunol 1980; 124:2828-33.
157. Rhodes J, Ivanyi J, Cozens P. Antigen presentation by human monocytes: effects of modifying major histocompatibility complex class II antigen expression and interleukin 1 production by using recombinant interferons and corticosteroids. Eur J Immunol 1986; 16:370-75.
158. Anderson R, Lukey P, Dippenaar U et al. Dithranol mediates pro-oxidative inhibition of polymorphonuclear leukocyte migration and lymphocyte proliferation. Br J Dermatol 1987; 117:405-18.
159. Kemény L, Michel G, Arenberger P et al. Down-regulation of epidermal growth factor receptors by dithranol. Acta Derm Venereol (Stockh) 1993; 73:37-40.

160. Gottlieb AB, Khandke L, Krane JF et al. Anthralin decreases keratinocyte TGF-α expression and EGF-receptor binding in vitro. J Invest Dermatol 1992; 98:680-5.
161. Milde P, Hauser U, Simon T, et al. Expression of 1,25-dihydroxyvitamin D_3 receptors in normal and psoriatic skin. J Invest Dermatol 97:230-6.
162. Kragballe K. Vitamin D_3 and skin diseases. Arch Dermatol Res 1992; 284 (suppl): S30-S36.
163. Rigby WFC, Denome S, Fanger MW. Regulation of lymphokine production and T lymphocyte activation by 1,25-dihydroxyvitamin D_3: specific inhibition at level of messenger RNA. J Clin Invest 1987; 70:1659-64.
164. Larsen CG, Kristensen M, Paludan K et al. 1,25(OH)$_2$ D_3 is a potent regulator of interleukin-8 expression and production. Biochem Biophys Res Commun 1991; 176:1020-6.
165. Reichel H, Koeffler HP, Tobler A et al. 1,25-dihydroxyvitamin D_3 inhibits gamma-interferon synthesis by normal peripheral blood lymphoyctes. Proc Natl Acad Sci USA 1987; 84:3385-9.
167. Bergstresser PR, Streilein JW. Ultraviolet radiation produces selective immune incompetence. J Invest Dermatol 1983; 81:85-6.
168. Baadsgaard O. In vivo ultraviolet irradiation of human skin results in profound perturbation of the immune system. Relevance to ultraviolet-induced skin cancer. Arch Dermatol 1991; 127:99-109.
169. Ashworth J, Kahan MC, Breathnach SM. PUVA therapy decreases HLA-DR⁺CD1a⁺ Langerhans cells and epidermal cell antigen-presenting capacity in human skin, but flow cytometrically-sorted residual HLA-DR⁺CD1a⁺ Langerhans cells exhibit normal alloantigen-presenting function. Br J Dermatol 1989; 120:329-39.
170a. Kurimoto I, Streilein JW. Deleterious effects of cis-urocanic acid and UVB radiation on Langerhans cells and on induction of contact hypersensitivity are mediated by tumor necrosis factor-alpha. J Invest Dermatol 1992; 99:69S-70S.
170b. Simon JC, Mosmann T, Edelbaum D et al. In vivo evidence that ultraviolet B-induced suppression of allergic contact sensitivity is associated with functional inactivation of Th_1 cells. Photodermatol Photoimmunol Photomed 1994; 10:206-11.
171. Okamoto H, Horio T, Maeda M. Alteration of lymphocyte functions by 8-methoxypsoralen and long-wave ultraviolet radiation. II. The effect of in vivo PUVA on IL-2 production. J Invest Dermatol 1987; 89:24-6.
172. Ellis CN, Fradin MS, Messana JM et al. Cyclosporine for plaque-type psoriasis: results of a multidose, double-blind trial. N Engl J Med 1991; 324:277-84.
173. Cooper KD, Voorhees JJ, Fisher GJ et al. Effects of cyclosporine on immunologic mechanisms in psoriasis. J Am Acad Dermatol 1990; 23:1318-28.
174. Wong RL, Winslow CM, Cooper KD. The mechanism of action of cyclosporin A in the treatment of psoriasis. Immunol Today 1993; 14:69-74.

175. Elder JT, Hammerberg C, Cooper KD et al. Cyclosporin A rapidly inhibits epidermal cytokine expression in psoriasis lesions, but not in cytokine-stimulated cultured keratinocytes. J Invest Dermatol 1993; 101:761-6.
176. Poizot-Martin I, Oliver C, Mawas C et al. Are CD4 antibodies and peptide T new treatments for psoriasis? Lancet 1991; 337:1477.
177. Prinz J, Braun-Falco O, Meurer M et al. Chimaeric CD4 monoclonal antibody in treatment of generalised pustular psoriasis. Lancet 1991; 338; 320-1.
178. Nicholas JF, Chamchick N, Thivolet J et al. CD4 antibody treatment of severe psoriasis. Lancet 1991; 338:321.
179. Debets R, Savelkoul HFJ. Cytokine antagonists and their potential therapeutic use. Immunol Today 1994; 15:455-8.

CHAPTER 10

WHAT CAN WE LEARN FROM 'GENE KNOCKOUT' MICE?

Andrew P. Cope

INTRODUCTION

Transgenic technology has provided us with a sophisticated approach for studying physiological and pathological processes in vivo. 'Knockout mice,' or more precisely mice with disrupted genes, are variations on a theme, being transgenic mice in their own right. The concept of mutational analysis was documented as early as the 18th century by the German physicist Georg Christoph Lichtenberg (1742-1791) who wrote, *"A good means to discovery is to take away certain parts of a system and to find out how the rest behaves"*. A remarkable number of studies utilizing this approach have been published over the last few years, driven by an increased understanding of the functions of genes in normal and pathological processes. In the field of immunology, systematic targeting of genes encoding key molecules of the immune system has already proved informative. For a comprehensive review, see Bluethmann and Ohashi.[1]

A unique advantage of gene knockout technology which distinguishes it from the alternative in vivo approaches is that it provides fundamental information about early embryonic development. At one extreme, mice homozygous for a mutation not developing to term would suggest that the gene under study is critical for implantation, embryonal cell differentiation and/or organ development. During subsequent maturation of the organism, information can be obtained about how organs function in the absence of proteins normally expressed in abundance in such tissues. Perhaps of greatest interest is that gene targeting in mice provides a tool for generating models of human disease, as well as opportunities to determine whether a gene is essential for inducing or sustaining pathophysiological processes in spontaneous disease

---

Cytokines in Autoimmunity, edited by Fionula M. Brennan and Marc Feldmann.
© 1996 R.G. Landes Company.

models. Depending on the model, it may be necessary to backcross the mutant animal of interest to the appropriate disease prone strain. The effects of the homozygous mutation can then be evaluated, bearing in mind the limitations in extrapolating mouse models to human pathology. Although an investigation of induced gene deficiency in rodents should cast considerable light on normal immune regulation and disease pathogenesis, the ultimate proof of the role of susceptibility genes in man rests on the correlation of its defect with the clinical picture.

Considering the time constraints involved in gene targeting, targets have been carefully selected. Given the widespread expression of many genes chosen as targets, it is remarkable how animals exhibit defects only in a subset of those tissues; further, many mutant mice develop normally. An extreme example is disruption of the hypoxanthine phosphoribosyl transferase gene that causes no clinical symptoms in mice, in sharp contradistinction to the Lesch-Nyhan syndrome characteristic of patients bearing the same deficiency.[2,3] There are several reasons why mutants may appear benign. Firstly, the protein's function may in fact be rather modest; some proteins are expressed at high levels in some tissues, yet have no obvious function at all. Secondly, inheritance of some genes may have become fixed in a population, conferring some small but nevertheless significant survival advantage whose phenotype may otherwise be undetectable in a laboratory animal. Thirdly, loss of protein function may induce major regulatory and compensatory pathways which do not occur under normal circumstances. In this regard, the functional importance of a protein in physiological processes may be grossly underestimated. Finally, the lack of a clear phenotype in mutant mice may suggest redundancy of function, indicating coexpression of proteins with duplicated functions.

WHY STUDY CYTOKINE KNOCKOUT MICE?

Cytokines are often discussed in terms of their potential pathogenic influence, and yet they play significant roles in embryonal development and normal physiological processes in the mature adult. Cytokines such as transforming growth factor-beta (TGFβ), leukemia inhibitory factor (LIF), interleukin (IL)-7 and stem cell growth factor are good examples.[4-7] One approach to study this in detail has been to inhibit cytokine bioactivity by injecting neutralizing antibodies (discussed in chapter 2). Although the half-life of antibodies is longer than that of many cytokines, the extent of blockade achieved in the adult mouse or during fetal development by maternal injections is unpredictable. Similarly, there are instances where selective blockade of a cell surface receptor protein may be desired. Since receptors are widely distributed on circulating and tissue cells, blockade using receptor specific antibodies in vivo can be difficult to achieve. Systematic gene disruption provides a unique opportunity to resolve these problems, and allows evaluation of systems in which a cytokine may bind and signal through two or more receptors (e.g., lymphotoxin),[8] or where receptor proteins transduce signals for several different ligands (e.g., gp130).[9] A genetic approach such as this provides opportunities to examine at a molecular level redundancy, pleiotropy and hierarchy, features highly characteristic of cytokine biology. Over more than a decade, our understanding of cytokine networks has reached the stage where defining which cytokines are involved in normal and pathological responses, and when and how they function in vivo, have become a priority. The answer to these and other key issues can now be addressed by gene targeting and the study of animals bearing these null mutations.

NATURE'S "KNOCKOUTS"

Are the best experiments of all those of Nature, as noted by Garrod in 1924?[10]

"..... Nature is nowhere accustomed more openly to display her secret mysteries than in cases where she shows traces of her workings apart from the beaten path;..... the study of nature's experiments and mistakes..... may throw a ray of light into some dark place..... "

The current pace of advancing technology has allowed some considerable light to be thrown upon cytokine networks and their complex hierarchies. Whilst a comprehensive review of spontaneously occurring gene mutations in mammals which give rise to distinct pathological phenotypes is beyond the scope of this chapter, examples of Nature's knockouts are worthy of brief discussion.

An important aspect of cloning novel mammalian genes, whatever their function, has been to define their chromosomal location. Sometimes the region of the chromosome corresponds to one within the genome to which genetic disease has been mapped. Recent advances using large sets of genetic markers based on simple sequence repeats (or microsatellites) that permit efficient and rapid mapping of mammalian genomes has begun already to compliment this approach.[11,12] Striking examples of mutations in cytokine ligands and coreceptors responsible for the induction of autoimmune syndromes have been described in recent years in the mouse. Thus, the *lpr* (lymphoproliferation) mutation in a substrain of MRL mice is recessive and determines an accumulation of T lymphocytes with the CD4-CD8-CD2-B220+ phenotype, and a lupus-like disease characterized by severe glomerulonephritis, vasculitis and autoantibody production.[13] The *lpr*[cg] and *gld* mutations induce a proliferative syndrome with an identical phenotype. By genetic mapping of backcrosses, the *lpr* mutation was assigned to chromosome 19, close to the gene encoding Fas antigen,[14] a transmembrane protein which when triggered by its ligand or antibody signals programmed cell death and apoptosis. Mice bearing the *lpr* mutation expressed no Fas mRNA in liver or thymus, and were found to display unique restriction fragment length polymorphisms in their genomic DNA due to integration of a retrotransposon sequence into the second intron of the *Fas* gene.[15,16] In mice bearing the *lpr*^cg mutation, the *Fas* gene was transcribed normally but showed a point mutation in a highly conserved region of the cytoplasmic domain, thereby abolishing the ability of Fas protein to transduce apoptotic signals.[15] The *gld* locus encodes the Fas ligand, so that mutations in this gene product prohibit signaling also.[17] When first reported, these data provided the first unequivocal evidence for defects in positive and negative selection contributing to autoimmunity, and indicated that spontaneously occurring mutations in cytokine/receptor genes could lead to disease. As mapping of the human genome progresses, it is likely that further examples of diseases caused by subtle defects in the functions of genes encoding immunoregulatory molecules or their receptors will be uncovered.[18]

"KNOCKOUT" TECHNOLOGY

CHOOSING THE TARGET

For studying the effects of disrupting cytokine function there are several options open to the investigator, each of which illustrates the complex nature of cytokine networks and cytokine/receptor families. Investigating the role of IL-1 in vivo, for example, could be approached by several different means.[19] Firstly, IL-1α or IL-1β genes can be targeted in embryonic stem cells. Chimeric mice can be produced and then bred to achieve germ-line transmission (see below). Alternatively, IL-1 bioactivity can be blocked by overexpressing the IL-1 receptor antagonist (IL-1ra) or soluble IL-1 receptors, introducing them as transgenes. A third approach is to target type I cell surface IL-1 receptors, since this receptor is responsible for transducing IL-1 signals.[20] Although disrupting the gene of interest by conventional gene targeting techniques more or less guarantees cytokine blockade, overexpressing inhibitors such as IL-1ra, or employing antisense transgene technology provides an opportunity to target specific tissues such as the thymus or the pancreas in a restricted fashion, at the expense of widespread cytokine inhibition. For the purpose of this chapter, however, I will focus exclusively on conventional gene targeting and how this technology has influenced concepts of the mechanisms of autoimmune disease.

CURRENT PROTOCOLS

Whilst in transgenic experiments expression constructs are employed, gene targeting strategies involve plasmids designed to inhibit or disrupt gene expression. A schematic of commonly used strategies for gene targeting and for generating mutant mice are outlined in Figures 10.1 and 10.2, respectively (see figure legends for details). Ultimately, the mutation should be transmitted in a Mendelian fashion. Any deviations from the expected numbers of homozygous mice derived

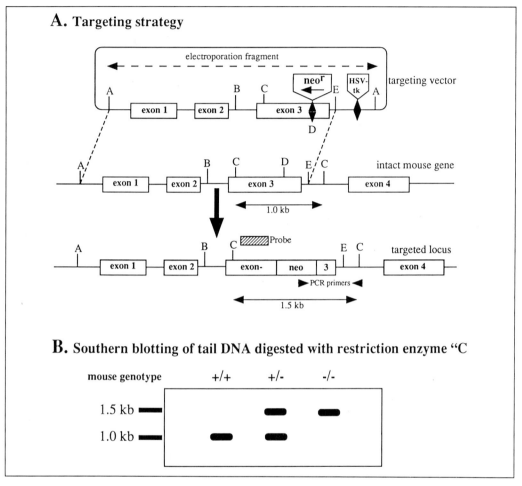

Fig. 10.1. Generation of targeting vectors. (A) Cloned and sequenced murine genomic DNA constructs in an appropriate targeting vector corresponding to the intact mouse gene are essential prerequisites for gene targeting. The critical event allowing gene disruption to be studied in vivo is homologous recombination (shown here to occur across arbitrary restriction enzyme sites "A" and "E"), a process first studied in yeast in which the targeting vector containing the same nucleotide sequence as a region in the target gene replaces one copy of an allele in a transfected cell.[21-23] The geometrical arrangement of sequences constituting the incoming DNA determines the outcome of the targeting event. Recombinants are screened before positive clones can be identified. Screening is facilitated by insertion into the targeting cassette of a selectable marker gene such as neomycin phosphotransferase (neo^r; often in reverse orientation). Alternatively, the hygromycin B resistance gene or the hprt gene may be used. Screening of G418 resistant colonies for the correct recombination event is performed by polymerase chain reaction (PCR; typical primer sites are shown), and (B) confirmed by Southern blotting using selected probes (shown here following a digest with restriction enzyme "C") which give clear patterns of hybridization for wild type mice, as well as for animals heterozygous and homozygous for the mutation. The herpes simplex virus thymidine kinase (TK) gene introduced at one or both ends of the construct, also facilitates selection of random integrants but by negative selection (Capecchi et al, 1989).[23] The TK genes are retained by random integrants, rendering cells sensitive to the TK inhibitor gancyclovir, whilst homologous recombination events lead to loss of the TK gene inserts; these cells are not killed by gancyclovir. Whichever selection strategy is employed, successful gene disruption is achieved by interrupting the reading frame of the cytokine gene by introducing frequent stop codons,[24-26] or by deleting a fragment of one or more exons.[27]

from heterozygous matings are noted, since the finding of marked reductions may imply lethality caused by the null mutation in some embryos. Such an observation may arise not only through disruption of critical stages in organogenesis, but also due to abnormalities in earlier events such as blastocyst implantation.[5] These unexpected outcomes may be in themselves of profound interest. Other examples have been reported in the literature.[32] Under such circumstances, the role of such genes in different tissues can be evaluated in chimeric mice.

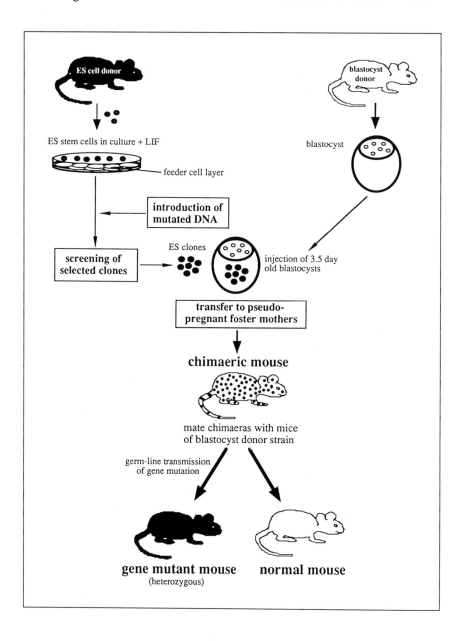

CYTOKINE GENE KNOCKOUTS AND AUTOIMMUNITY

We are still only beginning to understand the role of cytokines in autoimmune disease. Nevertheless, there are aspects to pathogenetic mechanisms of autoimmunity including those relating to central and peripheral tolerance, cell activation, growth and differentiation as well as cell trafficking which are hard to reconcile without casting cytokines in leading roles. I will now outline in turn some of the key elements of autoimmune responses, and discuss how disruption of specific cytokine genes has influenced our understanding of each process.

Regulating Tolerance

A role for IL-2

Several lines of evidence point to a role for interleukin-2 (IL-2) in the pathogenesis of autoimmune disease (reviewed in chapter 3). Local production of IL-2 can turn otherwise quiescent lymphocytes into autoaggressive effector cells, capable of destroying target tissues present in the host, or transplanted from naive recipients.[33] Such studies stem in part from studies of mouse or human T lymphocytes, which when rendered anergic through signals transduced exclusively through the T cell receptor, can be induced to proliferate in the presence of exogenous IL-2.[34-36] These observations may be of significance in the clinical context, since IL-2 has been employed in experimental therapy for cancer, immunodeficiency and infectious disease, and examples of flares of autoimmune disease following IL-2 therapy have been reported.[37,38] This mechanism could apply to the breaking of peripheral tolerance within multiple tissues. Accordingly, disruption of the IL-2 gene by homologous recombination in mice might prevent this process, rendering the host insensitive to autoimmune attack irrespective of the

---

Fig. 10.2 (opposite). Generation of mutant mice. Embryonic stem cells (ES cell) derived from the inner cell mass of mouse blastocysts are commonly derived from the 129/Ola mouse strain.[28] ES cells from C57Bl/6J have been used also with considerable success. Prior to electroporation of mutated DNA (see Fig.10.1), ES cells are maintained in tissue culture in the presence of mitomycin C-treated mouse embryo-derived fibroblasts as feeder cells, in LIF-supplemented media to prevent differentiation.[29,30] The ES cells are available for many but not all mouse strains, limiting to some extent the genetic background on which null mutations can be studied (at least until the appropriate number of backcrosses to disease prone strains have been obtained). Subsequently, 3.5 day old blastocysts injected with ES cells carrying the altered genome in the correct orientation are transferred to the uterus of pseudopregnant foster mothers.[31] Conventionally, derived chimeras are tested for germ-line transmission (frequencies range from 0 to 70%) by mating with normal mice. Those animals with the same coat color as the strain from which the ES cell line was derived can be tested to confirm the expression of the disrupted gene. Mice homozygous for the mutation are then obtained by interbreeding the progeny which are found to be heterozygous for the disrupted gene. In effect, predetermined alterations in the genome are derived in a culture dish and transferred to a "whole animal".

target organ. On the other hand, it has been shown that IL-2 is necessary both in vivo and in vitro for T lymphocytes to progress to the stage of the cell cycle permissive for programmed cell death.[39] Given these somewhat conflicting data, the phenotype of IL-2 knockout mice is of considerable interest. IL-2 deficient mice are normal at 3-4 weeks of age.[26,40] However, 50% of animals homozygous for the null mutation are dead by the age of 9 weeks chiefly from anemia. The remaining adult mice develop severe anemia, chronic diarrhea, intestinal bleeding and rectal prolapse. Enlargement of lymphoid organs is attributed in part to widespread amyloidosis, a feature characteristic of chronic inflammatory disease in man. That this phenotype has features of autoimmunity is suggested by the intense inflammatory infiltrates of activated CD44+, CD69+ T cells and antibody producing B lymphocytes in the lamina propria of the gut, aberrant MHC class II expression on colonic epithelium (ordinarily confined to small intestine) and the presence in serum of anticolon autoantibodies. This phenotype is accompanied also by raised levels of serum IgG1 and IgE, a finding consistent with increased levels of mRNA for IL-4, IL-6, and IL-10 as determined by ex vivo PCR analysis, although interferon-gamma (IFNγ) mRNA is also increased. Horak and colleagues believe that this striking phenotype exhibits features of ulcerative colitis in man, a disease thought to involve aberrant immune responses to environmental factors, including antigens present in the lumen of the gut.[40] Interestingly, loss of IL-2 production from CD4+ T cells is a recognized feature of the disease in man.[41] Significantly, no inflammatory bowel disease develops in mice retained in a germ free facility. Although the possibility cannot be excluded that IL-2 deficiency renders mice acutely susceptible to enterocolitis due to some as yet undefined gut pathogen, compartmentalization of inflammation to the bowel highlights the importance of the integrity and function of gut associated lymphoid tissue in inflammatory bowel disease, as well as the regulation of autoimmune responses in general. Why IL-2 deficient animals fail to limit clonal expansion of T lymphocytes is certainly worthy of further investigation. This animal model should allow a deeper analysis of mechanisms of inflammatory bowel disease in vivo. It is of interest that other knockout mice also develop inflammatory bowel disease, e.g., T cell receptor β chain or IL-10 (see later).

A role for TGFβ

Another cytokine whose role in peripheral tolerance has been the focus of long-standing in vitro and in vivo studies both in mice and in clinical trials in patients with autoimmune disease is the multifunctional regulatory factor transforming growth factor beta 1(TGFβ1).[42] Although the precise role of TGFβ in clonal inactivation has yet to be defined, there are several precedents for studying the role of this cytokine in the pathogenesis of autoimmune disease based on its potent immunoregulatory effects alone. For example, TGFβ inhibits both proliferation and differentiation of B cells,[43] and suppresses IL-2 or IL-6 dependent IgM and IgG secretion.[44] By inhibiting acquisition of κ and λ light chains induced by IFNγ, IL-1 or LPS, TGFβ may block the transition of pre-B cells to mature antigen-responsive B cells.[45] Powerful antiproliferative effects on the T cell compartment have been reported, findings of relevance in multiple sclerosis and rheumatoid arthritis, diseases in which it has been proposed that loss of functional suppressor-inducer or suppressor T cell subsets may contribute (discussed in chapters 2 and 4).[46,47] Indeed, both experiments in mice and clinical studies in which the effects of oral administration of autoantigens such as myelin basic protein or collagen type II have been evaluated in patients with multiple sclerosis and rheumatoid arthritis, respectively, suggest that CD8+ T lymphocytes contribute to maintaining oral tolerance through the production of TGFβ in the gut.[48-51] Finally, the role of TGFβ as a chemoattractant for monocytes, neutrophils and T lymphocytes,[52] as well as a potent inhibitor of the production of mediators of inflammation such as TNFα and IFNγ,[53] suggests that this cytokine may exert multiple effects in regulatory networks.

Targeted disruption of the murine TGFβ1 gene, including its precursor region, has revealed several interesting aspects of TGFβ1 function.[32,54] Mice lacking TGFβ1 activity suffer weight loss, but otherwise appear normal until 2-3 weeks of age. The phenotype thereafter is dominated by a severe inflammatory wasting syndrome in which the animals take on a disheveled, hunched appearance. Conjunctivitis and skin irritation are readily apparent, but death by cardiopulmonary disease is precipitous, occurring within days of the onset of visible signs. Whilst spleen and thymus are small, lymph nodes are enlarged compared to healthy littermates. The hallmark of mice homozygous for the mutation is revealed on histological analysis of multiple tissues. Features include widespread inflammatory infiltrates in heart, liver, stomach, lung, pancreas, muscle, salivary glands and brain, most of which appear lymphocytic. These findings confirm results implicating TGFβ1 as an important modulator of immune and inflammatory processes. Furthermore, the finding that the proportion of homozygous pups within litters was lower than expected (by up to 50%) suggests that the mutation may be lethal for a number of embryos.[32] Given that TGFβ1 is involved in pre- and postimplantation development,[4] the surprising number of animals which develop to term may reflect maternal rescue or compensation by other TGFβ isoforms, e.g., TGFβ2 or TGFβ3. Features of autoimmunity in TGFβ1 deficient mice other than lymphoid infiltrates have been reported more recently, including increased expression of MHC class I and II in young mutant mice prior to disease onset,[55] early leucocyte adherence and infiltration,[56] and the development of autoantibodies.[57] Furthermore, the inflammation of heart, blood vessels and striated muscle as well as disease affecting the eye and salivary glands resemble features common to systemic autoimmune syndromes such as mixed connective tissue disease and Sjögren's syndrome, and prompt further evaluations of TGFβ expression and regulation in these and related disorders. In addition, the wasting syndrome bears a striking resemblance to cachexia associated with chronic infection or malignancy, as well as to the phenotype characteristic of mice administered TNFα for prolonged periods.[58] These observations suggest that aberrant expression of proinflammatory cytokines such as TNFα and IL-1 may indeed contribute to the syndrome observed in TGFβ1 deficient mice, a concept supported by the finding of increased mRNA transcripts for TNFα and IFNγ in the liver and lung of these mutant animals,[32] and the finding that impaired immune responses in these mice bear a striking resemblance to those of T lymphocytes chronically exposed to TNFα in vitro and in vivo.[59,60]

A role for IL-10

There are substantial data to support important immunoregulatory roles for IL-10.[61] Such effects may serve indirectly to maintain homeostasis in the periphery by regulating the expression of factors capable of activating autoreactive T and B lymphocytes (see below), a concept supported by recent experiments which have confirmed the potent effects of IL-10 in models of established inflammatory disease.[62,63] Mice homozygous for an IL-10 null mutation develop normally.[64] Adult mice, on the other hand, develop gradual weight loss, accompanied by peripheral neutrophilia and microcytic hypochromic anemia with reductions in iron stores in the bone marrow. Although only a proportion of animals die, all mice develop chronic enterocolitis with features characteristic of ulcerative colitis and Crohn's disease in human patients.[64] The extent of bowel inflammation is variable, encompassing both small and large bowel; rectal prolapse is a common feature. In the absence of known pathogens, histological features include diffuse inflammatory infiltrates (of most cell types), desquamation and erosions, and pseudopolypoid structures. As noted for IL-2 deficient mice, levels of MHC class II expression are upregulated. Breeding into a pathogen free environment results in marked diminution of disease severity, although localized areas of colitis persist. Conceivably, responses to luminal antigens may play a role in the disease, since the disease can be noticed as early as weaning, when colonization of the gut with adult microflora occurs. Other secondary factors are likely also to be of significance. For example, it has been postulated that persistent antigen stimulation in the gut leads to overproduction of TNFα, IL-1 and IFNγ.[64] This would contribute to enhanced MHC class II expression which in turn further upregulates immune responses. Indeed, although TNFα cannot be detected in the serum of IL-10 deficient mice, a 20-fold increase in LPS induced cytokine production in vitro by splenocytes has been observed compared to control mice.[64]

It is intriguing how disruption of three immunoregulatory cytokine genes has highlighted an apparent susceptibility of organisms to gut inflammation. A less dramatic phenotype has been observed in I-Aβ, T cell receptor (TCR)β but not TCRδ or RAG-1 deficient mice, pointing to an important regulatory role for CD4+ lymphocytes in the gut.[65] The integrity and function of the gut in autoimmune disease clearly requires closer evaluation in terms of the effector role of autoantibodies and the complex relationship between innate resistance, acquired immunity, gut flora and nutrition. It remains to be seen whether the distribution of disease, particularly in IL-2 and IL-10 knockout mice, extends to other organs susceptible to autoimmune attack, such as the brain, pancreas, thyroid gland, kidney or synovial joint. These and related issues can be resolved by studies of the relevant null mutation on the genetic background of established autoimmune susceptible prone strains.

Lymphocyte Activation and Growth

Studies of mice expressing T cell receptor transgenes specific for self-antigens have demonstrated unequivocally that the presence of abundant specific autoreactive T cells and self antigen is insufficient to induce autoimmune responses.[66-68] The presence of inflammatory infiltrates in the absence of overt tissue destruction manifesting in failure of organ function is also well recognized, and implies that an autoimmune process follows a sequence of events, the outcome of which depends on the coordinate expression of soluble and cell surface molecules (discussed in chapter 3). On the other hand, aberrant expression of a single cytokine in target organs can be sufficient for disease induction, whilst sustained expression of others is not, suggesting that hierarchies exist.

Defining dominant players in cytokine hierarchies can be addressed by systematic gene disruption. Given the available data regarding the consequences of local expression of cytokines in the pancreas of transgenic mice (see chapter 3),[33,69,70] one might predict that disruption of IL-2, IFNγ or IFNα in the appropriate mouse strain may prevent the development of type I diabetes in nonobese diabetic (NOD) mice, whilst disease would persist despite deletion of TNFα or LT activity.[33,71-74] Moreover, recent evidence suggests that targeting overexpression of TNFα to the pancreatic islets in NOD mice protects rather than enhances the incidence of disease (R. Flavell, 1995 Midwinter Conference of Immunologists, Monterey, California), similar to effects observed following chronic administration of TNFα to adult NOD mice.[73] On the other hand, studies using neutralizing antibodies to TNF would seem to suggest that the reverse may be true.[74] Thus, administration of anti-TNF, but not control antibodies, from birth protects NOD mice from developing disease.[74] Almost complete absence of infiltrates in the islets, together with the loss of autoreactivity of T and B cells to a panel of islet cell autoantigens suggests that TNFα may influence lymphocyte maturation or development.[74] Might these findings reflect the fact that widespread expression, e.g., in the thymus, in addition to localized expression, of cytokines are of importance? The beneficial effects of neutralizing TNFα in patients with RA suggest that this may be the case (discussed in chapters 2 and 12). Thus, the effects of disrupting the TNFα gene on the development of collagen-induced arthritis (CIA) in DBA/1J mice or experimental autoimmune encephalomyelitis (EAE) in [SJL x PLJ] F1 mice as well as diabetes in NOD mice, will be of great interest. Disruption of GM-CSF in these background strains would also be worthy of study in view of the potent macrophage activating and MHC class II enhancing effects reported previously.[75,76] These studies will also serve to establish whether the cytokine-induced mechanisms of autoimmunity are similar in different diseases, findings likely to have profound therapeutic implications.

A role for TNF/LT

The phenotype of p55 and p75 TNF-R deficient mice have confirmed independently the roles of TNFα in septic shock and infection models.[77-79] Thus both receptor knockout mice exhibit varying degrees of resistance to LPS injection, although p55 TNF-R deficient mice are the more resistant. By contrast, these mice are more susceptible to *Listeria* and LCMV infection. Given the recent reports of the effects of TNF blockade in EAE, diabetes in NOD mice and CIA,[74,80,81] the effects not only of TNFα gene disruption, but of systematic receptor mutations will be important to investigate. Much emphasis has been placed on the role of the p55 TNF-R in transducing signals sufficient for most TNFα induced effects, including upregulating adhesion molecules such as ICAM-1, VCAM-1 and E-selectin,[82] and for inducing the production of proinflammatory cytokines such as IL-1, IL-6, IL-8 and GM-CSF (see chapter 2),[83] whilst p75 TNF-R plays a key role in the growth of thymocytes and mature T lymphocytes.[84] Experiments utilizing antagonistic antireceptor monoclonal antibodies indicate that proliferative responses may in fact be mediated through both receptors.[85] Thus an evaluation of the phenotype of autoimmune disease prone mice bearing disrupted p55 or p75 TNF-R genes may resolve these issues and provide clues as to the signaling pathway components involved in transducing signals necessary for the induction of specific aspects of autoimmune responses, such as cell activation and recruitment. It is anticipated that such an approach, already well advanced in the field of gp130 and IL-6 signaling events,[86] may help define novel targets both for subsequent gene disruption, and for therapeutic intervention. It is still possible that p55 and/or p75 TNF-R knockout mice will unravel a specific role for TNFα in T cell development, a finding consistent with its tissue expression and growth enhancing properties.[87,88] To date the mechanisms remain elusive.

Details documenting the biological effects of LT in vivo have been obscure until very recently, when the gene was disrupted by homologous recombination.[27] This was due in part to difficulties in expressing significant amounts of LT protein for injections in vivo, as well as for the production of high affinity neutralizing polyclonal and monoclonal antibodies. It was not until homozygous mutants were generated and immunized with soluble antigens to study immune function, that it become clear that LT deficient mice do not develop lymph nodes nor Peyer's patches, although both MHC class I and II restricted T cell responses are normal.[27] This unexpected characteristic of LT-/-mice has been reproduced in double knockout mice in which both TNFα and LT genes have been disrupted (B. Ryffel, unpublished data). Since lymph nodes are present in both p55 and p75 TNF-R deficient mice,[77-79] this striking anomaly suggests that structural development of lymphoid tissue occurs not only through LT mediated effects, but is likely to be transduced through a third TNF-R, now designated LTβ receptor.[8] This working hypothesis can be confirmed once the phenotype of p55 and p75 TNF-R double knockout mice have been studied. Crossing such mice to disease susceptible strains will provide unique opportunities to define the contribution of lymph node architecture, lymphocyte-lymphocyte and lymphocyte-dendritic cell interactions, and trafficking to and from lymph nodes to the induction and persistence of chronic immune and inflammatory responses. It is conceivable that vestigial lymphoid tissue present in the lungs of these mice is sufficient to carry out such functions.

A role for IL-6

The finding of abundant IL-6 in biological fluids of patients with cardiac myxoma, and subsequently those with autoimmune disease such as RA, glomerulonephritis and psoriasis, has provided evidence that this cytokine may have dominant proinflammatory effects in these patients.[89] Animal models support such a concept.[90] The B cell/plasma cell growth enhancing properties, and the finding of autoantibodies in these diseases is also significant. Furthermore, mice transgenic for the human IL-6 gene expressed under the influence of the human immunoglobulin heavy chain enhancer develop polyclonal plasmacytosis associated with mesangial cell proliferative glomerulonephritis.[91] On the other hand, anti-inflammatory effects have also been reported,[92] and induction of acute phase proteins could equally be viewed as regulatory and anti-inflammatory, as they could overtly proinflammatory. Disrupting the IL-6 gene and breeding the mutation onto strains such as the NOD mouse and [NZB x NZW] F1 mice provides one means of resolving this issue, and will define whether LIF, oncostatin M, CNTF, CT-1 or IL-11, which exhibit similar properties as a result of common receptor signaling pathways, can compensate for IL-6 deficiency in vivo.

It has become clear from preliminary reports that although IL-6 deficient mice develop normally, they fail to induce optimal acute phase responses after tissue damage or infection.[93] This appears to influence the outcome of challenge with vaccinia virus, *Listeria monocytogenes*, and antibody responses to vesicular stomatitis virus. Mice homozygous for the disrupted NFIL-6 gene also succumb to infection.[94] In contrast to TNF-R deficient mice, only modest reductions in responses to LPS challenge were observed.[93] Contrary to expectations, the B cell compartment in these mice is normal. On the other hand, mutant mice have only half the number of thymocytes and significantly lower numbers of T cells in the periphery. In the light of phenotypes described above for TGFβ mutant mice relating to bowel inflammation, the finding of markedly reduced IgA antibody responses of IL-6 mutant mice following mucosal challenge is of interest, suggesting a protective role for IL-6 in mucosal immunity.[95] Nevertheless, no spontaneous inflammatory diseases have been described in these mice to date, although a phenotype could be unmasked after an appropriate number of backcrosses onto relevant disease prone strains. Reports describing the effects of this mutation on the development of autoimmune disease in mouse models have yet to be described. The role of IL-6 in enhancing osteoclast formation and activity, on the other hand, suggests that overexpression of IL-6 may contribute to the bone loss characteristic of postmenopausal patients with chronic immune and inflammatory disease.[96]

There are no published studies describing mice homozygous for the IL-1 null mutation. Difficulties in deriving such mice initially raised the possibility that such mutations might be lethal.[19] However, several groups (L. Shornick, Washington University, USA; M. Tocci, Merck, USA) have reported normal fertility, growth, gross pathology, lymphoid organs and blood cellularity in IL-1β knockout mice, and the phenotype of type I IL-1 receptor deficient mice appears similar. Significantly, LPS-induced shock is not reduced, nor *Listeria* sensitivity increased (Proceedings of The International Cytokine Society Meeting, October 1994, Banff, Canada).

LYMPHOCYTE DIFFERENTIATION

The pioneering studies of Mosmann and Coffman have allowed differentiating murine CD4+ T lymphocytes to be defined in terms of the profiles of lymphokines they secrete.[97] Cells which encompass the two extremes of a spectrum of lymphokine production have been designated Th_1 and Th_2 helper cells.[98] Evidence suggests that similar phenotypes exist for CD8+ T cells.[99] The cytokine profiles become polarized, at least in vitro in terminally differentiated cells and are easy to distinguish; Th_1 cells produce IL-2, IFNγ and LT, whilst Th_2 lymphocytes secrete IL-4, IL-5, IL-6, IL-9 and IL-10. The factors involved in the pathways that drive the process to Th_1 or Th_2 are becoming clearer.

For example, IFNγ and IL-12 are particularly potent inducers of Th$_1$ phenotypes, and through interactions with B lymphocytes induce a restricted but nevertheless characteristic pattern of immunoglobulin isotype expression (IgG2a in the mouse, IgG1 in humans),[100-102] whilst IL-4 and IL-10 drive Th$_2$ responses with IgG1 and IgE production being predominant in the mouse.[103,104] Precisely how these factors influence signals within T lymphocytes, however, remains elusive. Nevertheless, their impact in conceptual terms has been as great on autoimmune disease as it has in infectious disease, and evidence has emerged for their contribution to human disease.[105] Thus, it is thought that some CD4+ T cell MHC class II restricted autoimmune diseases are Th$_1$ polarized diseases; recent evidence in TCR transgenic mice is consistent with this hypothesis.[67] The contribution of Th$_2$ cells to the pathogenesis of diseases in which autoantibodies play a significant role is less clear. Notwithstanding the biological effects of these cytokines on cell types other than T lymphocytes, knockout technology provides a unique opportunity to test the hypothesis that induction of polarized Th$_1$/Th$_2$-like phenotypes in vivo are pivotal for the progression of organ specific autoimmunity.

To date, mice bearing null mutations for IFNγ, LT, TNFα and LT, and their respective receptors have been reported in preliminary communications, as well as those for IL-12 and IL-4.[27,106-109] Since the effects of some of these mutations on autoimmune responses in vivo may be predicted to be protective (e.g., expression of mutant p55 TNF-R genes in the NOD mouse, or the mutant IFNγ gene in DBA1/J or SJL x PJL F1 mice), it will be necessary in many cases to cross these mutant mice onto appropriate autoimmune susceptible strains. Such studies are in progress. For example, recent evidence indicates that the development of EAE in B10.PL (H-2^k) mice with a disrupted IFNγ gene is almost identical in terms of kinetics and severity of disease to wild type mice (I.A. Ferber, C.G. Fathman, submitted). Unlike IL-4 deficient mice, IL-10 deficient mice described above provide an example where background strain appears not to influence the phenotype.[64] This may reflect the capacity of IL-10 to drive the development of Th$_2$ regulatory T cells in vivo,[110] as well as to inhibit the production of cytokines by Th$_1$ cells.[104] Alternatively, the anti-inflammatory effects of IL-10 on the expression of TNFα, IFNγ and IL-1 may be the dominant effect.[111,112] This could be formally tested by evaluating whether IDDM in NOD mice, CIA in DBA1/J mice and EAE in susceptible mice is aggravated in the absence of a functional IL-10 gene. The fact that local overexpression of IL-10 in pancreatic islets aggravates rather than protects against disease in NOD mice (discussed in chapter 3),[113] stresses the importance of such an analysis, and will allow further comparisons of local versus systemic effects of cytokine dysregulation.

Functional aspects of the balance of Th$_1$/Th$_2$ lymphokines have been facilitated greatly by the study of infectious disease models, in which the phenotype of mice known to exhibit polarized Th$_1$ or Th$_2$ responses following infectious challenge have been well characterised.[114] In IL-4 knockout mice, CD4⁺ T lymphocytes fail to produce significant levels of IL-3, IL-4, IL-5 and IL-10, although B cell help is unimpaired;[107,108] unlike IL-10 deficient mice whose immunoglobulin (Ig) profiles are normal,[64] levels of IgG1 are reduced in serum, whilst IgE levels are absent. Levels of IFNγ are raised in IL-4 mutant mice, and not surprisingly, these animals are highly susceptible to nematode infection.[107] These findings suggest that IL-4 may be critical for IgE responses, and may provide compensatory signals necessary for normal Ig levels in IL-10 knockout mice. The effects of this mutation on the development of spontaneous as well as induced autoimmune disease in mice should be evaluated, given that differentiation of Th$_2$ lymphocytes are suppressed on the one hand, whilst upregulation of MHC class II on B lymphocytes is prevented on the other.[108] It will be important to compare disease susceptibility and severity in autoimmune prone mice with either IL-4, IL-10, or both gene disruptions.

Analogous though contrasting data have emerged from studies of IFNγ and IFNγ-R deficient mice.[106,115] Although these animals appear normal in pathogen free animal facilities, significant phenotypes arise when animals are challenged. Responses to intracellular pathogens, such as *Mycobacterium tuberculosis* and *Listeria monocytogenes* are impaired, consequent in part upon a significant reduction in levels of inducible nitric oxide. A switch to Th$_2$ phenotype is apparent, manifest by the observation that normally resistant C57Bl/6 mice succumb to infection with *Leishmania*, and low levels of serum total and hapten specific IgG2a and to a lesser extent IgG3.[115,116] On the basis of these and other data, one might predict significant inhibition of diseases such as IDDM in the NOD mouse, CIA in DBA1/J mice or autoimmune nephritis in (NZB x NZW) F1 mice. This prediction would be consistent with the effects both on nephritis observed in mice treated with IFNγ or anti-IFNγ monoclonal antibodies,[117] and also with the effects of similar treatments on the development of IDDM in NOD mice.[118,119] Furthermore, the contribution of IFNγ to the induction and/or upregulation of MHC class II in vivo is still uncertain, since constitutive expression of class II molecules are normal in IFNγ deficient mice.[106] Studies under way in appropriate mouse strains should resolve these issues.

Mice bearing disrupted IL-12 genes have recently been reported.[109] These are of particular interest given the dominant role for macrophage/B cell derived IL-12 in driving Th$_1$ responses in vitro and in vivo.[102,120] Since IL-12 is a heterodimer comprising subunits of 35 (p35) and 40 (p40) kD respectively, both genes have been targeted and provisional data indicate that mutant animals have similar phenotypes. Despite the fact that targeting of the p40 gene included parts of exons 2 and 3, an 89 amino acid spliced product (out of a total of 390 for the mature protein) could be detected by ELISA in culture supernatants, although no bioactivity was apparent. Mice develop normally, and although proliferative responses to mitogens and IL-2 are normal, IL-12 mutant mice exhibit reductions in IFNγ production in vitro following stimulation with LPS or heat killed *Listeria* monocytogenes. IL-4 expression is unaffected, and in fact is increased under some circumstances. Delayed type hypersensitivity responses, as determined by paw swelling, are also reduced by 40-60% in IL-12 deficient mice; p35 knockout mice have similar responses. Interestingly, NK cell function is normal. It would appear that, as expected, skewing away from Th_1 responses is apparent. More detailed analyses are awaited.

These mutant animals are currently being backcrossed to autoimmune prone strains (L. Magram, personal communication). Since IL-12 or anti-IL-12 injections can enhance or slow the progression of EAE and diabetes,[120,121] disease manifestations in [SJL x PLJ] F1 mice as well as NOD mice expressing the IL-12 mutant gene will be of interest. Comparisons with IFNγ knockout mice on the same background should determine the relative contributions of these activating factors towards the development of Th_1 disease inducing T lymphocyte subsets, as well as providing a background on which to evaluate more precisely the mechanisms of such responses in vivo.

ADHESION AND MIGRATION TO TARGET TISSUES

It will not be surprising if many of the mutant mice described above will provide useful in vivo models for evaluating lymphocyte trafficking. Such studies have already been reported for TGFβ deficient mice, in whom early leucocyte adherence and infiltration is prominent.[56] It is anticipated that systematic disruption of members of the chemokine family of cytokines will be of great interest; studies are currently in their infancy, partly through lack of the availability of genomic clones for some members (e.g., murine IL-8). Given the widespread expression of adhesion molecules in multiple tissues, it is likely that selective trafficking to tissues arises through the action of chemokines in a cell and tissue specific fashion, in a manner suggested initially by the effects of IL-8, RANTES, and MIP-1α and MIP-1β on mononuclear cells in general, but T lymphocyte subsets in particular.[122,123] Targeting of these genes will be important for defining whether complete or partial redundancy exist and how trafficking to different tissues can be modulated. Interpretation of these studies will be facilitated considerably in spontaneous models of chronic immune and inflammatory disorders. The NOD mouse may prove to be a particularly good model in this regard, not just because autoimmunity affects multiple tissues in this strain, but because therapeutic intervention has demonstrated differential effects on disease progression in different tissues compared to the pancreatic islets.[74,124]

To date available data regarding mice expressing mutated chemokine/receptor genes are confined to that of the mouse IL-8R homologue.[125]

Mice develop normally, and as expected the migration responses of neutrophils after injection of thioglycollate are 20% those of wild type mice, although neutrophil functional studies revealed no obvious abnormalities. Somewhat surprisingly, IL-8R deficiency leads to enhanced extramedullary hemopoiesis with increases in numbers of neutrophils and of B cells in lymph nodes, spleen and bone marrow. Increased levels of IL-6 in the sera of mutant mice was considered a likely explanation for the B cell abnormalities. The effects of this phenotype in chronic inflammatory disease models is not entirely predictable. Nevertheless, it is probable that gene disruption of other members of this expanding family of small molecular weight proteins will uncover novel functions.

WHAT THE FUTURE HOLDS IN STORE

In the short term I believe that aspects of knockout technology will guide the way. The development of inducible or conditional knockout mice will provide powerful tools for studying the effects of gene disruption at different times in the evolution of spontaneous disease or following challenge.[126] This might more closely reflect pathophysiological conditions in which therapeutic intervention can be instituted only after the onset of disease. Moreover, such advances will allow evaluation of gene deficient animals in whom there has been insufficient time for compensatory or regulatory pathways to take effect, as well as those in whom the targeted mutation is lethal. Mice transgenic both for the gene encoding the Cre recombinase enzyme from bacteriophage P1 and for targeted genes flanked by loxP sites have demonstrated that cell-type specific gene inactivation is possible.[126,127] The analogous FLP/frt system in yeast may prove to be just as valuable. Dominant negative technology, especially appropriate for receptor and signaling molecules, is an alternative strategy which has allowed overexpression of mutant proteins to be directed to specific target tissues in transgenic mice. It is anticipated that knockout mice will also be useful in complementation experiments, in which mutant mice can be crossed to transgenic mice expressing the disrupted gene in a tissue specific fashion.

In the longer term, detailed knowledge of the nature of cytokine receptor signaling pathways may allow more focused targeting on intracellular components, providing a basis on which to selectively inhibit some aspects of cytokine function but not those which may be beneficial to the host. Eventually, it may be possible to direct therapy at these defined targets through the use of drugs, or in situations where components are found to be defective or deficient, by gene therapy.

ACKNOWLEDGMENTS

I am grateful to Drs. T.A. Stewart, T.J. Schall, M.W. Moore, L. Magram, Y. Chernajovsky and D. Rennick for helpful discussions.

REFERENCES

1. Bluethmann H, Ohashi P. Transgenesis and targeted mutagenesis in immunology. Academic Press, Inc., 1994.
2. Hooper M, Hardy K, Hyside A et al. HPRT-deficient (Lesch-Nyhan) mouse embryos derived from germline colonization by cultured cells. Nature 1987; 326:292-295.
3. Kuehn MR, Bradley A, Robertson EJ et al. A potential animal model for Lesch-Nyhan syndrome through introduction of HPRT mutations in mice. Nature 1987; 326:295-298.
4. Heine UI, Munoz EF, Flanders KC et al. Role of transforming growth factor-β in the development of the mouse embryo. J Cell Biol 1987; 105:2861-2876.
5. Stewart CL, Kaspar P, Brunet LJ et al. Blastocyst implantation depends on maternal expression of leukaemia inhibitory factor. Nature 1992; 388:76-79.
6. Namen AE, Lupton S, Hjerrild K et al. Stimulation of B-cell progenitors by cloned murine interleukin-7. Nature 1988; 333:571-573.
7. Saito S, Enomoto M, Sakakura S et al. Localization of stem cell factor (SCF) and c-kit mRNA in human placental tissue and biological effects of SCF on DNA synthesis in primary cultured cytotrophoblasts. Biochem Biophys Res Commun 1994; 205:1762-1769.
8. Crowe PD, VanArsdale TL, Walter BN et al. A lymphotoxin-β-specific receptor. Science 1994; 64:707-710.
9. Zhang XG, Gu JJ, Lu ZY et al. Ciliary neurotropic factor, interleukin-11, leukemia inhibitory factor and oncostatin M are growth factors for human myeloma cell lines using interleukin-6 signal transducer gp130. J Exp Med 1994; 179:1337-1342.
10. Garrod AE. The Harveian oration on the debt of science to medicine. Br Med J 1924; 2:747-752.
11. Dietrich W, Katz H, Lincoln SE et al. A genetic map of the mouse suitable for typing intraspecific crosses. Genetics 1992; 131:423-447.
12. Todd JA, Aitman TJ, Cornall RJ et al. Genetic analysis of autoimmune type-1 diabetes mellitus in mice. Nature 1991; 351:542-547.
13. Cohen PL and Eisenberg RA. *Lpr* and *gld*: single gene models of systemic autoimmunity and lymphoproliferative disease. Annu Rev Immunol 1991; 9:243-269.
14. Watanabe T, Sakai Y, Miyawaki S et al. Molecular genetic map of the mouse chromosome 19, including *lpr*, *Ly-44*, and *Tdt* genes. Biochem Genet 1991; 29:325-335.
15. Watanabe-Fukunaga R, Brannan CI, Copeland NG et al. Lymphoproliferative disorder in mice explained by defects in Fas antigen that mediates apoptosis. Nature 1992; 356:314-317.
16. Adachi M, Watanabe-Fukunaga R and Negata S. Aberrant transcription caused by the insertion of an early transposable element in an intron of the Fas antigen gene of *lpr* mice. Proc Natl Acad Sci USA 1993; 90:1756-1760.

17. Allen RD, Marshall JD, Roths JB et al. Differences defined by bone marrow transplantation suggest that *lpr* and *gld* are mutations of genes encoding an interacting pair of molecules. J Exp Med 1990; 172;1367-1375.
18. Noguchi M, Yi H, Rosenblatt HM et al. Interleukin 2 receptor γ chain mutation results in X-linked severe combined immunodeficiency in humans. Cell 1993; 73:147-157.
19. Csaikl FF, Csaikl UM, Durum SK. Strategies for modulation of interleukin-1 in vivo: knockout and transgenics. In: Jacob CO, ed. Overexpression and knockout of cytokines in transgenic mice. Academic Press Ltd, 1994:1-13.
20. Sims JE, Gayle MA, Slack JL et al. Interleukin 1 signaling occurs exclusively via the type I receptor. Proc Natl Acad Sci USA 1993; 90: 6155-6159.
21. Doetschman TC, Gregg RG, Maeda N et al. Targeted correction of a mutant HPRT gene in mouse embryonic stem cells. Nature 1987; 330:576-578.
22. Thomas KR, Capecchi MR. Site-directed mutagenesis by gene targeting in mouse embryo-derived stem cells. Cell 1987; 51:503-512.
23. Capecchi MR. Altering the genome by homologous recombination. Science 1989; 244:1288 1292.
24. Fuse A, Fujita T, Yasumitsu H et al. Organization and structure of the mouse interleukin-2 gene. Nucleic Acids Res 1984; 12: 9323-9331.
25. Zurawski SM, Zurawski G. Identification of three critical regions within mouse interleukin 2 by fine structural deletion analysis. EMBO J 1988; 7:1061-1069.
26. Schorle H, Holtsche T, Hunig T et al. Development and function of T cells in mice rendered interleukin-2 deficient by gene targeting. Nature 1991; 352:621-624.
27. De Togni P, Goellner J, Ruddle NH et al. Abnormal development of peripheral lymphoid organs in mice deficient in lymphotoxin. Science 1994; 264:703-707.
28. Evans MJ, Kaufman MH. Establishment or culture of pluripotential cells from mouse embryos. Nature 1981; 292:154-156.
29. Smith AG, Hooper ML. Buffalo rat liver cells produce a diffusible activity which inhibits the differentiation of murine embryonal carcinoma and embryonic stem cells. Devel Biol 1987; 121:1-9.
30. Williams RL, Hilton DJ, Pease S et al. Myeloid leukaemia inhibitory factor maintains the developmental potential of embryonic stem cells. Nature 1988; 336:684-687.
31. Bradley A. Production and analysis of chimaeric mice. In; Robertson EJ, ed. Terato-carcinomas and Embryonic Stem Cells: A Practical Approach. Oxford IRL Press, 1987:113-151.
32. Shull MM, Ormsby I, Kier AB et al. Targeted disruption of the mouse transforming growth factor-β1 gene results in mulitfocal inflammatory disease. Nature 1992; 359:693-699.
33. Heath WR, Allison J, Hoffman MW et al. Autoimmune diabetes as a consequence of locally produced interleukin-2. Nature 1992; 359:547-549.

34. Lamb JR, Skidmore BJ, Green N et al. Induction of tolerance in influenza virus-immune T lymphocyte clones with syngeneic peptides of influenza haemagglutinin. J Exp Med 1983; 157:1434-1447.
35. Schwartz RH. Acquisition of immunological self-tolerance. Cell 1989; 57:1073-1081.
36. Essery G, Feldmann M and Lamb JR. Interleukin-2 can prevent and reverse antigen-induced unresponsiveness in cloned human T lymphocytes. Immunology 1988; 64:413-417.
37. Lavelle-Jones M, Al-Hadrani A, Spiers EM et al. Reactivation of rheumatoid arthritis during continuous infusion of interleukin-2: evidence of lymphocytic control of rheumatoid disease. Br Med J 1990; 301:97.
38. Atkins MB, Mier JW, Parkinson DR et al. Hypothyroidism after treatment with interleukin 2 and lymphokine-activated killer cells. New Engl J Medicine 318:1557-1563.
39. Lenardo MJ. Interleukin-2 programs mouse α/β T lymphocytes for apoptosis. Nature 1992; 353:858-861.
40. Sadlack B, Merz H, Schorle H et al. Ulcerative colitis-like disease in mice with a disrupted interleukin-2 gene. Cell 1993; 75:253-261.
41. Kusugami K, Matsuura T, West GA et al. Loss of interleukin-2 producing intestinal CD4⁺ T cells in inflammatory bowel disease. Gastroenterology 1991; 101:1594-1605.
42. Roberts AB, Sporn MB. The transforming growth factors-β. In: Sporn MB, Roberts AB. Handbook of Experimental Pharmacology: Peptide growth factors and their receptors, volume 95/1. New York: Springer-Verlag, 1990:419-472.
43. Kehrl JH, Thevenin C, Rieckmann P et al. Transforming growth factor-beta suppresses human B lymphocyte Ig production by inhibiting synthesis and the switch from the membrane form to the secreted form of Ig mRNA. J Immunol 1991; 146:4016-4023.
44. Kehrl JH, Roberts AB, Wakefield LM et al. Transforming growth factor β is an important immunomodulatory protein for human B lymphocytes. J Immunol 1986; 137:3855-3860.
45. Lee G, Ellingsworth LR, Gillis S et al. β transforming growth factors are potential regulators of B lymphocytes. J Exp Med 1987; 166:1290-1299.
46. Goto M, Miyamoto T, Nihioka K et al. Selective loss of suppressor T cells in rheumatoid arthritis patients: analysis of peripheral blood lymphocytes by 2-dimensional flow cytometry. J Rheumatol 1986; 13:853-857.
47. Morimoto C, Hafler DA, Weiner HL et al. Selective loss of the suppressor-inducer T-cell subset in progressive multiple sclerosis. New Engl J Med 1987; 316:67-72.
48. Lider O, Santos LMB, Lee CSY et al. Suppressor T cells generated by oral tolerization to myelin basic protein suppress both in vitro and in vivo immune responses by the release of transforming growth factor beta after antigen-specific triggering. J Immunol 1989; 142:748-752.
49. Weiner HL, Friedman A, Miller A et al. Oral tolerance: immunologic mechanisms and treatment of animal and human organ-specific autoimmune diseases by oral admininstration of autoantigens. Annu Rev Immunol 1994; 12:809-837.

50. Weiner HL, Mackin GA, Matsui M et al. Double-blind pilot trial of oral tolerization with myelin antigens in multiple sclerosis. Science 1993; 259;1321-1324.
51. Trentham DE, Dynesius-Trentham RA, Orau EJ et al. Effects of oral administration of type II collagen on rheumatoid arthritis. Science 1993; 261:1727-1730.
52. Wahl SM, Hunt DA, Wakefield LM et al. Transforming growth factor type β induces monocyte chemotaxis and growth factor production. Proc Natl Acad Sci USA 1987; 84:5788-5792.
53. Espevik T, Figari IS, Shalaby MR et al. Inhibition of cytokine production by cyclosporin A and transforming growth factor β. J Exp Med 1987; 166:571-576.
54. Kulkarni AB, Huh C-G, Becker D et al. Transforming growth factor β1 null mutation in mice causes excessive inflammatory response and early death. Proc Natl Acad Sci USA 1993; 90:770-774.
55. Geiser AG, Letterio JJ, Kulkarni AB et al. TGF-β1 controls expression of major histocompatability genes in the postnatal mouse. Proc Natl Acad Sci USA 1993; 90:9944-9948.
56. Hines KL, Kulkarni AB, McCarthy JB et al. Synthetic fibronectin peptides interrupt inflammatory cell infiltration in TGF-β1 knockout mice. Proc Natl Acad Sci USA 1994; 91;5187-5191.
57. Talal N, Uang H, Geiser A et al. Generalized autoimmunity and lymphoproliferation in TGF-β1 "knockout" mice. Clinical Res 1994; 42:304 (Abstr.).
58. Tracey KJ, Wei H, Manogue KR et al. Cachectin/tumor necrosis factor induces cachexia, anorexia, and inflammation. J Exp Med 1988; 167:1211-1227.
59. Christ M, McCarteney-Francis NL, Kulkarni AB et al. Immune dysregulation in TGFβ1 deficient mice. J Immunol 1994; 153:1936-1946.
60. Cope AP, Londei M, Chu NR et al. Chronic exposure to TNF in vitro impairs the activation of T cells through the T cell receptor/CD3 complex; reversal in vivo by anti-TNF antibodies in patients with rheumatoid arthritis. J Clin Invest 1994; 94:749-760.
61. Moore KW, O'Garra A, de Waal Malefyt R et al. Interleukin-10. Annu Rev Immunol 1993;11:165-190.
62. Katsikis PD, Chu CQ, Brennan FM, Maini RN, Feldmann M. Immunoregulatory role of interleukin 10 in rheumatoid arthritis. J Exp Med 1994; 179:1517-1527.
63. Ishida H, Muchamuel T, Sakaguchis S et al. Continuous admininstration of anti-interleukin 10 antibodies delays onset of autoimmunity in NZB/W F1 mice. J Exp Med 994; 179:305-310.
64. Kuhn R, Lohler J, Rennick D et al. Interleukin-10-deficient mice develop chronic enterocolitis. Cell 1993; 75:263-274.
65. Mombaerts P, Mizoguchi E, Grusby MJ et al. Spontaneous development of inflammatory bowel disease in T cell receptor mutant mice. Cell 1993; 75:275-282.

66. Ohashi PS, Oehen S, Burki K et al. Ablation of "tolerance" and induction of diabetes by virus infection in viral antigen transgenic mice. Cell 1991; 65:305-317.
67. Scott B, Liblau R, Degermann S et al. A role for non-MHC genetic polymorphism in susceptibility to spontaneous autoimmunity. Immunity 1994; 1:78-84.
68. Schonrich G, Kalinke U, Momburg F et al. Downregulation of T cell receptors on self reactive T cells as a novel mechanism for extrathymic tolerance induction. Cell 1991; 65:293-304.
69. Sarvetnik N, Shizuru J, Liggitt D et al. Loss of pancreatic islet tolerance induced by β-cell expression of IFNγ. Nature 1990; 346:844-847.
70. Stewart TA, Hultgren B, Huang X et al. Induction of type I diabetes by interferon-alpha in transgenic mice. Science 1993; 260:1942-1946.
71. Picarella DE, Kratz A, Li C-B et al. Insulitis in transgenic mice expressing tumor necrosis factor beta (lymphotoxin) in the pancreas. Proc Natl Acad Sci USA 1992; 89;10036-10040.
72. Higuchi Y, Herrera P, Muniesa P et al. Expression of a tumor necrosis factor α transgene in murine pancreatic β cells results in severe and permanent insulitis without evolution towards diabetes. J Exp Med 1992; 176:1719-1731.
73. Jacob CO, Dadakazu A, Michie S et al. Prevention of diabetes in nonobese diabetic mice by tumor necrosis factor (TNF): similarities between TNFα and interleukin-1. Proc Natl Acad Sci USA 1990; 87:968-972.
74. Yang XD, Tisch R, Singer SM et al. Effect of tumor necrosis factor alpha on insulin dependent diabetes mellitus in NOD mice. I. The early development of autoimmunity and the diabetogenic process. J Exp Med 1994; 180:995-1004.
75. Elliott MJ, Strasser A, Metcalf D. Selective up-regulation of macrophage function in granulocyte-macrophage colony-stimulating factor transgenic mice. J Immunol 1991; 14:2957-2963.
76. Alvaro-Gracia JM, Zvaifler NJ, Firestein GS. Cytokines in chronic inflammatory arthritis. V. Mutual antagonism between interferon-gamma and tumor necrosis factor alpha on HLA-DR expression, proliferation, collagenase production and granulocyte macrophage colony-stimulating factor production by rheumatoid synoviocytes. J Clin Invest 1990; 86:1790-1798.
77. Pfeffer K, Matsuyama T, Kundig TM et al. Mice deficient for the 55 kd tumor necrosis factor receptor are resistant to endotoxic shock, yet succumb to *L. monocytogenes* infection. Cell 1993; 73:457-467.
78. Rothe J, Lesslauer W, Loetscher H et al. Mice lacking the tumour necrosis factor receptor 1 are resistant to TNF-mediated toxicity but highly susceptible to infection by *Listeria monocytogenes*. Nature 1993; 364:798-802.
79. Erickson SL, de Sauvage FJ, Kikly K et al. Decreased sensitivity to tumour necrosis factor but normal T cell development in TNF receptor-2-deficient mice. Nature 1994; 372:560-563.

80. Ruddle NH, Bergman CM, McGrath KN et al. An antibody to lymphotoxin and tumor necrosis factor prevents transfer of experimental allergic encephalomyelitis. J Exp Med 1990; 172:1193-1200.
81. Williams RO, Feldmann M, Maini RN. Anti-tumor necrosis factor ameliorates joint disease in murine collagen-induced arthritis. Proc Natl Acad Sci USA 1992; 89:9784-9788.
82. Mackay F, Loetscher H, Stueber D et al. Tumor necrosis factor alpha (TNF-alpha)-induced cell adhesion to human endothelial cells is under dominant control of one TNF receptor type, TNF-R55. J Exp Med 1993; 177:1277-1286.
83. Tartaglia LA, Pennica D, Goeddel DV. Ligand passing: The 75-kDa tumor necrosis factor (TNF) receptor recruits TNF for signaling by the 55-kDa TNF receptor. J Biol Chem 1993; 268:18542-18548.
84. Tartaglia LA, Weber RF, Figari IS et al. Two different receptors for tumor necrosis factor mediate distinct cellular responses. Proc Natl Acad Sci USA 1991; 88:9292-9296.
85. Gehr G, Gentz R, Brockhaus M et al. Both tumor necrosis factor receptor types mediate proliferative signals in human mononuclear cell activation. J Immunol 1992; 149:911-917.
86. Yawata H, Yasukawa K, Natsuka S et al. Structure-function analysis of human IL-6 receptor: dissociation of amino acid residues required for IL-6-binding and for IL-6 signal transduction through gp130. EMBO J 1993; 12:1705-1712.
87. Giroir BP, Brown T, Beutler B. Constitutive synthesis of tumor necrosis factor in the thymus. Proc Natl Acad Sci USA 1992; 89:4864-4868.
88. Ranges G, Zlotnik A, Espevick T et al. Tumor necrosis factor α/cachectin is a growth factor for thymocytes. Synergistic interactions with other cytokines. J Exp Med 1988; 67:1472-1478.
89. Hirano T, Kishimoto T. Biological and clinical aspects of interleukin-6. Immunology Today 1990; 11:443-449.
90. Hirano T. Interleukin-6 transgenic mouse: a model of chronic inflammatory proliferative disease. In: Jacob C, ed. Overexpression and knockout of cytokines in transgenic mice. New York: Academic Press Ltd, 1994:73-84.
91. Suematsu S, Matsuda T, Aozasa K et al. IgG1 plasmacytosis in interleukin 6 transgenic mice. Proc Natl Acad Sci USA 1989; 86:7547-7551.
92. Aderka D, Le J, Vilcek J. IL-6 inhibits lipopolysaccharide-induced tumor necrosis factor production in cultured human mononcytes, U937 cells, and in mice. J Immunol 1989; 143:3517-3523.
93. Kopf M, Baumann H, Freer G et al. Impaired immune and acute-phase responses in interleukin-6 deficient mice. Nature 1994; 368:339-342.
94. Tanaka T, Akira S, Yoshida K et al. Targeted disruption of the NF-IL-6 gene discloses its essential role in bacteria killing and tumor cytotoxicity by macrophages. Cell 1995; 80:353-361.
95. Ramsay AJ, Husband AJ, Ramshaw IA et al. The role of interleukin-6 in mucosal IgA antibody responses in vivo. Science 1994; 264:561-563.

96. Poli V, Balena R, Fattori E et al. Interleukin-6 deficient mice are protected from bone loss caused by estrogen depletion. EMBO J 1994; 13:1189-1196.
97. Mosmann TR and Coffman RL. Th$_1$ and Th$_2$ cells: different patterns of lymphokine secretion lead to different functional properties. Annu Rev Immunol 1989; 7:145-173.
98. Mosmann TR, Cherwinski H, Bond MW et al. Two types of murine helper T cell clone. I. Definition according to profiles of lymphokine activities and secreted proteins. J Immunol 1986; 136:2348-2357.
99. Fitch FW, McKisic MD, Lancki DW et al. Differential regulation of murine T lymphocyte subsets. Annu Rev Immunol 1993; 11:29-48.
100. Gajewski TF and Fitch FW. Anti-proliferative effect of IFNγ in immune regulation. I. IFNγ inhibits the proliferation of Th$_2$ but not Th$_1$ murine helper T lymphocyte clones. J Immunol 1988; 140:4245-4252.
101. Finkelman F, Katona IM, Mosmann TJ et al. IFNγ regulates the isotypes of Ig secreted during in vivo immune responses. J Immunol 1988; 140:1022-1027.
102. Seder RA, Gazzinelli R, Sher A et al. Interleukin-12 acts directly on CD4$^+$ T cells to enhance priming for interferon-γ production and diminishes interleukin-4 inhibition of such priming. Proc Natl Acad Sci USA 1993; 90:10188-10192.
103. Le Gros G, Ben-Sasson SZ, Seder R et al. Generation of interleukin-4 (IL-4)-producing cells in vivo and in vitro: IL-2 and IL-4 are required for in vitro generation of IL-4-producing cells. J Exp Med 1990; 172:921-929.
104. Fiorentino DF, Bond MW, Mossman TR. Two types of mouse T helper cell. IV. Th$_2$ clones secrete a factor that inhibits cytokine production by Th$_1$ clones. J Exp Med 1989; 170:2081-2095.
105. Maggi E, P Parronchi P, Manetti R et al. Reciprocal regulatory effects of IFN-γ and IL-4 on the in vitro development of human Th$_1$ and Th$_2$ clones. J Immunol 1992; 148:2142-2147.
106. Dalton D, Pitts-Meek S, Keshav S et al. Multiple defects of immune cell function in mice with disrupted interferon-γ genes. Science 1993; 259:1739-1742.
107. Kuhn R, Rajewsky K, Muller W. Generation and analysis of interleukin-4 deficient mice. Science 1991; 254:707-710.
108. Kopf M, Le Gros G, Bachmann M et al. Disruption of the murine IL-4 gene blocks Th$_2$ cytokine responses. Nature 1993; 362:245-248.
109. Magram L et al, 1995 Midwinter Conference of Immunologists, Monterey, California.
110. Hseih CS, Heimberger AB, Gold GS et al. Differential regulation of T helper phenotype development by interleukin 4 and 10 in an alpha beta T cell receptor transgenic system. Proc Natl Acad Sci USA 1992; 89: 6065-6069.
111. de Waal Malefyt R, Abrams J, Bennett B et al. IL-10 inhibits cytokine synthesis by human monocytes: an autoregulatory role of IL-10 produced by monocytes. J Exp Med 1991; 174:1209-1220.

112. Howard M, O'Garra A, Ishida H et al. Biological properties of interleukin-10. J Clin Immunol 1992; 12:239-247.
113. Wogensen L, Huang X, Sarvetnik N. Production of interleukin 10 by islet cells accelerates immune-mediated destruction of beta cells in nonobese diabetic mice. J Exp Med 1993; 178:175-185.
114. Heinzel FP, Sadick MD, Holaday BJ et al. Reciprocal expression of interferon γ or interleukin 4 during the resolution or progression of murine leishmaniasis: evidence for expansion of distinct helper T cell subsets. J Exp Med 1989; 169:59-72.
115. Huang S, Hendriks W, Althage A et al. Immune response in mice lacking the interferon-γ receptor. Science 1993; 259:1742-1745.
116. Wang Z-E, Reiner SL, Zheng S et al. CD4$^+$ effector cells default to the Th$_2$ pathway in interferon γ-deficient mice infected with Leishmania major. J Exp Med 1994; 179:1367-1371.
117. Jacob CO, Vander Meide P, McDevitt HO. In vivo treatment of (NZB x NZW)F1 lupus-like nephritis with monoclonal antibody to γ interferon. J Exp Med 1987; 166:798-802.
118. Campbell IL, Kay TW, Oxbrow L et al. Essential role for interferon-gamma and interleukin-6 in autoimmune insulin-dependent diabetes in NOD/Wehi mice. J Clin Invest 1991; 87:739-72.
119. Debray-Sachs M, Carnaud C, Boitard C et al. Prevention of diabetes in NOD mice treated with antibody to murine IFNγ. J Autoimmunity 1991; 4:237-248.
120. Trembleau S, Penna G, Bosi E et al. Interleukin 12 administration induces T helper type 1 cells and accelerates diabetes in NOD mice. J Exp Med 1995; 181:817-821.
121. Leonard JP, Waldburger KE, Goldman SJ. Prevention of experimental autoimmune encephalomyelitis by antibodies against interleukin 12. J Exp Med 1995; 181:381-386.
122. Schall TJ, Bacon K, Toy KJ et al. Selective attraction of monocytes and T lymphocytes of the memory phenotype by cytokine RANTES. Nature 1990; 347:669-671.
123. Schall TJ, Bacon K, Camp RDR et al. Human macrophage inflammatory protein α (MIP-1α) and MIP-1β chemokines attract distinct populations of lymphocytes. J Exp Med 1993; 177: 1821-1825.
124. Yang XD, Michie SA, Tisch R et al. A predominant role of integrin alpha 4 in the spontaneous development of autoimmune diabetes in nonobese diabetic mice. Proc Natl Acad Sci USA 1994; 91:12604-12608.
125. Cacalano G, Lee J, Kikly K et al. Neutrophil and B cell expansion in mice that lack the murine IL-8 receptor homology. Science 1994; 265:682-684.
126. Lakso M, Sauer B, Mosinger B Jr et al. Targeted oncogene activation by site-specific recombination in transgenic mice. Proc Natl Acad Sci USA 1992; 89:6232-6236.
127. Gu H, Marth JD, Orban PC et al. Deletion of a DNA polymerase beta gene segment in T cells using cell type-specific gene targeting. Science 1994; 265:103-106.

CHAPTER 11

WHAT CAN WE LEARN FROM TRANSGENIC MICE?

George Kollias

INTRODUCTION

A consensus hypothesis stemming from studies investigating autoimmunity, has been that the development of an autoimmune disease depends on the interaction of several pathogenic factors such as genetic or hormonal background, level of immune responsiveness, infectious agents and other exogenous factors.[1] Cytokines have been classically viewed as potent immunoregulatory factors and as such they are shown to be strong potential mediators of both the inductive and the effector phase of autoimmune disease. For example, the proinflammatory cytokines TNFα and IL-1 may act either directly to induce tissue destruction (and possibly autoantigen sequestration) or indirectly to upregulate MHC expression and induce leukocyte adhesion and activation. Chemokines such as IL-8 may be responsible for the influx of inflammatory cells in affected tissues, lymphokines such as IL-2 may mediate activation of autoreactive or cytotoxic T cells and regulatory cytokines such as IFNγ, IL-4 or IL-10 may bias the immune system towards pathogenic cellular or humoral responses. Moreover, inhibitory activities such as soluble cytokine receptors or cytokine antagonists also take part in the autoimmune cytokine milieu. A chronically imbalanced cytokine system would have the potential to initiate, enhance or perpetuate the development of autoimmune disease.

The power of a transgenic approach to the study of cytokine involvement in autoimmunity lies in the ability to design an in vivo situation where expression of a given cytokine or of a set of related factors is perturbed. In this way, the contribution of such a specific factor in the development of disease can be analyzed. Transgenic

Cytokines in Autoimmunity, edited by Fionula M. Brennan and Marc Feldmann.
© 1996 R.G. Landes Company.

animal models of cytokine over expression have proven invaluable to the study of the etiology, pathogenesis and treatment of autoimmune disease.

CYTOKINES AND THE T CELL COMPONENT IN AUTOIMMUNITY

One important hallmark in autoimmunity is the activation of self-reactive T cells, a process which may be accounted for by defects in mechanisms establishing and maintaining immunological self-tolerance. In the MRL-*lpr/lpr* mouse, the *lpr* genetic defect leading to systemic autoimmunity has been identified as a mutation in the *Fas* gene involved in apoptosis.[2] It has therefore been speculated that loss of tolerance in these mice is related to defective apoptosis of the CD4−CD8− subset of T cells in the thymus. To determine whether Fas dysfunction is directly responsible for the generalized autoimmune disease seen in the MRL-*lpr/lpr* mouse model, MRL-*lpr/lpr* mice were made transgenic for a *Fas* gene directed by the CD2 gene locus control region to express in their T cells.[3] Restoration of *Fas* expression in these CD2-*Fas* transgenic mice led to the abrogation of the lymphoproliferative defect and the systemic autoimmune disease, suggesting that abnormal *Fas* expression or, more generally, intrinsic defects of intrathymic T cell development, may be major determinants in the development of autoimmunity.

The existence of peripheral T cell clones which do not become tolerized to self antigens has also been demonstrated by several studies.[4-6] Potentially, these autoreactive T cells would circulate in the periphery but normally remain silent. If such cells exist in a quiescent state then what determines their activation? Are cytokines involved in this process?

IL-2, a potent T cell growth factor, has been implicated as a causal factor in autoimmunity.[7] This hypothesis was tested in transgenic mice engineered to overexpress IL-2 in several of their tissues, under the control of a MHC class I promoter,[8] or in pancreatic β cells under the control of a rat insulin promoter.[9] In both cases, although general inflammatory lesions and tissue damage were apparent, autoimmunity could not be established. However, autoimmunity could be induced in a triple transgenic background where β islet cells are forced to express IL-2 and H-2K^b (RIP-K^b), and T cells a K^b-specific T cell receptor transgene.[10] In this system, mice carrying the rearranged K^b-specific T cell receptor transgene show a T cell repertoire which is highly skewed (by allelic exclusion) for the transgene-encoded specificity. Measurements of K^b-specific TCR densities in peripheral T cells from double RIP-K^b x K^b-specific TCR transgenic mice, showed that deletion of T cells with high K^b-specific TCR densities had occurred. However, despite the presence of large numbers of "low avidity" T cells, β islet cells expressing K^b restricted antigens remained unaffected until IL-2 was also co-expressed in β islet cells. These results indicate that large numbers of "low-avidity" self reactive T cells can produce a self destructive response if sufficient help is provided, as for example in the form of IL-2. This finding highlights the importance of chronically produced cytokines (e.g., in the course of chronic infectious or inflammatory diseases) as triggering factors in the development of autoimmune disease.

TNFα may also serve as a factor providing help in the activation of large numbers of autoreactive T cells. This has been established in a transgenic mouse model of autoimmune diabetes in which a lymphocytic choriomeningitis virus (LCMV) glycoprotein gene linked to the rat insulin promoter (RIP-gp) is expressed in the β cells of the pancreas.[4] Such mice do not become diabetic unless they are infected by LCMV. Viral infection may lead to the "breaking" of tolerance in some systems.[11] However in the LCMV infected mice splenic T cells could respond to macrophages presenting LCMV-gp without in vivo priming, suggesting that these T cells have not become anergic and indicating that autoimmunity in this model results from the activation of naive self-reactive T cells rather than from the breaking of self-tolerance. Interestingly, immunization of the RIP-gp transgenic mice with a recombinant vaccinia virus expressing the LCMV-gp (vacc-gp) did not induce diabetes, indicating that limited activation of self reactive T cells, in this case by vaccinia-gp and also by nonprofessional antigen presenting cells,, e.g., β islet cells, is not sufficient to induce an autoimmune attack. What other factors are then needed to induce autoimmunity? TNFα transgenic mice expressing TNFα in their islets (RIP-TNFα) do not become diabetic although they suffer a permanent insulitis[12] (see also below). Strikingly, when RIP-gp x RIP-TNFα double transgenic mice are immunized with vaccinia-gp, diabetes does develop,[13] indicating that recruitment of a threshold number of activated LCMV-gp-specific T cells to the islets (effected in this case by TNFα) may be critical to the triggering of an autoimmune response.

CYTOKINES AND THE B CELL COMPONENT IN AUTOIMMUNITY

Several recent reports support the earlier concept that systemic autoimmune disease may be explained on the basis of a defect in B cell tolerance or B cell activation.[14] Probably the most convincing in vivo evidence for a possible role of a biased B cell repertoire in the induction of autoimmunity has been provided by transgenic studies addressing the role of autoantibody overproduction in the development of disease.[15] However, limited evidence for the involvement of cytokines in the induction of "B cell driven" autoimmunity has been obtained in cytokine transgenic systems. With reference to the CD2-*Fas* transgenic MRL-*lpr/lpr* mice which are rescued from the lymphoproliferative defect and the systemic autoimmune disease (see above), it still remains possible that abrogation of disease development is due to a corrected Fas expression in a subpopulation of B cells as well as T cells.[3] In such a case, defective B cell apoptosis could also be taking part in the development of the autoimmune phenotype.

Cytokines such as IL-4 or IL-6 have been implicated in the development of a range of autoimmune diseases, both being described as growth factors for B cells.[16,17] However, results with transgenic mice expressing either of these transgenes in several different tissues have not yet provided conclusive evidence for a dominant role of these factors in the triggering or maintenance of autoimmunity.[18,19]

CYTOKINE OVEREXPRESSION CAN BE CAUSAL IN THE DEVELOPMENT OF CHRONIC INFLAMMATORY DISEASE

There is now a wealth of supportive evidence that cytokines may be critical factors in the triggering and maintenance of the chronicity of autoimmune diseases. The in vivo accuracy of this statement has been confirmed in several cytokine transgenic systems.

In addition to its antiviral activities, IFN-α has been strongly implicated in the local activation of macrophages and NK cells.[20] The possibility that IFNα, found to be overexpressed in autoimmune diabetes,[21] could be causal in the development of this disease in humans was tested in transgenic mice in which expression of IFNα was targeted in pancreatic β islet cells.[22] These mice develop a syndrome resembling type I diabetes associated with a mixed inflammation centered on the β islet cells. Chronicity of inflammation in this model is easy to explain since transgenic IFNα is constitutively produced. Similarly, in human disease, persistence of high levels of IFNα expression may be explained by positive mechanisms involving either continuous stimulation (e.g., chronic nonproductive viral infections) or feedback loops consisting of different cell types and factors. For example, it may be suggested that persistent IFNα expression may stimulate macrophages to release nitric oxide which could lead directly to the destruction of β cells in the pancreas.[23] Professional antigen presenting cells attracted in the area could pick up and represent the sequestered self antigens to T cells in lymphoid organs, allowing for their activation. Sufficient numbers of autoreactive T cells may recirculate in the affected tissue and a further local activation step could take place in the presence of self-antigen presenting cells (e.g., macrophages, B cells) or other activating factors (e.g., TNFα, IL-2) leading to the perpetuation of the initial destructive process.

Autoimmunity also develops as a consequence of overexpression of IFNγ in the islets of transgenic mice.[24,25] Although IFNγ is not detected in human diabetes, it can be suggested that in these transgenic mice a pathogenic process similar to the one proposed for the IFNα transgenics might have been operating. Additionally, IFNγ may also act as a potent inducer of T cell costimulatory activity,[26] enhance class I and class II MHC expression[27] and synergize with cytokines such as TNFα or IL-1 in the induction of destructive inflammatory cascades.[28]

Considering the possibility that local TNFα overproduction may also lead to autoimmune destruction, transgenic mice expressing TNFα[12] or LT[29] in their islets have been generated. In both cases permanent insulitis would develop but progression to autoimmunity would not follow. Even when perfusion of IFNγ or mild β cell damage has been attempted diabetes failed to develop,[12] indicating that insulitis and autoimmune diabetes are distinct pathogenic processes and that progression from the one stage to the other necessitates the contribution of additional specific factors. Interestingly, autoimmunity develops when B7-1, a T cell costimulatory factor, is co-expressed in transgenic islets with the TNFα molecule.[30] This finding supports the hypothesis that an inflammatory stimulus (such as TNFα) may not be sufficient to induce an autoimmune attack in a local environment where activation of autoreactive T cells cannot be sustained. In contrast, the presence of B7-1 on the β cells may substitute for professional antigen presenting cells which may be required for the amplification of the autoimmune response. Consistent with this hypothesis, it has been recently shown that, unlike normal keratinocytes, psoriatic keratinocytes express a B7-1 like molecule.[31]

TUMOR NECROSIS FACTOR SPECIFICALLY TRIGGERS INFLAMMATORY ARTHRITIS IN TRANSGENIC MICE

TNFα and IL-1 share many biological activities which may directly implicate them in the arthritic process. Perhaps the most telling activity of these molecules has been their ability to trigger activation and proliferation of synovial cells in vitro.[32,33] Other activities, including their interference with cartilage and bone metabolism, the induction of cytokine cascades and the triggering of adhesion molecules on endothelial cells enabling lymphocytes to home in the site of inflammation, are also considered to be decisive in the pathogenesis of arthritis[34] (reviewed in chapter 2 and its clinical implications in chapter 12.)

The pivotal role of TNFα in the development of chronic inflammatory arthritis has been recently confirmed in transgenic mice.[35] Transgenic mice engineered to overexpress a human TNFα gene, under the influence of its own wild-type promoter, progressively develop chronic inflammatory polyarthritis with 100% phenotypic penetrance, timed onset and histological characteristics typical of human rheumatoid arthritis.[36] Hyperproliferation of synovial cells, inflammatory infiltrates of the synovial space, fibrous tissue and pannus formation, articular cartilage destruction and bone resorption are observed. Development of arthritis in these transgenic mice can be completely suppressed by treatment with antibodies against human TNFα, confirming that the pathology observed is effected by the in vivo deregulated production of the human TNFα protein.

TNFα action in this model may be direct, for example by inducing destructive processes in the joint tissues (e.g., cartilage) and consequently immune reactivity against sequestered antigens, or indirect, possibly by inducing synovial cell activation and proliferation which in turn may be causal in the development of arthritic disease. For example, it may be speculated that proliferating activated synoviocytes may act directly to destroy cartilage (e.g., through excessive production of matrix metalloproteinases), even in the absence of antigen-specific mature T and B cells. This hypothesis is supported by preliminary experiments showing that full blown arthritis still develops in immunodeficient double transgenic TNFα x RAG-/- mice (our unpublished observations, RAG-/- mice provided by E. Spanopoulou, Rockefeller University). The specific triggering of arthritis by TNFα overexpression in the joint comes in contrast to the inability of the same factor to cause autoimmune destruction of β islets when expressed in the pancreas (see above). This probably reflects existing molecular and cellular differences between the two anatomical compartments. For example, it may be that in compartments such as the joint, where circulation is less prevalent, rates of clearance of specific factors are altered[37] and initial cytokine imbalances are much more easily maintained or even amplified.

CHEMOKINE TRANSGENICS

Inflammation is characterized by the influx of leukocytes from the peripheral blood into the tissue. This site-specific accumulation is thought to be induced by chemotactic factors produced by various stimulated cells. IL-8, a most extensively studied cytokine, is produced by monocytes, endothelial cells, fibroblasts and many other cells of epithelial origin. It has been implicated as an important chemotactic attractant of neutrophil and T cell infiltrates in a range of autoimmune/inflammatory diseases such as rheumatoid arthritis,[38] psoriasis[39] and ulcerative colitis.[40] However, additional anti-inflammatory activities have also been reported and an anti-inflammatory role for IL-8 in serum has also been suggested, e.g., inhibition of neutrophil adhesion.[41] This could be explained by disruption of IL-8 gradients in the tissues by high serum IL-8.

It has been therefore of interest to assess the in vivo potential of constitutive IL-8 overexpression in a transgenic mouse system; a recent report addressed this question.[42] Interestingly, transgenic mice overexpressing IL-8 in their serum show an increased intravascular accumulation of neutrophils which is not followed by enhanced neutrophil migration into the tissues. The latter was correlated with a decreased expression of L-selectin on the surface of the transgenic neutrophils, an observation supported by earlier in vivo studies.[43] It may therefore be suggested that in vivo, IL-8, although acting to induce neutrophil accumulation at sites of inflammation, by itself is not sufficient to induce neutrophil extravasation into tissues and that a more complex regulation involving additional chemokines, adhesion molecules and/or other factors may be required. However, as chemokines act locally, firm conclusions await transgenic mice expressing IL-8 in a restricted site, e.g., islets.

IMMUNOREGULATORY CYTOKINE TRANSGENICS

Several in vitro studies have suggested that IL-10, a T helper type 2 (Th$_2$) cell product, may act as an immunossuppressive cytokine, by directly inhibiting the proliferation and function of Th$_1$ lymphocytes and macrophages. This has raised the possibility of the therapeutic use of IL-10 in situations requiring inhibition of cell-mediated responses. Indeed, IL-10 pretreatment prevents mortality in mice at an LD50 challenge with LPS by reducing the amount of macrophage mediators, particularly TNFα.[44] However, despite the apparent immunosuppressive activities of IL-10, transgenic mice expressing IL-10 in the β islet cells develop inflammatory lesions but not diabetes.[45] Moreover, when they are back-crossed to the nonobese diabetic genetic background (the NOD strain of mice which develops a macrophage and T cell dependent diabetes), an acceleration of the immune-mediated destruction of β cells is observed.[46] In additional studies, when IL-10 x LCMV-gp double transgenic mice were produced (for the LCMV-gp system, see above) and infected with LCMV, development of diabetes could not be inhibited.[47] These data, taken together, suggest that at least in the pancreas IL-10 exerts powerful immunostimulatory activities and indicate that autoimmune diabetes may be a Th$_2$-mediated phenomenon.[48] The effects of IL-10 in several other autoimmune diseases remain to be evaluated.

CONCLUDING REMARKS

The cellular and molecular basis of autoimmunity is complex and multifactorial. Immunogenetic susceptibility, physical stress or injury, infectious agents and endogenous substances have all been implicated in the triggering and perpetuation of the primary immune response. The evaluation of the relative contribution of each of these components in the development of autoimmunity has been effectively addressed in relevant transgenic mouse models. In general, it may be suggested that the loss of tolerance to an autoantigen or the aberrant expression of an MHC molecule in a certain tissue, are not sufficient by themselves to trigger disease. Cytokines have emerged as key molecules in the regulation of the immune response and evidence so far suggests that at least some of them (e.g., Fas, IFNα, IFNγ, TNFα) may be directly involved in both the inductive and the effector phase of autoimmunity. Other cytokines such as IL-2 and IL-10 may also provide essential help for autoreactive T cells to multiply and perform their destructive scenario. Yet, although several studies have indisputably identified the role of cytokines such as IL-4 and IL-6 in autoimmunity, transgenic studies have not been too revealing, reminding us that we have a lot more to learn before we are able to faithfully simulate and understand autoimmunity as it develops in vivo.

ACKNOWLEDGMENTS

I wish to thank David Plows for critical reading of the manuscript. Research in the author's laboratory is supported in part by the Greek Secreteriat of Research and Technology and by Research Grants SCI-CT91-0653, BIO2-92-0002-GR, CHRX-CT-930182 and BIO2-CT94-2092 from the Commission of the European Communities.

REFERENCES

1. Rose NR. Pathogenetic mechanisms in autoimmune diseases. Clin Immunol Immunopathol 1989; 53:S7-16.
2. Watanabe-Fukunaga R, Brannan CI, Copeland NG et al. Lymphoproliferation disorder in mice explained by defects in *Fas* antigen that mediates apoptosis. Nature 1992; 356:314-7.
3. Wu J Zhou T, Zhang J et al. Correction of accelerated autoimmune disease by early replacement of the mutated lpr gene with the normal *Fas* apoptosis gene in the T cells of transgenic MRL-lpr/lpr mice. Proc Natl Acad Sci USA 1994; 91:2344-2348.
4. Ohashi PS, Oehen S, Burki K et al. Ablation of "tolerance" and induction of diabetes by virus infection in viral antigen transgenic mice. Cell 1991; 65:305-17.
5. Oldstone MB, Nerenberg M, Southern P et al. Virus infection triggers insulin-dependent diabetes mellitus in a transgenic model: role of anti-self (virus) immune response. Cell 1991; 65:319-31.
6. Katz JD, Wang B, Haskins K et al. Following a diabetogenic T cell from genesis through pathogenesis. Cell 1993; 74:1089-100.
7. Kroemer G, Wick G. The role of interleukin 2 in autoimmunity. Immunol Today 1989; 10:246-51.
8. Ishida Y, Nishi M, Taguchi O et al. Effects of the deregulated expression of human interleukin-2 in transgenic mice. Int Immunol 1989; 1:113-7.
9. Allison J, Malcolm L, Chosich N, Miller JFAP. Inflammation but not autoimmunity occurs in transgenic mice expressing constitutive levels of interleukin-2 in islet β cells. Eur J Immunol 1992; 22:1115-21.
10. Heath WR, Allison J, Hoffmann MW et al. Autoimmune diabetes as a consequence of locally produced interleukin-2. Nature 1992; 359:547-9.
11. Rocken M, Urban JF, Shevach SM. Infection breaks T cell tolerance. Nature 1992; 359:79-82.
12. Higuchi Y, Herrera P, Muniesa P et al. Expression of a tumor necrosis factor α transgene in murine pancreatic β cells results in severe and permanent insulitis without evolution towards arthritis. J Exp Med 1992; 176:1719-31.

13. Ohashi PS, Oehen S, Aichele P et al. Induction of diabetes is influenced by the infectious virus and local expression of MHC class I and tumour necrosis factor α. J Immunol 1993; 150:5185-94.
14. Nemazee D. Promotion and prevention of autoimmunity by B lymphocytes. Curr Op Immunol 1993; 5:866-72.
15. Murakami M, Tsubata T, Okamoto M et al. Antigen-induced apoptotic death of Ly-1 B cells responsible for autoimmune disease in transgenic mice. Nature 1992; 357:77-80.
16. Paul WE, Ohara J. B-cell stimulatory factor-1/interleukin 4. Annu Rev Immunol 1987; 5:429-59.
17. Hirano T. Interleukin-6 and its relation to inflammation and disease. 1992; 62:S60-5.
18. Muller W, Kuhn R, Rajewsky K. Major histocompatibility complex class II hyperexpression on B cells in interleukin-4 transgenic mice does not lead to B cell proliferation and hypergammaglobulinemia. Eur J Immunol 1991; 21:921-5.
19. Kimura T, Suzuki K, Inada S et al. Induction of autoimmune disease by graft-versus-host reaction across MHC class II difference: modification of the lesions in IL-6 transgenic mice. Clin Exp Immunol 1994; 95:525-9.
20. Schattner A. Review: Interferons and autoimmunity. Am J Med Sci 1988; 31:532-44.
21. Foulis AK, Farquharson MA, Meager A. Immunoreactive alpha-interferon in insulin-secreting beta cells in type 1 diabetes mellitus. Lancet 1987;ii:1423-7.
22. Stewart TA, Hultgren B, Huang X et al. Induction of Type I diabetes by interferon α in transgenic mice. Science 1993; 260:1942-6.
23. Appels B, Burkart V, Kantwerk-Funke G et al. Spontaneous cytotoxicity of macrophages against pancreatic islet cells. J Immunol 1989; 142:3803-8.
24. Sarvetnick N, Liggitt D, Pitts SL et al. Insulin-dependent diabetes mellitus induced in transgenic mice by ectopic expression of class II MHC and interferon γ. Cell 1988; 52:773-82.
25. Sarvetnick N, Shizuru J, Liggitt D et al. Loss of pancreatic islet tolerance induced by β-cell expression of interferon γ. Nature 1990; 346:844-7.
26. Hawrylowicz CM, Unanue ER. Regulation of antigen presentation-I: IFNγ induces antigen-presenting properties on B cells. J Immunol 1988; 141:4083-8.
27. Campbell IL, Oxbrow L, West J et al. Regulation of MHC protein expression in pancreatic β-cells by interferon gamma and tumour necrosis factor alpha. Mol Endocrinol 1988; 2:101-7.
28. Pukel C, Baquerizo H, Rabinovitch A. Destruction of rat islet cell monolayers by cytokines. Synergistic interactions of interferon γ, tumor necrosis factor, lymphotoxin and interleukin-1. Diabetes 1988; 37:133-42.
29. Picarella E, Kratz A, Chang-Ben L et al. Insulitis in transgenic mice expressing tumor necrosis factor β (lymphotoxin) in the pancreas. Proc Natl Acad Sci USA 1992; 89:10036-40.

30. Guerder S, Picarella DE, Linsley PS et al. Costimulator B7-1 confers antigen-presenting-cell function to parenchymal tissue and in conjuction with tumor necrosis factor α leads to autoimmunity in transgenic mice. Proc Natl Acad Sci USA 1994; 91:5138-42.
31. Nickoloff BJ, Mitra RS, Lee K et al. Discordant expression of CD28 ligands, BB-1, and B7 on keratinocytes in vitro and psoriatic cells in vivo. Am J Pathol 1993; 142:1029-40.
32. Butler DM, Piccoli DS, Hart PH et al. Stimulation of human synovial fibroblast DNA synthesis by recombinant human cytokines. J Rheumatology 1988; 15:1463-70.
33. Gitter BD, Labus JM, Lees SL et al. Characteristics of human synovial fibroblast activation by IL-1β and TNFα Immunology 1989; 66:196-200.
34. Kollias G. Tumour necrosis factor: a specific trigger in arthritis. Res Immunol 1993; 144:342-7.
35. Keffer J, Probert L, Cazlaris H et al. Transgenic mice expressing human tumour necrosis factor: a predictive genetic model of arthritis. EMBO J 1991; 10:4025-31.
36. Harris ED Jr. Rheumatoid arthritis: pathophysiology and implications for therapy. New Engl J Med 1990; 322:1277-89.
37. Aderka D, Engelmann H, Maor Y et al. Stabilization of the bioactivity of tumor necrosis factor by its soluble receptors. J Exp Med 1992; 175:323-9.
38. Brennan FM, Zachariae COC, Chantry D et al. Detection of interleukin 8 biological activity in synovial fluids from patients with rheumatoid arthritis and production of interleukin 8 mRNA by isolated synovial cells. Eur J Immunol 1990; 20:2141-4.
39. Sticherling ME, Bornscheuer E, Schroder JM et al. Localization of neutrophil-activating peptide 1/interleukin-8 immunoreactivity in normal and psoriatic skin. J Invest Dermatol 1991; 96:26-30.
40. Izzo RS, Witkon K, Chen AI et al. Interleukin-8 and neutrophil markers in colonic mucosa from patients with ulcerative colitis. Am J Gastroenterol 1992; 87:1447-52.
41. Hechtman DH, Cybulski MI, Fuchs HJ et al. Intravascular IL-8: Inhibitor of polymorphonuclear leukocyte accumulation at sites of acute inflammation. J Immunol 1991; 147:883-92.
42. Simonet WS, Hughes TM, Nguyen HQ et al. Long-term impaired neutrophil migration in mice overexpressing human interleukin-8. J Clin Invest 1994; 94:1310-19.
43. Kishimoto TK, Jutila MA, Berg EL et al. Neutrophil Mac-1 and MEL-14 adhesion proteins inversely regulated by chemotactic factors. Science 1989; 245:1238-41.
44. Gerard C, Bruyns C, Marchant A et al. Interleukin 10 reduces the release of tumour necrosis factor and prevents lethality in experimental endotoxemia. J Exp Med 1993; 177:547-50.
45. Wogensen L, Huang X, Sarvetnick N. Leukocyte extravasation into the pancreatic tissue in transgenic mice expressing interleukin-10 in the islets of Langerhans. J Exp Med 1993; 178:175-85.

46. Wogensen L, Lee MS, Sarvetnick N. Production of interleukin 10 by islet cells accelerates immune-mediated destruction of β cells in nonobese diabetic mice. J Exp Med 1994; 179:1379-84.

47. Lee MS, Wogensen L, Shizuru J et al. Pancreatic islet production of murine interleukin-10 does not inhibit immune mediated tissue destruction. J Clin Invest 1994; 93:1332-8.

48. Anderson JT, Cornelius JG, Jarpe AJ et al. Insulin-dependent diabetes in the NOD mouse model II. β cell destruction in autoimmune diabetes is a Th_2 and not a Th_1 mediated event. Autoimmunity 1993; 15:113-22.

CHAPTER 12

WHAT ARE THE PROSPECTS FOR THERAPY BASED ON CYTOKINES AND ANTICYTOKINES IN RHEUMATOID ARTHRITIS?

Michael J. Elliott and Ravinder N. Maini

INTRODUCTION

The expansion of knowledge concerning the role of cytokines in autoimmune disease has been documented in detail elsewhere in this book. Clinical exploitation of this knowledge is most advanced in rheumatoid arthritis (RA), the commonest autoimmune disease in man and one in which standard therapies have made little difference to long-term outcomes such as progression of joint damage, locomotor function or mortality.[1] Cytokine related therapies which have been tested in RA are described in two sections: first, those which block cytokine action (or production) and second, hemopoietic growth factors used in the management of systemic features of RA or in the treatment of complications arising from standard antirheumatic therapy. With the exception of antitumor necrosis factor (anti-TNFα) therapy for short-term disease control and erythropoietin (EPO) for the treatment of RA-associated anemia, none of these therapies are yet proven in clinical trials.

Cytokines in Autoimmunity, edited by Fionula M. Brennan and Marc Feldmann.
© 1996 R.G. Landes Company.

CYTOKINE BLOCKADE IN RA

Anti-TNFα Therapy

Rationale

The in vitro and animal model data linking TNFα with disease pathogenesis in RA are compelling and are presented in detail in chapter 2. The anti-TNFα clinical trial program which we established in 1992 aimed to extend our experience to the final and most relevant frontier, namely the patient. The studies exploited the properties of a chimeric (human/mouse) neutralizing monoclonal anti-TNFα antibody (cA2). The generation and biological properties of cA2 were recently described,[2] with improved binding characteristics seen compared with the original murine reagent and evidence of good in vitro functional activity.

cA2 is effective therapy in RA

The cA2 dose range used was derived by extrapolation from studies using similar reagents in murine collagen induced arthritis (CIA). In our pilot study, in which 20 patients received 20 mg/kg cA2 (by intravenous infusion, 2-4 infusions, over 2 weeks), therapeutic levels of antibody (>10 µg/ml) were detectable in sera taken up to 6 weeks postcommencement of treatment (unpublished data). This favorable pharmacokinetic profile most likely results from reduced antibody clearance as a result of chimerisation.[3]

The patients recruited for the trials had disease at the more severe end of the clinical spectrum: long standing RA; a history of failed treatment with disease modifying antirheumatic drugs (DMARDs); active inflammation. Most also showed erosions on X-rays of hands or feet and were seropositive for rheumatoid factor. Patients were permitted to continue on stable doses of prednisolone and nonsteroidal anti-inflammatory drugs (NSAIDs), but DMARD therapy was withdrawn at least 1 month prior to trial entry. In the pilot study, each of the patients who completed the treatment program experienced improvement in multiple clinical assessments of disease activity, including the duration of morning stiffness, the pain score, the Ritchie articular index and the swollen joint count.[4] These changes were matched by statistically significant improvements in the acute phase measures, including C-reactive protein (CRP) and serum amyloid-A (SAA). The median CRP level fell to the normal range by 1 week and remained low for the 8 week duration of the trial.

The mechanism of control of the acute phase response by cA2 may be in part due to regulation of IL-6 production. Serum IL-6 fell significantly at weeks 1 and 2 post-treatment and detailed studies in individual patients confirmed that the fall in IL-6 preceded falls in CRP and SAA (ref. 4 and unpublished data). Trends to improvement were also seen in the ESR, hemoglobin, white cell and platelet counts and the rheumatoid factor titer. Using a composite clinical and laboratory index,[5] all patients achieved a response (median duration 14 weeks).

We followed with a randomized, placebo controlled, double-blind multicenter trial conducted on four European sites. Seventy-three patients received a single infusion of cA2 (1 or 10 mg/kg) or placebo (human serum albumin), revealing clear differences in both primary and secondary study endpoints between the groups. Seventy-nine percent of patients treated with high dose cA2 achieved a response at week 4, compared with only 8% treated with placebo. Forty-four percent of those treated with the intermediate dose of cA2 (1 mg/kg) achieved a response at this time.[6] Using a more stringent definition of response (Paulus 50%) almost 60% of patients treated with high dose cA2 were responders, demonstrating that the quality of clinical response was mostly good. Analysis of individual disease activity measures including the tender and swollen joint counts, the ESR and CRP showed impressive improvements, supporting the composite data. Four clinical assessments contributing to quality of life in RA patients are shown in Figure 12.1. Statistically significant and clinically important improvements can be seen for pain, morning stiffness, a measure of hand function (the grip strength) and fatigue. Improvement in fatigue was of particular interest: although not often recorded, the latter may be a debilitating feature of RA and evidence from trials of TNFα administration in patients with cancer suggests that it may result, at least in part, from direct actions of TNFα.[7]

Also of interest was the improvement in hemoglobin in patients treated with high-dose cA2, contrasting with a fall in patients receiving placebo (Fig. 12.2). The absolute changes were small but occurred over a period of only 4 weeks despite significant venesection for research purposes and cessation of standard DMARD therapy. The changes are therefore clinically important as well as statistically significant. TNFα is known to suppress erythroid burst forming- and colony forming-units (BFUe and CFUe) growth in bone marrow cultures in vitro[8] and its abnormal expression in nude mice in vivo results in a reticulocytopenia followed by profound anemia.[9] cA2 may act directly to prevent TNFα-induced suppression of erythropoiesis in the marrow. Alternatively, it may allow an appropriate erythropoietin response to anemia, normally suppressed in RA.[10-12]

The safety profile in the short term for cA2 in these studies has been good. Although about 12% of cA2-treated patients experienced infections in the placebo trial, these were for the most part minor and occurred predominantly in the low-dose group. Other minor events were equally scattered throughout the three treatment groups.

Repeated administration of cA2 was studied in patients originally enrolled in the open label pilot study. Patients were treated with up to four cycles of cA2, counting the infusion program from the open

Available Free Titles

*Please check three titles in order of preference.
Your request will be filled based on availability. Thank you.*

- ☐ Water Channels
  Alan Verkman,
  University of California-San Francisco

- ☐ The Na,K-ATPase:
  Structure-Function Relationship
  J.-D. Horisberger, University of Lausanne

- ☐ Intrathymic Development of T Cells
  J. Nikolic-Zugic,
  Memorial Sloan-Kettering Cancer Center

- ☐ Cyclic GMP
  Thomas Lincoln, University of Alabama

- ☐ Primordial VRM System and the Evolution
  of Vertebrate Immunity
  John Stewart, Institut Pasteur-Paris

- ☐ Thyroid Hormone Regulation
  of Gene Expression
  Graham R. Williams, University of Birmingham

- ☐ Mechanisms of Immunological Self Tolerance
  Guido Kroemer, CNRS Génétique Moléculaire et
  Biologie du Développement-Villejuif

- ☐ The Costimulatory Pathway
  for T Cell Responses
  Yang Liu, New York University

- ☐ Molecular Genetics of Drosophila Oogenesis
  Paul F. Lasko, McGill University

- ☐ Mechanism of Steroid Hormone Regulation
  of Gene Transcription
  M.-J. Tsai & Bert W. O'Malley, Baylor University

- ☐ Liver Gene Expression
  François Tronche & Moshe Yaniv,
  Institut Pasteur-Paris

- ☐ RNA Polymerase III Transcription
  R.J. White, University of Cambridge

- ☐ src Family of Tyrosine Kinases in Leukocytes
  Tomas Mustelin, La Jolla Institute

- ☐ MHC Antigens and NK Cells
  Rafael Solana & Jose Peña,
  University of Córdoba

- ☐ Kinetic Modeling of Gene Expression
  James L. Hargrove, University of Georgia

- ☐ PCR and the Analysis of the T Cell Receptor
  Repertoire
  Jorge Oksenberg, Michael Panzara & Lawrence
  Steinman, Stanford University

- ☐ Myointimal Hyperplasia
  Philip Dobrin, Loyola University

- ☐ Transgenic Mice as an In Vivo Model
  of Self-Reactivity
  David Ferrick & Lisa DiMolfetto-Landon,
  University of California-Davis and Pamela Ohashi,
  Ontario Cancer Institute

- ☐ Cytogenetics of Bone and Soft Tissue Tumors
  Avery A. Sandberg, Genetrix & Julia A. Bridge,
  University of Nebraska

- ☐ The Th1-Th2 Paradigm and Transplantation
  Robin Lowry, Emory University

- ☐ Phagocyte Production and Function Following
  Thermal Injury
  Verlyn Peterson & Daniel R. Ambruso,
  University of Colorado

- ☐ Human T Lymphocyte Activation Deficiencies
  José Regueiro, Carlos Rodríguez-Gallego
  and Antonio Arnaiz-Villena,
  Hospital 12 de Octubre-Madrid

- ☐ Monoclonal Antibody in Detection and
  Treatment of Colon Cancer
  Edward W. Martin, Jr., Ohio State University

- ☐ Enteric Physiology of the Transplanted Intestine
  Michael Sarr & Nadey S. Hakim, Mayo Clinic

- ☐ Artificial Chordae in Mitral Valve Surgery
  Claudio Zussa, S. Maria dei Battuti Hospital-Treviso

- ☐ Injury and Tumor Implantation
  Satya Murthy & Edward Scanlon,
  Northwestern University

- ☐ Support of the Acutely Failing Liver
  A.A. Demetriou, Cedars-Sinai

- ☐ Reactive Metabolites of Oxygen and Nitrogen
  in Biology and Medicine
  Matthew Grisham, Louisiana State-Shreveport

- ☐ Biology of Lung Cancer
  Adi Gazdar & Paul Carbone,
  Southwestern Medical Center

- ☐ Quantitative Measurement
  of Venous Incompetence
  Paul S. van Bemmelen, Southern Illinois University
  and John J. Bergan, Scripps Memorial Hospital

- ☐ Adhesion Molecules in Organ Transplants
  Gustav Steinhoff, University of Kiel

- ☐ Purging in Bone Marrow Transplantation
  Subhash C. Gulati,
  Memorial Sloan-Kettering Cancer Center

- ☐ Trauma 2000: Strategies for the New Millennium
  David J. Dries & Richard L. Gamelli,
  Loyola University

the infusion procedures were mostly well tolerated, one patient experienced a procedure-related vasovagal syncope requiring withdrawal and a second patient experienced a mild postinfusion reaction. Several patients withdrew early for other safety reasons, including sinusitis, urticaria and the development of anti-dsDNA antibodies. The latter event was of particular interest and experience now suggests that about 8% of patients treated with cA2 develop such autoantibodies, accompanied in some cases by other laboratory changes normally associated with systemic lupus erythematosus (refs. 4, 14 and unpublished data). These phenomena remain unexplained, but accord with experimental data from NZB/NZW F1 (lupus prone) mice, where TNFα has been shown to protect against the development of autoimmunity and anti-TNF accelerates the development of autoimmune nephritis in mice whose disease had been suppressed by anti-IL-10 (reviewed in ref. 14). We would speculate that in patients with an appropriate genetic predisposition, TNFα blockade may predispose to the development of lupus.

Other TNFα-blocking biologicals

The overall findings with cA2 have been supported by the results of TNFα blockade with other TNFα-blocking biological agents. In one study, 36 patients with active RA were randomized to receive

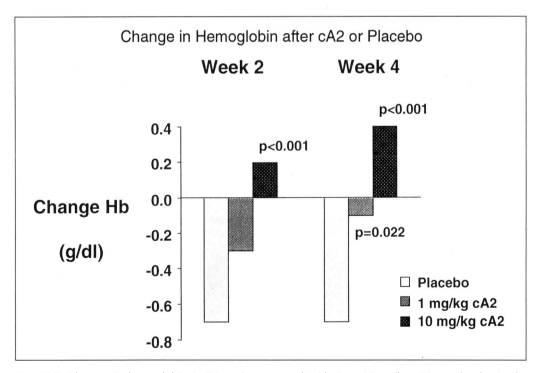

Fig. 12.2. Changes in hemoglobin in RA patients treated with 1 or 10 mg/kg cA2 or placebo in the randomized, controlled, double-blind trial. p values show the significance of changes in the cA2 groups, compared to placebo, by ANOVA.

a humanized (human/mouse) monoclonal anti-TNFα antibody (CDP571) or placebo in a dose escalation study.[15] The best responses were seen in the high dose group (10 mg/kg), with significant improvements relative to placebo at weeks 1 or 2 for the pain score, the tender joint score, the ESR and in a composite measure of disease activity. Nonsignificant trends towards improvement were seen in other parameters, including the patient's global assessment of disease activity, the number of swollen joints, the CRP and the platelet count. No consistent adverse events attributable to CDP571 were reported. The data from this study suggest that although effective, CDP571 has lower potency at equivalent dose levels than cA2.

A preliminary report describing the use of a recombinant human soluble TNF receptor Ig:Fc (sTNFR:Fc) fusion protein has also appeared.[16] In a phase I, dose escalation study, 16 patients with active RA were administered an IV loading dose of sTNFR:Fc or placebo at doses ranging from 4-32 mg/m^2, followed by twice weekly subcutaneous maintenance dosing for a period of 4 weeks. Compared to baseline, significant improvements in the ESR, swollen and tender joint counts, patient and physician global assessments and duration of morning stiffness were seen in the fusion protein treated patients, without evidence of a dose response relationship. The improvements in sTNFR:Fc treated patients were greater than those seen in the placebo group for both the joint score and the CRP, although they did not reach statistical significance. Adverse events were mild and included injection site reactions.

Clinical application of TNFα-blockers in RA

From the point of view of patient management, the data suggest that TNFα blocking therapy may be useful in the short term control of RA synovitis. Clinical situations where this may be relevant include the induction of remission in patients at first presentation or the management of disease flares. We have not yet tested cA2 in the setting of rheumatoid vasculitis, but evidence implicating TNFα in other forms of systemic vasculitis[17,18] raises the possibility that anti-TNFα may be useful in this clinical setting. The intra-articular use of anti-TNFα antibody or sTNF:Fc for the control of synovitis in individual joint remains to be tested.

Although these areas are of interest, the major challenge for a new therapeutic agent in RA is in the long term management of disease and in the achievement of altered disease outcomes. The promotion of tissue destruction by TNFα, both directly and through the induction of other mediators such as IL-1, together with the preliminary data showing the feasibility of repeated use of cA2 in vivo[13] provide strong justification for testing this agent in long-term trials.

Other disorders where TNFα may have an important role include inflammatory bowel disease, multiple sclerosis and asthma. The use of cA2 in patients with Crohns disease resulted in impressive improvements in both clinical and laboratory measures of disease[19] and it is likely that trials of other TNFα-blocking agents will follow.

ANTI-IL-1 THERAPY

Rationale

IL-1 shares many of the biological functions of TNFα and its particular importance in cartilage and bone metabolism[20] has led many to consider it the prime cytokine target in RA. Increased IL-1 production was seen in fresh or cultured RA peripheral blood cells[21,22] and in situ hybridization and immunohistological studies have demonstrated its expression in RA synovium.[23-25] Although IL-1 detection in RA synovial fluid has been controversial, careful analysis revealed low levels in a minority of samples.[26] In contrast, levels of the competitive IL-1 receptor antagonist (IL-1ra) in RA synovial fluid were high in the majority of patients, produced both by synovial fluid cells (predominantly neutrophils) and within the synovium itself.[24,27-29] Overall the data suggest that there is overexpression of IL-1 and its receptors in RA, with inadequate modulation of IL-1 activity by inhibitors such as IL-1ra.[30]

Animal model data also support the contention that IL-1 may be a good therapeutic target. Repeated injections of IL-1 into rat limb joints resulted in acute synovitis with fibroblast proliferation and bone and cartilage damage,[31] while systemic administration lead to marked acceleration of onset and progression of diverse arthritis models.[32,33] In experiments testing the role of IL-1 inhibitors in various forms of experimental arthritis, neutralizing antimurine IL-1 antibodies were able to prevent the onset of murine CIA and were also effective in the treatment of established disease.[34,35] Systemic administration of a blocking monoclonal antibody directed to the IL-1 receptor in mice with established CIA resulted in impressive amelioration of disease. The improvement in paw swelling exceeded 60% in mice treated with anti-IL-1R, similar to that seen in mice treated with combination anti-TNF and anti-CD4.[36] IL-1ra was also effective in preventing the development of CIA in mice and in the amelioration of LPS induced arthritis in rabbits[37,38] but was ineffective in preventing antigen induced arthritis in either mice or rabbits.[39,40]

In addition, inhibition of IL-1 with neutralizing antibodies or IL-1ra has been shown to block the adverse changes in connective tissue metabolism and the cartilage destruction seen in diverse animal models of arthritis (for review see ref. 20).

Clinical experience with IL-1 Blockade

Information about the clinical utility of the various IL-1-blocking strategies in man is sparse, with published data limited to meeting abstracts. On the basis of these abstracts however, it seems that both soluble (s)IL-1R and IL-1ra may have anti-inflammatory activity in vivo.

In a phase I, randomized, single center study, recombinant human sIL-1R was administered by intra-articular injection to patients with active RA.[41] Four doses were evaluated, with three patients receiving sIL-1R and one receiving placebo at each dose level. A dose related reduction in knee circumference was observed, which reached significance at an intermediate dose, and other parameters showed a nonsignificant trend towards improvement at higher sIL-1R dose levels (50 ft walk time and ESR). In a follow up study, the mode of administration of sIL-1R was changed to daily subcutaneous injection for 28 consecutive days.[42] This was a randomized, placebo controlled, double blind, dual center study of 23 patients with active RA. Trends to improvement in individual disease activity measures were noted, but no patients met predetermined criteria for significant clinical improvement. In both studies, sIL-1R was mostly well tolerated, although injection site reactions occurred in some patients.

The use of IL-1ra in RA has also been reported. In a small, open label pilot study of recombinant human IL-1ra, daily subcutaneous injection for 28 days led to a reduction in the tender joint count by about 50%, with smaller improvements in the ESR and CRP. Adverse events were frequent and included gastrointestinal disturbance, 'flu'-like illnesses and injection site reactions. There were three withdrawals, one due to a distant fungal infection, the second due to Felty's syndrome and the third due to an injection reaction.[43] In a subsequent, double blind, multicenter trial, IL-1ra was self administered by subcutaneous injection in 175 patients with active RA on a background of stable concomitant NSAIDS and/or prednisolone.[44] Patients were randomized to receive either 20, 70 or 200 mg of IL-1ra either daily, 3 times a week or once a week for a 3 week period. This administration was followed by a once weekly maintenance injection of the same dose for 4 weeks. The 3 week data revealed a statistically significant frequency/response, but no significant dose/response relationship. Improvements in some groups were maintained during the subsequent, once weekly administration. Dose dependent injection site reactions were frequent in this study (58%) but were mostly mild and resulted in discontinuation in 5% of patients. Serious adverse events were uncommon.

ANTI-IL-6 THERAPY

Rationale

The actions of IL-6 in promoting humoral immunity and autoantibody production provide the most convincing arguments linking this cytokine to disease pathogenesis in RA.[45-48] Other relevant properties include T cell activation and the stimulation of hepatic acute phase protein synthesis (in common with IL-1 and TNFα) and effects on hemopoiesis.[46] IL-6 lacks many of the other disease promoting functions of TNFα and IL-1, however, including the activation of endothelial cells and synoviocytes, the stimulation of fibroblast proliferation and the induction of TNFα and IL-1 synthesis. In addition, IL-6 induces the production of hepatic protease inhibitors such as α1-antitrypsin,[49] molecules which may play protective roles in inflammation. The data suggest that IL-6 may have both potentiating and protective roles in autoinflammatory disease.

IL-6 levels are raised in the majority of RA synovial fluid samples.[50-52] Local production within the joint is suggested by lower levels in matched sera[51,52] and synovial cell culture and immunohistochemical studies.[53,54] Double staining techniques revealed that the majority of IL-6 positive cells were macrophages, often found in close proximity to immunoglobulin producing plasma cells, suggesting a role for locally produced IL-6 in the stimulation of immunoglobulins in RA.[54] Discrepancies between different authors on the relationship between serum levels and disease activity may be explained in part by the presence of a marked diurnal variation in serum IL-6.[55]

Published arthritis model studies with IL-6 are limited and do not support the use of IL-6-blocking therapy in RA, since systemic administration of IL-6 led not to worsening, but inhibition, of antigen induced arthritis in rats.[56]

Clinical experience with anti-IL-6

Clinical experience specifically targeting IL-6 in RA is limited to an open label study in which a murine anti-IL-6 monoclonal antibody (B-E8) was administered at a dose of 10 mg/day IV for 10 days to five patients.[57] The pain score, duration of morning stiffness and the number of tender and swollen joints showed trends to improvement by day 15 and remained improved at day 30. Similar changes were noted for CRP and ESR with normalization of the former value by day 15. No significant side effects were observed. Although the data are encouraging, the small patient group, the open label administration and most importantly, the long period of hospitalization which itself may have induced some clinical improvement all argue for caution in interpretation. At a recent meeting, the results of an extension of this study to a total of eight patients were reported, with similar findings to those described above.[58]

WHAT ARE THE PROSPECTS FOR LONG-TERM CYTOKINE BLOCKADE?

The development of a host antiglobulin response following repeated administration is likely to limit long-term use of monoclonal anticytokine antibodies. Although anti-isotypic responses may be largely avoided by antibody chimerization (as employed in the construction of cA2), anti-idiotypic responses may still develop and lead to accelerated clearance, interference with antibody/target interaction, or allergy.[3] How important these phenomena will be in practice is unclear, but preliminary data from the repeated use of cA2, where a 50% incidence of anti-idiotypic human antichimeric antibody (HACA) responses was seen, is not encouraging. Although the magnitude of the responses to repeated cycles of cA2 remained impressive, shortening of response duration was seen in some patients.[13] In theory, the development of anti-idiotypic responses may be reduced by complementarity determining region (CDR) grafting, in which only the antigen binding site from the murine antibody is grafted onto a human Ig framework.[3] Experience with such a CDR grafted monoclonal antibody to the pan leukocyte antigen CDw52 (CAMPATH;[59]) in RA has shown that antiglobulin responses still occur, although their clinical significance is unclear. CDP571 is also CDR-grafted, but no data on the immunogenicity of this reagent have yet been presented.

Means of circumventing the development of antiglobulin responses may need to be sought. The coadministration of a cytokine blocking antibody together with a T cell directed reagent such as anti-CD4 is one such approach. Experiments performed in mice showed that T cell directed immunotherapy resulted in tolerance to a coadministered antigen.[60] More recently, coadministration of anti-CD4 and a hamster antimurine-anti-TNF (TN3) was beneficial in CIA, resulting in an enhancement of the clinical efficacy of suboptimal doses of TN3, a prolongation of the response duration and of most importance, a reduction in the murine anti-TN3 antiglobulin response[36]

Problems of a different type may limit the long-term use of soluble cytokine receptors or receptor antagonists. Soluble receptors are generally small, with a poor pharmacokinetic profile, leading to difficulty in maintaining adequate blocking levels in vivo. Coupling a carrier molecule to such IgG may improve pharmacokinetics, but lead to antibody responses to new epitopes created at the site of receptor:IgG fusion. No information on the incidence or clinical importance of such responses has been presented. The therapeutic use of sIL-6R may well be contraindicated for other reasons. IL-6/sIL-6R complexes formed outside the cell may insert into cell membranes and associate with gp130, resulting in intracellular signaling and cell activation.[61]

IL-1ra is also a small molecule and its short half life in vivo,[62] together with the need to maintain high tissue levels in order to effectively block IL-1R,[63] present problems in long-term use. The fusion of IL-1ra to a larger, carrier protein or the development of a mutant inhibitor with higher affinity for the membrane bound receptor might overcome these problems.

Other means of delivering cytokine inhibitors in vivo are under investigation. In a recent example, gene therapy was used to express human IL-1ra in rabbit knee joints.[64] Inhibitors of cytokine production may also be developed; peptide inhibitors of the IL-1β converting enzyme, a protease responsible for the conversion of the 31 kD inactive precursor of IL-1β to the 17 kD active form, show high activity and selectivity in vitro.[65]

Cytokines such as IL-4, IL-10 and TGFβ inhibit inflammatory cytokine synthesis in vitro and may provide new means of treating RA. IL-10 shows a particular promise in this regard, acting to reduce TNFα and IL-1 synthesis in RA synovial cultures while upregulating the expression of cytokine inhibitors.[66,67] IL-10 appears to be effective in reducing disease expression in murine CIA,[68] providing justification for its application in man. No clinical data are yet available.

The importance of IL-1, IL-6 and TNFα in specific immune events such as T and B cell activation and immunoglobulin secretion and in nonspecific resistance to infection[63] suggests that long-term cytokine blockade may be achieved at a price. There is good evidence that TNFα in particular has an important role in resistance to bacterial infection[69,70] arguing for caution in the use of therapies blocking TNFα function. In practice, only one serious infection (pneumonia) has been reported amongst more than 100 patients so far treated with anti-TNFα,[4,6,13,15] and other infective events occurring in cA2 treated patients have been mild. These results are reassuring, but greater experience will be required before the effect of anti-TNFα on infection incidence can be clarified.

CYTOKINES AS THERAPY

Interferon γ has been tested extensively as a therapeutic agent in RA. The scientific justification for its application in this disease is arguable and results of trials unimpressive. For a review, see ref. 71 Other cytokines administered in RA include the colony-stimulating factors (CSF) and erythropoietin (EPO).

COLONY STIMULATING FACTORS IN RA

The therapeutic use of CSF in RA has been restricted to the management of leukopenia, caused either by Felty's syndrome or induced by antirheumatic drugs such as sulphasalazine or methotrexate. Case reports describing the use of granulocyte (G)-CSF and granulocyte macrophage (GM)-CSF in patients with methotrexate- and sulphasalazine-induced neutropenia have suggested benefit, although the use of GM-CSF was associated with systemic side effects including fever.[72,73] The use of GM-CSF in a patient with RA complicated by Felty's syndrome and in a second patient who received GM-CSF following chemotherapy for a coincident neoplasm also lead to correction of the granulocytopenia, but resulted in disease flares.[74,75] In both cases, the clinical disease flare was accompanied by increases in serum cytokines, including IL-6 and TNFα. These changes most likely result from the stimulation of mature myeloid cell function by GM-CSF[76] and support the notion that hemopoietic growth factors have a role in the basic disease processes in RA.[77] The exact place of CSF in the management of RA—associated leukopenia and the risk/benefit ratio—remains to be established.

ERYTHROPOIETIN

Hypoproliferative anemia of chronic disease (ACD) is a common systemic feature of RA. Erythropoiesis is controlled by erythropoietin (EPO), a lineage specific hemopoietic growth factor, which stimulates growth of BFUe and CFUe. Serum EPO has been shown to be inappropriately low in RA patients with ACD compared with non-RA patients with iron deficiency anemia.[10-12] The concept has risen that ACD in RA results at least in part from deficient EPO production, possibly due to high TNFα expression, and that the administration of EPO may be of clinical benefit. Clinical experience so far appears to confirm this view with good hematological responses in RA patients treated with recombinant human EPO, without significant toxicity.[78,79] In contrast to the experience with GM-CSF, no meaningful change in RA disease activity was noted with EPO administration, in keeping with the tight lineage specificity of this cytokine.

SUMMARY

Attention has focused on the use of biologicals which inhibit cytokine function. The specificity of action of such agents means that the choice of cytokine target is critical; the scientific justification for targeting TNFα and IL-1 in RA is strong, while the rationale for using IL-6-blocking therapies is equivocal. The available data confirm that anti-TNFα strategies are safe and effective in the short-term control of both clinical and laboratory manifestations of RA. The data from the placebo controlled trial of chimeric anti-TNFα (cA2) are particularly convincing: cA2 was administered in a study of rigorous design and led to improvements which were statistically significant and clinically important, with clear dose response relationships. Falls in serum IL-6 following treatment with cA2 support the contention that TNFα is regulatory for other cytokines in RA. The published data on the use of IL-1ra and sIL-1-R are sparse and clear evidence of clinical efficacy is yet to be presented, but the preliminary data look encouraging. An uncontrolled trial of anti-IL6 in RA produced interesting preliminary results.

Repeated treatment with cA2 was feasible in some patients, suggesting that long-term disease suppression may be achievable. Likely problems in long-term therapy include the development of sensitization with monoclonal antibodies and pharmacokinetic problems with smaller inhibitors (IL-1ra, soluble receptors). New means of inhibiting cytokine production may include delivery of inhibitory molecules by gene therapy and treatment with inhibitory cytokines such as IL-10.

Hemopoietic growth factors may find a niche in the management of systemic complications of RA, or in the treatment of complications of standard antirheumatic therapy. G-CSF may be useful for managing neutropenia, while GM-CSF should probably be avoided. EPO has been proven effective in the control of anemia of chronic disease in RA and may improve quality of life, as it has in other diseases.

Acknowledgment

The Kennedy Institute is supported by the Arthritis and Rheumatism Council of Great Britain.

References

1. Kushner I, Dawson NV. Aggressive therapy does not substantially alter the long-term course of rheumatoid arthritis. Rheum Dis Clin N Amer 1993; 19:163-172.
2. Knight DM, Trinh H, Le J et al. Construction and initial characterization of a mouse-human chimeric anti-TNFα antibody. Mol Immunol 1993; 30:1443-1453.
3. Winter G, Harris WJ. Humanized antibodies. Immunol Today 1993; 14:243-246.
4. Elliott MJ, Maini RN, Feldmann M et al. Treatment of rheumatoid arthritis with chimeric monoclonal antibodies to tumor necrosis factor α. Arthritis Rheum 1993; 36:1681-1690.
5. Paulus HE, Egger MJ, Ward JR et al. Analysis of improvement in individual rheumatoid arthritis patients treated with disease-modifying antirheumatic drugs, based on the findings in patients treated with placebo. Arthritis Rheum 1990; 33:477-484.
6. Elliott MJ, Maini RN, Feldmann M et al. Randomised double-blind comparison of chimeric monoclonal antibody to tumour necrosis factor α (cA2) versus placebo in rheumatoid arthritis. Lancet 1994; 344:1105-1110.
7. Barbuto JAM, Hersh EM. Role of cytokines in cancer therapy. In: Aggarwal BB, Puri RK, ed. Human Cytokines: their role in disease and therapy. Cambridge MA. USA: Blackwell Science, 1995:503-524.
8. Roodman GD. Mechanisms of erythroid suppression in the anemia of chronic disease. Blood Cells 1987; 13:171-184.
9. Johnson RA, Waddelow TA, Caro J et al. Chronic exposure to tumor necrosis factor in vivo preferentially inhibits erythropoiesis in nude mice. Blood 1989; 74:130-138.
10. Vreugdenhil G, Wognum AW, van Eijk HG et al. Anaemia in rheumatoid arthritis: the role of iron, vitamin B_{12}, and folic acid deficiency, and erythropoietin responsiveness. Ann Rheum Dis 1990; 49:93-98.
11. Boyd HK, Lappin RJ, Bell AL. Evidence for impaired erythropoietin response to anaemia in rheumatoid disease. Br J Rheumatol 1991; 30:255-259.
12. Remacha AF, Rodriguez-De La Serna A, Garcia-Die F et al. Erythroid abnormalities in rheumatoid arthritis: the role of erythropoietin. J Rheumatol 1992; 19:1687-1691.

13. Elliott MJ, Maini RN, Feldmann M et al. Repeated therapy with monoclonal antibody to tumour necrosis factor α (cA2) in patients with rheumatoid arthritis. Lancet 1994; 344:1125-1128.
14. Maini RN, Elliott MJ, Charles PJ et al. Immunological intervention reveals reciprocal roles for tumor necrosis factor-α and IL-10 in rheumatoid arthritis and systemic lupus erythematosus. Springer Semin Immunopathol 1994; 16:327-336.
15. Rankin ECC, Choy EHS, Kassimos D et al. The therapeutic effects of an engineered human anti-tumour necrosis factor alpha antibody (CDP571) in rheumatoid arthritis. Br J Rheumatol 1995; 34:334-342.
16. Moreland LW, Margolies GR, Heck LW et al. Soluble tumor necrosis factor receptor (sTNFR): results of a phase I dose-escalation study in patients with rheumatoid arthritis. Arthritis Rheum 1994; 37:S295.
17. Deguchi Y, Shibata N, Kishimoto S. Enhanced expression of the tumour necrosis factor/cachectin gene in peripheral blood mononuclear cells from patients with systemic vasculitis. Clin Exp Immunol 1990; 81:311-314.
18. Cook A, Gallagher G, Field M. Localisation of tumour necrosis factor α and its receptors in temporal arteritis. Clin Rheumatol 1994; 13:162.
19. Derkx B, Taminiau J, Sandra R et al. Tumour-necrosis-factor antibody treatment in Crohn's disease. Lancet 1993; 342:173-174.
20. Arend WP, Dayer J-M. Inhibition of the production and effects of interleukin-1 and tumor necrosis factor α in rheumatoid arthritis. Arthritis Rheum 1995; 38:151-160.
21. Barkley DEH, Feldmann M, Maini RN. Cells with dendritic morphology and bright interleukin-1 staining circulate in the blood of patients with rheumatoid arthritis. Clin Exp Immunol 1990; 80:25-31.
22. Goto M, Fujisawa M, Yamada A et al. Spontaneous release of angiotensin converting enzyme and interleukin 1β from peripheral blood monocytes from patients with rheumatoid arthritis under a serum free condition. Ann Rheum Dis 1990; 49:172-176.
23. Firestein GS, Alvaro-Garcia JM, Maki R. Quantitative analysis of cytokine gene expression in rheumatoid arthritis. J Immunol 1990; 144:3347-3353.
24. Deleuran BW, Chu CQ, Field M et al. Localization of interleukin-1α, type 1 interleukin-1 receptor and interleukin-1 receptor antagonist in the synovial membrane and cartilage/pannus junction in rheumatoid arthritis. Br J Rheumatol 1992; 31:801-809.
25. Chu CQ, Field M, Allard S et al. Detection of cytokines at the cartilage/pannus junction in patients with rheumatoid arthritis: implications for the role of cytokines in cartilage destruction and repair. Br J Rheumatol 1992; 31:653-661.
26. Holt I, Cooper RG, Denton J et al. Cytokine inter-relationships and their association with disease activity in arthritis. Br J Rheumatol 1992; 31:725-733.
27. Malyak M, Swaney RE, Arend WP. Levels of synovial fluid interleukin-1 receptor antagonist in rheumatoid arthritis and other arthropathies. Arthritis Rheum 1993; 36:781-789.

28. Firestein GS, Berger AE, Tracey DE et al. IL-1 receptor antagonist protein production and gene expression in rheumatoid arthritis and osteoarthritis synovium. J Immunol 1992; 149:1054-1062.
29. Koch AE, Kunkel SL, Chensue SW et al. Expression of interleukin-1 and interleukin-1 receptor antagonist by human rheumatoid synovial tissue macrophages. Clin Immunol Immunopathol 1992; 65:23-29.
30. Firestein GS, Boyle DL, Yu C et al. Synovial interleukin-1 receptor antagonist and interleukin-1 balance in rheumatoid arthritis. Arthritis Rheum 1994; 37:644-652.
31. Chandrasekhar S, Harvey AK, Hrubey PS et al. Arthritis induced by interleukin-1 is dependent on the site and frequency of intraarticular injection. Clin Immunol Immunopathol 1990; 55:382-400.
32. Hom JT, Bendele AM, Carlson DG. In vivo administration with IL-1 accelerates the development of collagen-induced arthritis in mice. J Immunol 1988; 141:834-841.
33. Staite ND, Richard KA, Aspar DG et al. Induction of an acute erosive monarticular arthritis in mice by interleukin-1 and methylated bovine serum albumin. Arthritis Rheum 1990; 33:253-260.
34. Geiger T, Towbin H, Cosenti-Vargas A et al. Neutralization of interleukin-1β activity in vivo with a monoclonal antibody alleviates collagen-induced arthritis in DBA/1 mice and prevents the associated acute-phase response. Clin Exp Rheumatol 1993; 11:515-522.
35. Van den Berg WB, Joosten LAB, Helsen M et al. Amelioration of established murine collagen-induced arthritis with anti-IL-1 treatment. Clin Exp Immunol 1994; 95:237-243.
36. Williams RO, Mason LM, Feldmann M et al. Synergy between anti-CD4 and anti-tumor necrosis factor in the amelioration of established collagen-induced arthritis. Proc Natl Acad Sci USA 1994; 91:2762-2766.
37. Wooley PH, Whalen JD, Chapman DL et al. The effect of an interleukin-1 receptor antagonist protein on type II collagen-induced arthritis and antigen-induced arthritis in mice. Arthritis Rheum 1993; 36:1305-1314.
38. Matsukawa A, Ohkawara S, Maeda T et al. Production of IL-1 and IL-1 receptor antagonist and the pathological significance in lipopolysaccharide-induced arthritis in rabbits. Clin Exp Immunol 1993; 93:206-211.
39. Wooley PH, Dutcher J, Widmer MB et al. Influence of a recombinant human soluble tumor necrosis factor receptor Fc fusion protein on type II collagen-induced arthritis in mice. J Immunol 1993; 151:6602-6607.
40. Lewthwaite J, Blake SM, Hardingham TE et al. The effect of recombinant human interleukin 1 receptor antagonist on the induction phase of antigen induced arthritis in the rabbit. J Rheumatol 1994; 21:467-472.
41. Drevlow B, Capezio J, Lovis R et al. Phase I study of recombinant human interleukin-1 receptor (RHUIIL-1R) adinistered intra-articularly in active rheumatoid arthritis. Arthritis Rheum 1993; 36:S39.
42. Drevlow B, Lovis R, Haag MA et al. Phase I study of recombinant human interleukin-1 receptor (RHUIL-1R) administered subcutaneously in patients with active rheumatoid arthritis. Arthritis Rheum 1994; 37:S339.

43. Lebsack ME, Paul CC, Bloedow DC et al. Subcutaneous IL-1 receptor antagonist in patients with rheumatoid arthritis. Arthritis Rheum 1991; 34:S45.
44. Lebsack ME, Paul CC, Martindale JJ et al. A dose- and regimen-ranging study of IL-1 receptor antagonist in patients with rheumatoid arthritis. Arthritis Rheum 1993; 36:S39.
45. Lipsky PE. The control of antibody production by immunomodulatory molecules. Arthritis Rheum 1989; 32:1345-1355.
46. Kishimoto T, Akira S, Taga T. Interleukin-6 and its receptor: a paradigm for cytokines. Science 1992; 258:593-597.
47. Hirano T, Taga T, Yasukawa K et al. Human B-cell differentiation factor defined by an anti-peptide antibody and its possible role in autoantibody production. Proc Natl Acad Sci USA 1987; 84:228-231.
48. Jourdan M, Bataille R, Seguin J et al. Constitutive production of interleukin-6 and immunologic features in cardiac myxomas. Arthritis Rheum 1990; 33:398-402.
49. Baumann H, Gauldie J. The acute phase response. Immunol Today 1994; 15:74-80.
50. Hirano T, Matsuda T, Turner M et al. Excessive production of interleukin 6/B cell stimulatory factor-2 in rheumatoid arthritis. Eur J Immunol 1988; 18:1797-1801.
51. Houssiau FA, Devogelaer J-P, Van Damme J et al. Interleukin-6 in synovial fluid and serum of patients with rheumatoid arthritis and other inflammatory arthritides. Arthritis Rheum 1988; 31:784-788.
52. Swaak AJ, Van Rooyen A, Nieuwenhuis E et al. Interleukin-6 (IL-6) in synovial fluid and serum of patients with rheumatic diseases. Scand J Rheumatol 1988; 17:469-474.
53. Rosenbaum JT, Cugnini R, Tara DC et al. Production and modulation of interleukin 6 synthesis by synoviocytes derived from patients with arthritic disease. Ann Rheum Dis 1992; 51:198-202.
54. Field M, Chu C, Feldmann M et al. Interleukin-6 localisation in the synovial membrane in rheumatoid arthritis. Rheumatol Int 1991; 11:45-50.
55. Arvidson NG, Gudbjörnsson B, Elfman L et al. Circadian rhythm of serum interleukin-6 in rheumatoid arthritis. Ann Rheum Dis 1994; 53:521-524.
56. Mihara M, Ikuta M, Koishihara Y et al. Interleukin 6 inhibits delayed-type hypersensitivity and the development of adjuvant arthritis. Eur J Immunol 1991; 21:2327-2331.
57. Wendling D, Racadot E, Wijdenes J. Treatment of severe rheumatoid arthritis by anti-interleukin 6 monoclonal antibody. J Rheumatol 1993; 20:259-262.
58. Wendling D, Racadot E, Wijdenes J. Serum levels of IL6, CRP, IL6 receptor and cortisol under anti IL6 monoclonal antibody therapy in rheumatoid arthritis. Arthritis Rheum 1994; 37:S382.
59. Issacs JD, Watts RA, Hazleman BL et al. Humanised monoclonal antibody therapy for rheumatoid arthritis. Lancet 1992; 340:748-752.

60. Waldmann H, Cobbold S. The use of monoclonal antibodies to achieve immunological tolerance. Immunol Today 1993; 14:247-251.
61. Taga T, Hibi M, Hirata Y et al. Interleukin-6 triggers the association of its receptor with a possible signal transducer, gp130. Cell 1989; 58:573-581.
62. Granowitz EV, Porat R, Mier JW et al. Pharmacokinetics, safety and immunomodulatory effects of human recombinant interleukin-1 receptor antagonist in healthy humans. Cytokine 1992; 4:353-360.
63. Dinarello CA. Interleukin-1 and interleukin-1 antagonism. Blood 1991; 77:1627-1652.
64. Bandara G, Mueller GM, Galea-Lauri J et al. Intraarticular expression of biolocally active interleukin 1-receptor-antagonist protein by ex vivo gene transfer. Proc Natl Acad Sci USA 1993; 90:10764-10768.
65. Thornberry NA, Peterson EP, Zhao JJ et al. Inactivation of interleukin-1β converting enzyme by peptide (acyloxy)methyl ketones. Biochemistry 1994; 33:3934-3940.
66. Katsikis PD, Chu CQ, Brennan FM et al. Immunoregulatory role of interleukin 10 in rheumatoid arthritis. J Exp Med 1994; 179:1517-1527.
67. Joyce DA, Gibbons DP, Green P et al. Two inhibitors of pro-inflammatory cytokine release, interleukin-10 and interleukin-4, have contrasting effects on release of soluble p75 tumor necrosis factor receptor by cultured monocytes. Eur J Immunol 1994; 24:2699-2705.
68. Walmsley M, Katsikis PD, Abney ER et al. IL-10 inhibits progression of established collagen-induced arthritis. Arth & Rheum 1995; (submitted).
69. Havell EA. Evidence that tumor necrosis factor has an important role in antibacterial resistance. J Immunol 1989; 143:2894-2899.
70. Pfeffer K, Matsuyama T, Kündig TM et al. Mice deficient for the 55 kd tumor necrosis factor receptor are resistant to endotoxic shock, yet succumb to L. monocytogenes infection. Cell 1993; 73:457-467.
71. Elliott MJ, Maini RN. Anticytokines and cytokines in rheumatoid arthritis. Rheumatol Eur 1995; 24/3:96-98.
72. Ellman MH, Telfer MC, Turner AF. Benefit of G-CSF for methotrexate-induced neutropaenia in rheumatoid arthritis. Am J Med 1992; 92:337-338.
73. Kuipers EJ, Vellenga E, de Wolf JTM et al. Sulfasalazine induced agranulocytosis treated with granulocyte-macrophage colony stimulating factor. J Rheumatol 1992; 19:621-622.
74. Hazenberg BPC, Van Leeuwen MA, Van Rijswijk MH et al. Correction of granulocytopenia in Felty's syndrome by granulocyte-macrophage colony stimulating factor, simultaneous induction of interleukin-6 release and flare-up of the arthritis. Blood 1989; 74:2769-2770.
75. De Vries EGE, Willemse PHB, Biesma B et al. Flare-up of rheumatoid arthritis during GM-CSF treatment after chemotherapy. The Lancet 1991; 338:517-518.
76. Vadas MA, Lopez AF, Gamble JR et al. Role of colony-stimulating factors in leucocyte response to inflammation and infection. Curr Opin Immunol 1991; 3:97-104.

77. Hamilton JA. Rheumatoid arthritis: opposing actions of haemopoietic growth factors and slow-acting anti-rheumatic drugs. Lancet 1993; 342:536-539.
78. Means RTJ, Olsen N J., Krantz SB et al. Treatment of the anemia of rheumatoid arthritis with recombinant human erythropoietin: clinical and in vitro studies. Arthritis Rheum 1989; 32:638-642.
79. Pincus T, Olsen NJ, Russell IJ et al. Multicenter study of recombinant human erythropoietin in correction of anemia in rheumatoid arthritis. Am J Med 1990; 89:161-168.

INDEX

Page numbers in italics denote figures (f) or tables (t).

A
Abraham D, 156
Adhesion molecules, 31, 81, 83-84, 154, 156, 158-160, 165, 181, 183-184
Allison J, 56
Antibodies. *See also* B cells/Ig.
   anti-cytokine, 29, *30f*, 33, 40, 63, *85f*, 88, 158, 211, 240-245, 247-249
   anti-cytokine receptor, *35f*
   anti-differentiation marker, 50, 124, 188
   autoantibodies, 58-59, 77, 86, 105, 108, 137, 140, *144f*, 153-154
      La (SSB), 122-123, 125
      Ro (SSA), 122-123, 125

B
B cells, 84, 229-230
   hyperactivity. *See* Sjögren's syndrome; Systemic lupus erythematosus.
   Ig (immunoglobulins), 38, 84
   neoplasia. *See* Sjögren's syndrome.
Baker D, 87
Bluethmann H, 201
Boumba D, 126
Bowman MA, 51
Brennan FM, 29, 31

C
c-fos, 122
c-jun, 122
c-myc, 110, 122, 131
Carswell EA, 1
Cerami A, 2
Charlton B, 50
Chemokines, *11-12t*, 30-31, 217, 232-233. *See also* IL-8, RANTES.
Coffman RL, 18, 214

Cytokines, 1-21. *See also individual cytokines.*
   anti-inflammatory, *10t*
   families, 3-6, *4t*
   macrophage/monocyte activators, 37, 86, 142
   networks, 2-3, 6, 31-32, *32f*, 82, *157f*
   proinflammatory, *8-9t*, 17, 40, 61, 65, 142
   receptors, 2, 6-17, *7f*, *13-18f*
      antagonists, 34
         IL-ra, 34-37, 167, 184, 246
      IFNγ-R, 216
      IL-1R, 35-36, 167, 246
      IL-2R, 81-82, 124-125, *125t*, 131, 139
      IL-8R, 218
      PDGF-R (α, β), 163
      TGFβ-R, 162
      TNF-R, 34, 36-38, *35-37f*, 40-41, 84, *143-144f*, 165, 212-213
   regulation, 19-21, *21f*, 33-38, 88
      inhibitors, 25, 34-40, 59
      overexpression, 230-231

D
Dayer JM, 34
Deguchi Y, 163
Diabetes, 49-68, 229
   β cell destruction, 50-51, 54, 59-61, 65
   BB rat, 49
   cytokines in, 51-67
   IDDM (Insulin dependent diabetes mellitus), 49, 59, 62, 65
   insulin secretion, 52, 59
   NOD mouse, 49-50, 55, 59-61, 66, 211-212, 217
   pancreatic regeneration, 62-63

F
Falanga V, 161
Fas/lpr, 56, 129, 138-140, 142, 203-204, 228
Fathman CG, 215
Feghali CA, 158, 167
Ferber IA, 215
Flavell RA, 66, 211
Fox RI, 126, 128
Free oxygen radicals, 49, 52, 54

G

Gabrielli A, 161
Garrod AE, 203
Gay S, 161-162, 164
Growth factors
  EGF (Epidermal growth factor), 164
  FGF (a, b Fibroblast growth factors), 164, 168
    bFGF in systemic sclerosis, 168
  GM-CSF (Granulocyte monocyte colony stimulating factor)
    multiple sclerosis, 86
    psoriasis, 185-186
    rheumatoid arthritis, 29, 249
  M-CSF (Macrophage colony stimulating factor), 86
  PDGF, 163-164
    systemic sclerosis, 157, 163-165
  TGFα (Transforming growth factor α)
    psoriasis, 185-186
  TGFβ (Transforming growth factor β), 38-39, 109, 129, 208-210, 217
    HTLV-1 transactivation, 130
    multiple sclerosis, 89
    psoriasis, 185-186
    systemic sclerosis, 158, 161-163
    thyroid inhibition, 106
Gruschwitz M, 162

H

Hamano H, 129
Harrison NK, 165
Heath WR, 57
Hirano T, 58
Horak I, 208

I

Interferons, 140, 166
  IFNα, 63, 130-131, 230
    diabetes, 63
    multiple sclerosis, 90
    psoriasis, 185
    Sjögren's syndrome, 131
    systemic sclerosis, 166
  IFNβ
    multiple sclerosis, 90, *91f*
  IFNγ, 40, 61, 108, 230-231, 249
    diabetes, 61-63
    multiple sclerosis, 82, 86, 88
    psoriasis, 185
    Sjögren's syndrome, 126-127
    systemic lupus erythematosus, 140, *141f*
    tolerance abrogation, 62

Interleukins. See also Cytokines/receptors.
  IL-1, 108
    diabetes, 51-52
    multiple sclerosis, 83, 87
    psoriasis, 184
    rheumatoid arthritis, 29-32, *31f*, 240-245
    systemic lupus erythematosus, 145
    systemic sclerosis, 158, 166-167
  IL-10, *37f*, 39-40, 59, 210-211, 233
    diabetes, 59-61
    multiple sclerosis, 89
    Sjögren's syndrome, 128
    systemic lupus erythematosus, 140-141
  IL-12, 216-217
  IL-13, 88-89
  IL-2, 52-53, 108-109, 139, 230
    diabetes, 52-58
    multiple sclerosis, 80-82
    Sjögren's syndrome, 124-125, *126f*, 129
    systemic lupus erythematosus, 139-140
    tolerance reversal, 53, 207, 228-229
  IL-4, *5f*, 39, 84
    multiple sclerosis, 80, 88
    Sjögren's syndrome, 127
    systemic lupus erythematosus, 140
    thyroid disease, 105
  IL-6, 58, 108, 213-214, 246-247
    diabetes, 58-59
    multiple sclerosis, 84, 86-87, *87f*
    psoriasis, 185
    rheumatoid arthritis, 29-30
    Sjögren's syndrome, 129, *130f*
    systemic lupus erythematosus, 145-146
    systemic sclerosis, 158, 167-168
  IL-8, *5f*, 232-233
    psoriasis, 185
    rheumatoid arthritis, 29-30
    systemic sclerosis, 165
Ishida Y, 53

J

Jolicoeur C, 57
Julien J, 161

K

Keystone E, 161
Kikuchi K, 163
Klareskog L, 164
Kollias G, 33
Kulozik M, 162

L

Lafferty KJ, 63
LeRoy EC, 157
Liblau RS, 65
Lichtenberg GC, 201
Lo D, 50
LT (Lymphotoxin), 67, 84, 86, 128, 213

M

Magram L, 217
Manoussakis MN, 124
Markmann J, 63
Miller JPAP, 66
Miyasaka N, 124
MMP (Matrix metalloproteases), 39, 86
Moreland LW, 163
Mosmann TR, 18, 214
Mozes E, 140
Multiple sclerosis (MS), 77-92
    cytokines in, 78t, 79f, 80-92
    EAE (experimental autoimmune encephalitis), 77, 80-83, 85f, 87f, 88-90, 212

N

Needleman BW, 162, 167
Nitric oxide (NO), 49, 52, 54

O

Ogawa N, 126, 128
Ohashi PS, 57-58, 201
Oldstone MB, 57
Olsson I, 34

P

Peltonen J, 162
Psoriasis, 175-188
    cytokines in, 184-188
    dermal lesion/plaque, 175, 176-178f, 177
    HLA component, 176-177
    keratinocytes, 178-179
        cytokines, 179-181, 180t
    superantigens, 182-183
    therapy, 186-188

R

RANTES (Regulated upon activation, T cell expressed and secreted), 30, 83
ras, 164
Rheumatoid arthritis (RA), 25-41
    cytokines in, 26
    synovial tissue, 27-33, 28t, 30f
    DBA/1 mouse, 33
    HLA component, 26
    therapy, 239-251
        anti-IL-1, 245-246
        anti-IL-6, 246-247
        anti-TNFα, 240-245
        CSF, 249-250
        erythropoietin, 250
        IFNγ, 249
Ryffel B, 213

S

Saito I, 131
Scleroderma. *See* Systemic sclerosis.
Scott B, 54
Shehadah NN, 66
Shornick L, 214
Sjögren's syndrome (SS), 121-131
    B cell hyperactivity, 122-123
    cytokines in, 124-131, 126t
    HLA component, 123
    salivary gland lesion, 121-122, 123f
Systemic lupus erythematosus (SLE), 137-146
    bcl-2, 138, 141
    cytokines in, 138-146, 142t
    HLA component, 137
Systemic sclerosis (SSc, scleroderma), 153-169, 154t
    abnormal dermal fibroblast phenotype, 155, 155t, 157-158
    cytokines in, 155-169, 156t, 157f, 159f
    Raynaud's phenomenon, 153, 162

T

T cells, 18, 49, 52, 84, 86-87
    autoantigen reactive, 26, 49-57, 61-62, 64, 77, 81-82, 108, 228
    CD4
        diabetes, 49-50, 60, 66
        psoriasis, 182
    CD8, 40
        diabetes, 49-51, 55, 66
        Graves' disease, 111
        psoriasis, 182
    hyperactivity in SLE, 138, 141
    inhibition, 38, 41
    rheumatoid arthritis, 27
    Th_0, 19-20, 20t, 82, 138, 142
    Th_1, 18-20, 20t, 52, 59, 65-66, 82, 88, 106, 127-128, 131, 138, 142, 214-216
    Th_2, 18-20, 20t, 49, 65-66, 82, 88, 106, 109, 127-128, 138, 214-216

Takeda K, 165
Takehara K, 168
Talal N, 130
Tan EM, 168
Thyroid, 101-112
  cytokines in, 102-112, *103t, 105t*
    thyroid disease, 103-112, *105t, 107t*
      carcinoma, 104, 107
      Graves' disease (GD), 103-106, 109-111, *112f*
      Hashimoto's thyroiditis (HT), 103-106, 108
      nontoxic goiter, 104, 107
      subacute thyroiditis (de Quervain's), 106-107
Tocci M, 214
Transgenic mice, 227-234
  'Gene knockout', 201-218, *205-206f*
    IFNγ, 216
    IL-10, 210-211
    IL-12, 216-217
    IL-2, 207-208
    IL-6, 213-214
    IL-8R, 218
    LT, 213
    TGFβ, 208-210, 217
    TNF-R, 212-213
  Fas, 228
  IFNα, 230
  IFNγ, 230-231
  IL-10, 233
  IL-2, 228-229
  IL-8, 232-233
  TNFα, 229, 231-232

Tumor necrosis factors, *5f*. See also Cytokines/receptors/TNF-R.
  TNFα, 63, 142, 229, 231-232
    diabetes, 52, 63-64
    multiple sclerosis, 82-84, *85f*, 86-88
    psoriasis, 184-185
    rheumatoid arthritis, 25, 29-33, 40-41, 240-245
    systemic lupus erythematosus, 142-145, *143-144f*
    systemic sclerosis, 165-166
  TNFβ, 64
    diabetes, 63-65

V
von Herrath MG, 58

W
Wallach D, 34
Wang Y, 50

Y
Yamakage A, 163

MOLECULAR BIOLOGY INTELLIGENCE UNIT
AVAILABLE AND UPCOMING TITLES

- Organellar Proton-ATPases
  Nathan Nelson, Roche Institute of Molecular Biology
- Interleukin-10
  Jan DeVries and René de Waal Malefyt, DNAX
- Collagen Gene Regulation in the Myocardium
  M. Eghbali-Webb, Yale University
- DNA and Nucleoprotein Structure In Vivo
  Hanspeter Saluz and Karin Wiebauer, HK Institut-Jena and GenZentrum-Martinsried/Munich
- G Protein-Coupled Receptors
  Tiina Iismaa, Trevor Biden, John Shine, Garvan Institute-Sydney
- Viroceptors, Virokines and Related Immune Modulators Encoded by DNA Viruses
  Grant McFadden, University of Alberta
- Bispecific Antibodies
  Michael W. Fanger, Dartmouth Medical School
- Drosophila Retrotransposons
  Irina Arkhipova, Harvard University and Nataliya V. Lyubomirskaya, Engelhardt Institute of Molecular Biology-Moscow
- The Molecular Clock in Mammals
  Simon Easteal, Chris Collet, David Betty, Australian National University and CSIRO Division of Wildlife and Ecology
- Wound Repair, Regeneration and Artificial Tissues
  David L. Stocum, Indiana University-Purdue University
- Pre-mRNA Processing
  Angus I. Lamond, European Molecular Biology Laboratory
- Intermediate Filament Structure
  David A.D. Parry and Peter M. Steinert, Massey University-New Zealand and National Institutes of Health
- Fetuin
  K.M. Dziegielewska and W.M. Brown, University of Tasmania
- Drosophila Genome Map: A Practical Guide
  Daniel Hartl and Elena R. Lozovskaya, Harvard University
- Mammalian Sex Chromosomes and Sex-Determining Genes
  Jennifer A. Marshall-Graves and Andrew Sinclair, La Trobe University-Melbourne and Royal Children's Hospital-Melbourne
- Regulation of Gene Expression in *E. coli*
  E.C.C. Lin, Harvard University
- Muscarinic Acetylcholine Receptors
  Jürgen Wess, National Institutes of Health
- Regulation of Glucokinase in Liver Metabolism
  Maria Luz Cardenas, CNRS-Laboratoire de Chimie Bactérienne-Marseille
- Transcriptional Regulation of Interferon-γ
  Ganes C. Sen and Richard Ransohoff, Cleveland Clinic
- Fourier Transform Infrared Spectroscopy and Protein Structure
  P.I. Haris and D. Chapman, Royal Free Hospital-London
- Bone Formation and Repair: Cellular and Molecular Basis
  Vicki Rosen and R. Scott Thies, Genetics Institute, Inc.-Cambridge
- Mechanisms of DNA Repair
  Jean-Michel Vos, University of North Carolina
- Short Interspersed Elements: Complex Potential and Impact on the Host Genome
  Richard J. Maraia, National Institutes of Health
- Artificial Intelligence for Predicting Secondary Structure of Proteins
  Xiru Zhang, Thinking Machines Corp-Cambridge
- Growth Hormone, Prolactin and IGF-I as Lymphohemopoietic Cytokines
  Elisabeth Hooghe-Peters and Robert Hooghe, Free University-Brussels
- Human Hematopoiesis in SCID Mice
  Maria-Grazia Roncarolo, Reiko Namikawa and Bruno Péault DNA Research Institute
- Membrane Proteases in Tissue Remodeling
  Wen-Tien Chen, Georgetown University
- Annexins
  Barbara Seaton, Boston University
- Retrotransposon Gene Therapy
  Clague P. Hodgson, Creighton University
- Polyamine Metabolism
  Robert Casero Jr, Johns Hopkins University
- Phosphatases in Cell Metabolism and Signal Transduction
  Michael W. Crowder and John Vincent, Pennsylvania State University
- Antifreeze Proteins: Properties and Functions
  Boris Rubinsky, University of California-Berkeley
- Intramolecular Chaperones and Protein Folding
  Ujwal Shinde, UMDNJ
- Thrombospondin
  Jack Lawler and Jo Adams, Harvard University
- Structure of Actin and Actin-Binding Proteins
  Andreas Bremer, Duke University
- Glucocorticoid Receptors in Leukemia Cells
  Bahiru Gametchu, Medical College of Wisconsin
- Signal Transduction Mechanisms in Cancer
  Hans Grunicke, University of Innsbruck
- Intracellular Protein Trafficking Defects in Human Disease
  Nelson Yew, Genzyme Corporation
- apoJ/Clusterin
  Judith A.K. Harmony, University of Cincinnati
- Phospholipid Transfer Proteins
  Vytas Bankaitis, University of Alabama
- Localized RNAs
  Howard Lipschitz, California Institute of Technology
- Modular Exchange Principles in Proteins
  Laszlo Patthy, Institute of Enzymology-Budapest
- Molecular Biology of Cardiac Development
  Paul Barton, National Heart and Lung Institute-London
- RANTES, *Alan M. Krensky, Stanford University*
- New Aspects of V(D)J Recombination
  Stacy Ferguson and Craig Thompson, University of Chicago

Neuroscience Intelligence Unit

Available and Upcoming Titles

- Neurodegenerative Diseases and Mitochondrial Metabolism
  M. Flint Beal, Harvard University

- Molecular and Cellular Mechanisms of Neostriatum
  Marjorie A. Ariano and D. James Surmeier, Chicago Medical School

- Ca^{2+} Regulation By Ca^{2+}-Binding Proteins in Neurodegenerative Disorders
  Claus W. Heizmann and Katharina Braun, University of Zurich, Federal Institute for Neurobiology, Magdeburg

- Measuring Movement and Locomotion: From Invertebrates to Humans
  Klaus-Peter Ossenkopp, Martin Kavaliers and Paul Sanberg, University of Western Ontario and University of South Florida

- Triple Repeats in Inherited Neurologic Disease
  Henry Epstein, University of Texas-Houston

- Cholecystokinin and Anxiety
  Jacques Bradwejn, McGill University

- Neurofilament Structure and Function
  Gerry Shaw, University of Florida

- Molecular and Functional Biology of Neurotropic Factors
  Karoly Nikolics, Genentech

- Prion-related Encephalopathies: Molecular Mechanisms
  Gianluigi Forloni, Istituto di Ricerche Farmacologiche "Mario Negri"-Milan

- Neurotoxins and Ion Channels
  Alan Harvey, A.J. Anderson and E.G. Rowan, University of Strathclyde

- Analysis and Modeling of the Mammalian Cortex
  Malcolm P. Young, University of Oxford

- Free Radical Metabolism and Brain Dysfunction
  Irène Ceballos-Picot, Hôpital Necker-Paris

- Molecular Mechanisms of the Action of Benzodiazepines
  Adam Doble and Ian L. Martin, Rhône-Poulenc Rorer and University of Alberta

- Neurodevelopmental Hypothesis of Schizophrenia
  John L. Waddington and Peter Buckley, Royal College of Surgeons-Ireland

- Synaptic Plasticity in the Retina
  H.J. Wagner, Mustafa Djamgoz and Reto Weiler, University of Tübingen

- Non-classical Properties of Acetylcholine
  Margaret Appleyard, Royal Free Hospital-London

- Molecular Mechanisms of Segmental Patterning in the Vertebrate Nervous System
  David G. Wilkinson, National Institute of Medical Research-UK

- Molecular Character of Memory in the Prefrontal Cortex
  Fraser Wilson, Yale University